DRINKING WATER *and* INFECTIOUS DISEASE

Establishing the Links

DRINKING WATER *and* INFECTIOUS DISEASE

Establishing the Links

Edited by
Paul Raymond Hunter
Mike Waite
Elettra Ronchi

CRC PRESS
Boca Raton London New York Washington, D.C.

IWA Publishing

Library of Congress Cataloging-in-Publication Data

Drinking water and infectious disease : establishing the links / editors, Paul R. Hunter, Mike Waite, Elettra Ronchi.
p. ; cm.
"Based on the Organisation for Economic Cooperation and Development expert group meeting--Basingstoke 2000."
Includes bibliographical references and index.
ISBN 0-8493-1259-0
1. Drinking water--Microbiology--Congresses. 2. Communciable diseases--Environmental aspects--Congresses. 3. Drinking water--Contamination--Congresses. 4. Waterborne infection--Congresses. I. Hunter, Paul R. II. Waite, Mike. III. Ronchi, Elettra. IV. Organisation for Economic Co-operation and Development.
[DNLM: 1. Water Microbiology--Congresses. 2. Water Supply--analysis--Congresses. 3. Communicable Diseases--epidemiology--Congresses. 4. Disease Outbreaks--Congresses. WA 686 D781 2002]
RA1216 .D74 2002
614.4--dc21 2002025936

Co-published by IWA Publishing, Alliance House, 12 Caxton Street, London, SW1H 0QS, UK
Tel. +44 (0) 20 7654 5500, Fax. +44 (0) 20 7654 5555
publications@iwap.co.uk
www.iwapublishing.com
ISBN 1-84339-027-2

No claim to original U.S. Government works
International Standard Book Number 0-8493-1259-0
Library of Congress Card Number 2002025936
Printed in the United States of America 1 2 3 4 5 6 7 8 9 0
Printed on acid-free paper

Foreword

An increasing number of countries can be considered water-stressed.[1] Of all environmental questions, those related to water are perhaps the most far-reaching in their long-term consequences, and the most difficult to tackle from a scientific point of view. In many parts of the world there is widespread scarcity, gradual destruction, and increased pollution of fresh water resources, and many nations face growing problems associated with guaranteeing an adequate drinking water supply. Today in the developing world, one person in three lacks safe drinking water and sanitation, the basic requirements for survival, health, and dignity. The prospects for the future do not look any better.

At the turn of the millennium there were approximately 6.2 billion people alive on this planet. By 2025 this number will have risen to somewhere between 7.9 and 9.1 billion.[1] The provision of safe drinking water for all these people will be one of the major challenges facing humanity. Waterborne pathogens represent a serious and growing hazard, and infectious diseases continue to affect populations throughout the world. Other problems exist as well, such as aging of water treatment infrastructures and the increasing occurrence, or perhaps the increasing recognition and detection, of organisms resistant to conventional disinfection treatments. Diarrheal illness thus remains the sixth leading cause of death worldwide, responsible for an estimated 2,219,000 deaths in 1998, some 4.1% of all deaths, mostly among children under the age of five.[2] Diarrheal illness makes an even bigger contribution, 5.3%, to disease burden.[2] Most of this burden of illness falls onto the residents of the world's less well-developed regions, where it is responsible for 8.1% of the disease burden, ranked second only to respiratory illness (9.1%).[3]

Diarrheal illness is often attributed to contaminated water consumption, although the percentage specifically due to waterborne pathogens is still unknown. The problem is that many countries, including the most advanced Organization for Economic Cooperation and Development (OECD) countries, do not have effective surveillance systems in place to detect waterborne disease. Even in those countries with effective disease surveillance systems, the systems often fail to identify the sources of infection. There is, therefore, still considerable uncertainty about the proportion of waterborne disease outbreaks detected and the burden of such disease not associated with outbreaks (sporadic disease). Further research is needed to determine rates of illness and, where rates are elevated, to determine whether illness is caused by inadequately treated waters or by water that has deteriorated in the distribution system. A major challenge, as discussed in this book, is to collect meaningful data on water quality and to improve data sharing between water suppliers and the public health community. Water data are in general comprehensive but are under-utilized, especially by the public health community. In contrast, health data are often relatively unstandardized, reactive, and limited in respect to identifying risks relating to waterborne disease.

For all these reasons, particularly the need to develop better methods for assessing the safety of drinking water and to monitor and respond to adverse events, the OECD, in cooperation with the World Health Organization (WHO), has devoted its attention to water.

The need to achieve a better understanding of the role of water in the transmission of infectious disease was first officially acknowledged by the international community in 1996 at the OECD Workshop on Biotechnology for Water Use and Conservation in Cocoyoc, Mexico. At the end of this workshop, the government of Switzerland proposed to continue to address this issue with the ultimate goal of bringing about the policy changes required by public health. In 1998 a Workshop on Molecular Technologies for Safe Drinking Water was organized in Interlaken, Switzerland to review the effectiveness of drinking water plants in preventing the passage of microbial contaminants and the reliability of current indicators as means to guarantee microbiologically safe water to consumers. A number of key conclusions were reached at this workshop, leading to the following recommendations:

- Development of a guidance document on microbiological testing of drinking water
- International coordination and promotion of molecular methods in the field of drinking water microbiology
- International coordination for improved surveillance and outbreak investigation

In 1999 a drafting group was formed to address the first of the three recommendations, namely the preparation of a guidance document, *Improving Microbiological Safety of Drinking Water.* In July 2000, the U.K. government hosted an OECD expert group meeting, "Approaches for Establishing Links between Drinking Water and Infectious Disease," to address the third recommendation, and from which this book originates. The executive summary of the Basingstoke meeting is reproduced in full as an appendix to this introduction.

This renewed interest in the potentially adverse public health consequences of drinking water has also stimulated a number of initiatives by the WHO, one of which led to the publication of *Water Quality: Guidelines, Standards and Health. Risk Assessment and Management for Water-Related Infectious Disease,* edited by Lorna Fewtrell and Jamie Bartram and published by IWA Publishing in 2001. Our book and the WHO book complement each other in that the WHO book gives a broad view on the public health issues regarding water (including recreational water contract) and health, whereas the Basingstoke meeting and our book concentrate on the question of how the link between drinking water and infectious disease can be demonstrated and proven.

The layout of this book does not exactly follow the structure of the Basingstoke meeting. Instead of the five sessions at Basingstoke, we have organized this book into three sections. Section I deals with surveillance, Section II with the investigation and management of outbreaks of disease that may be linked to drinking water, and Section III with methods for determining the contribution of drinking water to sporadic disease. Each section is introduced by the relevant session chair.

To conclude this introduction we felt it would be appropriate to remind readers of the basis of epidemiological proof as first discussed by Bradford-Hill in 1965.[4] He suggested nine epidemiological criteria to be used in assessing whether an environmental factor was associated with human disease. These criteria were:

1. *Strength of association* as determined by statistical methods of association
2. *Consistency* of results between different researchers using different approaches
3. *Specificity* of association between a particular type of exposure and a particular disease
4. *Temporality,* in that disease should follow exposure, rather than the other way around
5. *Biological gradient,* as shown when risk of disease becomes greater with increasing exposure
6. *Plausibility,* when the association described in epidemiological studies is compatible with existing knowledge of the biology or toxicity of the proposed disease agent
7. *Coherence,* when the epidemiological data do not conflict with what is already known about the epidemiology of the disease agent
8. *Experiment,* when the hypothesis can be subject to some form of experimental study such as a randomized controlled trial (see Chapter 18)
9. *Analogy,* when the proposed epidemiology can be shown to be similar to another comparable illness

When considering the methods discussed in subsequent chapters, the reader may wish to consider how these approaches add to the knowledge of the criteria for epidemiological proof discussed above.

REFERENCES

1. Hunter, P.R., *Waterborne Disease: Epidemiology and Ecology*, Wiley, Chichester, 1997.
2. WHO, The World Health Report, Making a Difference, World Health Organization, Geneva, 1999.
3. Murray, C.J.L. and Lopez, A.D., *The Global Burden of Disease and Injury Series. Volume 1. The Global Burden of Disease*, Harvard School of Public Health, World Bank, World Health Organization, 1996.
4. Bradford-Hill, A., The environment and disease: association or causation?, *Proc. R. Soc. Med.*, 58, 295, 1965.

Appendix

Executive Summary of the Basingstoke 2000 Expert Group Meeting on Approaches for Establishing Links between Drinking Water and Infectious Diseases

Poor quality drinking water and inadequate sanitation are among the world's major preventable causes of early mortality. According to World Health Organization estimates, contaminated drinking water is responsible for some five million deaths each year. Risk of death is particularly high for children. A child dies every eight seconds from a preventable water- or sanitation-related disease. The problem is not limited to developing countries. Even in OECD countries, waterborne outbreaks occur all too frequently, without necessarily being recognized as such. During the years 1991–98, there were 35 outbreaks of disease linked to drinking water in the United Kingdom and 113 in the United States. Yet despite the clear importance of drinking water as a cause of infectious disease, very little consideration has been given to how best to investigate the relationship between the two.

The need to achieve a better understanding of water's role in the transmission of infectious disease was officially acknowledged by the international community in 1996 at the OECD Workshop on Biotechnology for Water Use and Conservation in Cocoyoc, Mexico. Then, in 1998, the OECD Interlaken Workshop on Molecular Technologies for Safe Drinking Water reviewed the effectiveness of drinking water plants in preventing the passage of microbial contaminants and the reliability of current indicators as means to guarantee microbiologically safe water to consumers. Recommendations from that workshop highlighted the need for better approaches and methods to assess the safety of drinking water and to monitor and respond to adverse events.

In response, the U.K. Government hosted in July 2000 an OECD expert group meeting, "Approaches for Establishing Links between Drinking Water and Infectious Disease," to address the following questions in particular:

- What is the minimum appropriate surveillance system for member countries to have in place to "identify outbreaks or incidents of water-related disease or significant threats of such outbreaks"?
- What are appropriate "indicators or technical developments to monitor system performance in preventing, controlling or reducing water-related disease" for member countries to use?
- What are the "appropriate comprehensive national and local contingency plans for responses to such outbreaks" to be developed by member countries?

Accordingly, 26 presentations were made on four key topics:

- Surveillance of waterborne disease
- Outbreak investigation
- Use of water quality, treatment, and distribution data to assess human health risk
- Epidemiological approaches to assessing endemic waterborne disease burden

Participants agreed on a number of important conclusions:

- They recognized that there were two main sources of data on the risk to health from drinking water: *i)* epidemiological data from surveillance systems and other studies, and

TABLE 1
Issues that Might Affect Efficient Utilization of Water and Health Data

Water Data	Health Data
Comprehensiveness varies between countries	Non-standardized
Usually geared towards statutory reporting	Need to maintain flexible methodological approach
Under-utilized	Frequently reactive
Not easily accessible to public health community	Lack of geographical resolution
Commercial sensitivity	Incomplete
Might underestimate health risks	Not timely
Much data may not be timely	Potentially subject to significant bias

Source: OECD Biotechnology Unit.

ii) data on water quality collected by the water utility. The advantages and disadvantages of these sources differ in terms of assessing risk to health (Table 1).

In addressing these differences the following general considerations apply:

- Current water quality data are mainly driven by statutory standards, which may or may not relate to health risks.
- Water quality data is often comprehensive but under-utilized by the public health community.
- Data sharing between water suppliers and the public health community should be encouraged and each should take account of the other's needs when collecting data.

In addition, in devising surveillance systems for waterborne diseases the following general criteria should be considered:

- Surveillance systems for waterborne diseases are only valuable if they lead to improved protection of public health or confirm the adequacy of current practices.
- Surveillance and outbreak investigation must inform policy so that mistakes leading to outbreaks are not repeated.
- Surveillance information should inform economic analyses of costs and benefits of changes in water treatment regimens.
- Consideration needs to be given to how the public health benefits of surveillance can be balanced with individual human rights to privacy. Countries are invited to examine approaches to improve security of data flows.
- Most surveillance systems are disease-specific or symptom-complex-specific. Appropriate additional information needed to aid linkages with water as a risk factor should be considered. The multidisciplinary nature of such systems should be recognized.

Outbreaks probably represent only a small proportion of cases of infectious disease caused by drinking water. Existing surveillance systems may not detect sporadic cases. Even if sporadic cases are identified by current surveillance systems, the role of drinking water may be far from clear. This is likely to be a particular problem for emerging waterborne infectious diseases. To improve the detection of the links between sporadic cases and drinking water, the following issues should be addressed:

- Vigilance should be maintained on the surveillance of emerging and chronic infectious diseases, including disease in populations at particular risk of infection or severe outcomes of illness. Appropriate epidemiological tools and surrogate indicators are needed to determine levels of waterborne disease, including the potential consequences of infrequent adverse events (e.g., floods, sudden contamination, treatment failures, and conflicts).

- It is crucial to develop adequate real-time measurement or predictive models in order to understand the link between water safety and health.
- Public health protection should focus on critical control points throughout the water supply chain and on developing adequate indicators to assess the health impacts of water quality in distribution systems.
- When assessing any of the various types of studies of sporadic disease and water, it is important to acknowledge the intrinsic advantages and disadvantages of the proposed study design.
- Consideration needs to be given to how studies of waterborne disease can be adapted for use in developing countries.

Finally, participants agreed that there is great variation in the nature of surveillance systems across OECD countries, which makes country-to-country comparisons difficult, and that international initiatives are urgently needed to:

- Identify the best approaches to surveillance and outbreak investigation.
- Strengthen the linkage of current international disease-based surveillance systems and environmental surveillance networks to integrate data on surveillance of waterborne diseases (the current review of the International Health Regulations should be encouraged to achieve this).
- Develop new surveillance tools, such as neural networks and Geographical Information Systems.
- Encourage data sharing on outbreaks across the OECD area, in particular to address adverse events with transboundary health and environmental impacts.

Acknowledgments

The editors and the OECD wish to thank all those whose efforts made possible this book and the expert group meeting on which it is based. The contributors to the book are listed on the following pages. Thanks are also due to Doranne LeCercle of OECD for help with editing several of the chapters.

In addition we would like to thank the U.K. Department of Health, the OECD Working Party on Biotechnology and its chairman, Dr. David Harper. We are very grateful to Dr. Sarah Woodhouse, who acted as rapporteur at the expert meeting and played an important role in writing its report. We also wish to thank the staff and management of Water Training International, Tadley Court, Basingstoke for their care and attention during the Basingstoke 2000 meeting.

Special thanks are due to the Drinking Water Inspectorate of the U.K. Department for the Environment, Food and Rural Affairs for providing financial support for the expert group meeting.

Paul R. Hunter
University of East Anglia

Mike Waite
Drinking Water Inspectorate

Elettra Ronchi
OECD Biotechnology Unit

Acknowledgments

Editors

Paul R. Hunter is professor of health protection in the School of Medicine, Health Policy and Practice, University of East Anglia, U.K. He graduated in medicine from Manchester University in 1979 and went on to specialize in medical microbiology. He earned his M.D. for research into the epidemiology of *Candida albicans* infections. From 1988 to 2001 he was director of the Chester Public Health Laboratory. Professor Hunter also worked as a consultant in Communicable Disease Control and as a regional epidemiologist. He chairs the Public Health Laboratory Service Advisory Committee on Water and the Environment and sits on several other national and international expert committees. Professor Hunter developed an early interest in infection related to food and water and has been involved in the investigation of many food and waterborne outbreaks. He has published over 100 articles in the scientific literature, and his first book, *Waterborne Disease-Epidemiology and Ecology,* was published by John Wiley & Sons in 1997. His second book, *Microbiological Aspects of Biofilms in Drinking Water* (co-authored with S. Percival and J. Walker), was published by CRC Press in 2000.

Mike Waite graduated with an honors degree in bacteriology from Edinburgh University in 1966. After working in the food industry for 4 years, he has spent over 30 years in the water industry, the last 11 as a principal inspector with the U.K. Drinking Water Inspectorate. He has published a number of papers on bacteriology, virology, mutagenicity, and parasitology in relation to water supply and waste disposal and has contributed to the activities of a number of expert working groups including the production of *The Microbiology of Water 1994 Part 1 — Drinking Water.* He has been instrumental in the move from a culture-based to a genotypic definition of coliforms.

Elettra Ronchi is Coordinator of Health and Biotechnology Activities at the OECD, Directorate for Science, Technology and Industry. She earned a Ph.D. from the Rockefeller University/Cornell Medical School, New York. Dr. Ronchi has held research, teaching, and assistant appointments at the Howard Hughes Medical Institute in New York and the Ecole Normale Superieure in Paris. She has lectured and published extensively on a variety of topics linked to new developments in molecular genetics and biotechnology and their impact on health care systems. Dr. Ronchi has also acted as consultant and science adviser on biotechnology, health system management, and technology transfer for human health to the United Nations and the OECD since 1992. In 1995 Dr. Ronchi joined the OECD to lead a program of work on emerging technologies related to human health, particularly new biotechnologies. She sits as expert and as OECD representative on a number of committees and advisory boards, including the UNESCO International Bioethics Committee and the Bioethics Committee of the Council of Europe.

Contributors

Yvonne Andersson
Swedish Institute for Infectious Disease Control
Solna, Sweden
E-mail: yvonne.andersson@smi.ki.se

Jamie Bartram
World Health Organization
Geneva, Switzerland
E-mail: bartramj@who.int

Pascal Beaudeau
Département Santé Environnement
Institut de Veille Sanitaire
Saint-Maurice, France
E-mail: p.beaudeau@invs.sante.fr

Jim Black
Department of Epidemiology and Preventive Medicine
Monash University
Melbourne, Victoria, Australia
E-mail: jim.black@med.monash.edu.au

Carl-Henrik von Bonsdorff
Department of Virology
Helsinki University
Helsinki, Finland
E-mail: carl-henrik.vonbonsdorff@helsinki.fi

Rebecca L. Calderon
U.S. Environmental Protection Agency
Research Triangle Park, North Carolina
United States
E-mail: Calderon.Rebecca@epamail.epa.gov

Gunther Craun
Gunther F. Craun and Associates
Staunton, Virginia, United States
E-mail: gfcraun@cfw.com

Friederike Dangendorf
Institute of Hygiene and Public Health
University of Bonn
Bonn, Germany
E-mail: Friedang@mailer.meb.uni-bonn.de

Al P. Dufour
U.S. Environmental Protection Agency
Cincinatti, Ohio, United States
E-mail: dufour.alfred@epamail.epa.gov

Martin Exner
Institute of Hygiene and Public Health
University of Bonn
Bonn, Germany
E-mail: Martin.Exner@ukb.uni-bonn.de

Christopher K. Fairley
Department of Public Health
The University of Melbourne
Victoria, Australia
E-mail: cfairley@unimelb.edu.au

Kim Fox
U.S. Environmental Protection Agency
Cincinnati, Ohio, United States
E-mail: fox.kim@epa.gov

Floyd J. Frost
Lovelace Clinic Foundation
Albuquerque, New Mexico, United States
E-mail: ffrost@lrri.org

James Gibson
Department of Health and Environmental Control
Columbia, South Carolina, United States
E-mail: GIBSONJJ@columb60.dhec.state.sc.us

Leila Gofti-Laroche
TIMC-SIIM Laboratory, School of Medicine
Grenoble University
La Tronche, France
E-mail: leila.gofti@imag.fr or leila.gofti@ujf-grenoble.fr

Susanne Herbst
Institute of Hygiene and Public Health
University of Bonn
Bonn, Germany
E-mail: susanne.herbst@ukb.uni-bonn.de

Paul R. Hunter
School of Medicine, Health Policy and Practice
University of East Anglia
Norwich, United Kingdom
E-mail: paul.hunter@uea.ac.uk

Peter Jiggins
Drinking Water Inspectorate
London, United Kingdom
E-mail: Peter.Jiggins@defra.gsi.gov.uk

Thomas Kistemann
Institute of Hygiene and Public Health
University of Bonn
Bonn, Germany
E-mail: Thomas.Kistemann@ukb.uni-bonn.de

Twila Kunde
Lovelace Clinic Foundation
Albuquerque, New Mexico, United States
E-mail: twila@lcfresearch.org

Deborah Levy
Centers for Disease Control and Prevention
Atlanta, Georgia, United States
E-mail: del7@cdc.gov

Jim McLauchlin
Central Public Health Laboratory
London, United Kingdom
E-mail: jmclauchlin@phls.org.uk

Leena Maunula
Department of Virology
Helsinki University
Helsinki, Finland
E-mail: Leena.Maunula@Helsinki.Fi

Christine Moe
Department of International Health
Rollins School of Public Health of Emory University
Atlanta, Georgia, United States
E-mail: clmoe@sph.emory.edu

Tim Muller
Lovelace Clinic Foundation
Albuquerque, New Mexico, United States
E-mail: tmuller@lrri.org

Gordon Nichols
PHLS Communicable Disease Surveillance Centre
London, United Kingdom
E-mail: GNichols@phls.org.uk

Nena Nwachuku
U.S. Environmental Protection Agency
Washington, D.C., United States
E-mail: nwachuku.nena@epa.gov

Pierre Payment
INRS-Institut Armand-Frappier
Université du Quebec
Laval, Québec, Canada
E-mail: pierre.payment@inrs-iaf.uquebec.ca

Catherine Quigley
Sefton Health Authority
Liverpool, United Kingdom
E-mail: Catherine.Quigley@sefton-ha.nhs.uk

Brent Robertson
Department of Epidemiology and Preventive Medicine
Monash University
Melbourne, Victoria, Australia
E-mail brent.robertson@med.monash.edu.au

William Robertson
Health Canada
Ottawa, Ontario, Canada
E-mail: will_robertson@hc-sc.gc.ca

Elettra Ronchi
OECD Biotechnology Unit
Paris, France
E-mail: elettra.ronchi@oecd.org

Martha Sinclair
Department of Epidemiology and Preventive Medicine
Monash University
Melbourne, Victoria, Australia
E-mail: Martha.Sinclair@med.monash.edu.au

Rosalind Stanwell-Smith
Independent Consultant
London, United Kingdom
E-mail: RStanwellSmith@aol.com

Alan Thompson
Lyonnaise des Eaux France
Paris, France
E-mail: alan.thompson@lyonnaise-des-eaux.fr

Mike Waite
Drinking Water Inspectorate
London, United Kingdom
E-mail: mike.waite@defra.gsi.gov.uk

Denis Zmirou
Public Health Department
School of Medicine of Nancy University
INSERM U420
Vandoeuvre les Nancy, France
E-mail: denis.zmirou@nancy.inserm.fr

Disclaimer

The opinions expressed in this publication are the opinions of the authors and do not necessarily reflect the views or policies of the Organization for Economic Cooperation and Development or the World Health Organization. Furthermore, the mention of specific manufacturers' products does not imply that they are endorsed or recommended in preference to others of a similar nature that are not mentioned.

List of Figures

Figure 1.1 Basic diagram of a negative feedback control loop such as a simple thermostat. 4
Figure 1.2 Data flow for *Salmonella* surveillance in England and Wales. 7
Figure 2.1 Laboratory reports of cryptosporidiosis in Cheshire and Wirral, by month, 1996–1999. 16
Figure 2.2 Probable waterborne outbreak in Wirral and Ellesmere Port, April 1996. Cases by week of report. 16
Figure 2.3 Communicable disease case reporting in the U.S.: a three-tiered system. 17
Figure 3.1 Outbreaks of waterborne disease associated with public water supplies in England and Wales from 1980–2000. 27
Figure 3.2 Outbreaks of waterborne disease associated with private water supplies in England and Wales from 1991–2000. 27
Figure 3.3 Waterborne disease outbreaks associated with drinking water by year and etiologic agent, United States 1971–1998 (N = 689). 29
Figure 3.4 Waterborne disease outbreaks associated with drinking water by year and type of water system, United States 1971–1998 (N = 689). 30
Figure 3.5 Organization of the epidemic surveillance in Sweden in case of food and waterborne outbreaks. 34
Figure 3.6 Conditions for a pathogenic microorganism to be diagnosed and reported in a waterborne outbreak. 34
Figure 3.7 Outbreaks and cases of waterborne disease in Sweden, 1980–1999. 36
Figure 3.8 Microbial agents associated with waterborne outbreaks in Sweden, 1980–1999. 36
Figure 4.1 Cholera, reported number of cases and case fatality rates, 1950 to 1998. 44
Figure 4.2 Reports made to European Working Group on *Legionella* infection surveillance scheme for travel-associated *Legionella*. 45
Figure 5.1 A systems map of an outbreak of waterborne disease. 54
Figure 5.2 The learning curve for outbreak investigations, showing important iterations. 55
Figure 5.3 Outbreak of cryptosporidiosis, Wirral and Ellesmere Port, 1996: cases by week of onset (n = 51). 58
Figure 5.4 Outbreak of cryptosporidiosis, Wirral and Ellesmere Port, 1996: geographical distribution. 59
Figure 6.1 The MMWR method. (Source: *MMWR*, 50, 10, March 16, 2001.) 70
Figure 6.2 An example of a CUSUM chart. 71
Figure 6.3 Structure of a feed-forward neural network. 74
Figure 6.4 Execution of a single hypothetical neuron with 5 inputs and logistic activation function. 75
Figure 7.1 General properties of human caliciviruses. 80
Figure 7.2 Tree diagram based on the amplicon sequence obtained from patient samples of NLV outbreaks that occurred in Finland during 1997–99. (Source: v. Bonsdorff C-H, Maunula, L., *Duodecim* 116: 70, 2000. With permission.) 83
Figure 8.1 Western blot of *Cryptosporidium* isolates using FITC-labeled monoclonal antibody MAB C1 and alkaline phosphatase-labeled anti FITC. 88

Figure 8.2 DNA extraction (method 2) from 218 patients diagnosed as having cryptosporidiosis. (Source: Nichols, G.L., McLauchlin, J., and Samuel, D., *J. Protozool.*, 38, 2375, 1991. With permission.) 89
Figure 8.3 *Cryptosporidium* types by month including outbreaks. 90
Figure 8.4 *Cryptosporidium* types in people returning from outside the U.K. 91
Figure 8.5 *Cryptosporidium* types in travellers. 92
Figure 9.1 Gideon, Missouri propagation map 99
Figure 9.2 Karl Meyer Hall storage tank. 100
Figure 9.3 Maximum daily turbidity and number of cases during Milwaukee outbreak 102
Figure 12.1 The elements of surveillance 132
Figure 12.2 Cryptosporidiosis in England and Wales, 1983–1997. 133
Figure 12.3 *Cryptosporidium* reports in England and Wales by reporting date, 1983–2000 134
Figure 12.4 Age distribution of patients with cryptosporidiosis 135
Figure 12.5 Cryptosporidiosis cases per day in England and Wales, 1989–1997. Total travel-related cases. 135
Figure 12.6 Incidents of cryptosporidiosis in cattle and sheep in the U.K. 137
Figure 12.7 Cryptosporidiosis in England and Wales by region, 1989–1997. 138
Figure 12.8 Geographical incidence of cryptosporidiosis by health authority in England and Wales, 1983–1998. 139
Figure 13.1 Concept of GIS processing concerning epidemiological surveillance of waterborne infectious diseases. 145
Figure 13.2 Origin of drinking water in the study area of Rhein-Berg District, Germany 146
Figure 13.3 Purification facilities and drinking water delivery in Rhein-Berg District, Germany. 147
Figure 13.4 Spatial patterns of the enteritis incidence in the subdistricts of Rhein-Berg, Germany (1988-1998). 148
Figure 14.1 Hypothetical scheme of infectious waterborne risk in rural sectors of Eastern Normandy 158
Figure 14.2 Precipitation, raw water turbidity, and treated water turbidity at a karstic spring in Eastern Normandy. The treatment alternates filtration and flocculation/settling and filtration, according to the level of the raw water turbidity. 159
Figure 14.3 Free residual chlorine in finished water from a karstic spring in Eastern Normandy. Water is distributed without filtration 160
Figure 14.4 Assessment of the contamination of a raw karstic water. Available sources of relevant information. 161
Figure 17.1 Time trend of acute digestive conditions incidence rates among children in a prospective study. 185

List of Tables

Table 3.1 Criteria for the Strength of Association of Water with Human Infectious Disease and How They Are Applied in the National Surveillance for Water-Related Disease in England and Wales 26
Table 3.2 Causes of Outbreaks of Waterborne Disease in England and Wales. 28
Table 3.3 Classification of Investigations of Waterborne Disease Outbreaks in the United States 31
Table 4.1 Countries Reporting Cases to EWGLI in 1999 45
Table 8.1 Genotyping of Human Isolates of *Cryptosporidium* in Outbreaks of Cryptosporidiosis Linked to Water 90
Table 10.1 Waterborne Outbreaks Reported in U.S. Drinking Water Systems by Type of System and Water Source, 1991–1998 107
Table 10.2 Etiology of Waterborne Outbreaks, 1991–1998; Number of Outbreaks by Type of Water System and Water Source 107
Table 10.3 Etiology of Waterborne Outbreaks; Cases of Illness by Type of Water System and Water Source, 1991–1998 108
Table 10.4 Waterborne Outbreaks and Deficiencies in Public Water Systems, Surface-Water Sources, 1991–1998 109
Table 10.5 Waterborne Outbreaks and Deficiencies in Public Water Systems, Groundwater Sources, 1991–1998 109
Table 10.6 Total Coliform Data Collected during Waterborne Outbreak Investigations, Public Water Systems, 1991–1998d 110
Table 10.7 Etiology of Waterborne Outbreaks in Individual Water Systems Outbreaks and Cases of Illness by Water Source, 1991–1998 111
Table 10.8 Etiology of Recreational Waterborne Outbreaks, Outbreaks, and Cases of Illness by Type of Water Source, 1991–1998 112
Table 10.9 Causes of Waterborne Disease Outbreaks Associated with Recreational Water 113
Table 11.1 Notification Requirements of the Water Undertakers (Information) Direction 1992 121
Table 11.2 Water Undertakers (Information) Direction 1992 Requires a Report within 72 Hours Which Must Include: 121
Table 11.3 Water Undertakers (Information) Direction 1992 Requires a Full Report within 1 Month, Which Must Include: 121
Table 12.1 Outbreaks and Cases of Cryptosporidiosis in England and Wales 1983 to 1997 136
Table 13.1 Product–Moment Correlation of Water Supply Structures and Incidence of Enteritis 149
Table 13.2 Results of the Partial Correlation of the Influence of Surfacewater Supply on the Variance in the Incidence of Enteritis 149
Table 14.1 Statistical Models for Time Series Modeling 156
Table 15.1 Serological Responses to 15/17-kDa Antigen as a Percent of Positive Control Responses for Surface-Water (SW) or Groundwater (GW) Systems 167
Table 15.2 Serological Responses to 27-kDa Antigen as a Percent of Positive Control Responses for Surface-Water (SW) or Groundwater (GW) Systems 168

Table 15.3 Results of Paired City Comparisons (Surface-Water [SW] or Groundwater [GW] Systems) — Response as a Percent of Positive Control Responses for the 15/17-kDa Antigen Group....170
Table 15.4 Comparisons of Surface- vs. Groundwater Sources — Significance Level Under Different Definitions of a Positive Response....171
Table 19.1 Global Burden of Diarrheal Diseases in Children < 5 Years....198
Table 19.2 Reported Microbiological Quality of Domestic Water Sources in Developing Countries....199

Contents

SECTION 1 Surveillance of Waterborne Disease 1
Pierre Payment

Chapter 1 Principles and Components of Surveillance Systems..3
Paul R. Hunter

Chapter 2 Local Surveillance Systems 13
Catherine Quigley, James J. Gibson, and Paul R. Hunter

Appendix A: Developing an Integrated System of Health and Technical Data 21
Alan Thompson

Chapter 3 National Surveillance Systems...25
Rosalind Stanwell-Smith, Yvonne Andersson, and Deborah A. Levy

Chapter 4 International Surveillance...41
Paul R. Hunter

SECTION 2 Investigation of Outbreaks of Waterborne Disease 49
Will Robertson and Al Dufour

Chapter 5 A Systems Approach to the Investigation and Control of Waterborne Outbreaks ...53
Catherine Quigley and Paul R. Hunter

Chapter 6 Early Detection of Water-Related Disease Outbreaks 67
Jim Black and Christopher K. Fairley

Chapter 7 Microbiology and the Investigation of Waterborne Outbreaks: Typing of Norwalk-Like Virus 79
Carl-Henrik von Bonsdorff and Leena Maunula

Chapter 8 Microbiology and the Investigation of Waterborne Outbreaks: The Use of *Cryptosporidium* Typing in the Investigation of Waterborne Disease 87

Gordon Nichols and Jim McLauchlin

Chapter 9 Engineering Considerations in the Investigation of Waterborne Outbreaks 97

Kim R. Fox

Chapter 10 Causes of Waterborne Outbreaks Reported in the United States, 1991–1998........105

Gunther F. Craun, Rebecca L. Calderon, and Nena Nwachuku

Chapter 11 *Cryptosporidium* in England and Wales 119

Mike Waite and Peter Jiggins

SECTION 3 Investigation of Sporadic Waterborne Disease.. 127

Jamie Bartram

Chapter 12 Using Existing Surveillance-Based Data 131

Gordon Nichols

Chapter 13 Geographical Information Systems 143

Friederike Dangendorf, Susanne Herbst, Martin Exner, and Thomas Kistemann

Chapter 14 Time Series Analyses 155

Pascal Beaudeau

Chapter 15 Seroepidemiology 165

Floyd J. Frost, Tim Muller, Twila Kunde, Gunther Craun, and Rebecca Calderon

Chapter 16 Case-Control Studies 175

Brent Robertson, Christopher K. Fairley, Jim Black, and Martha Sinclair

Chapter 17 Prospective Epidemiological Studies 183

Denis Zmirou and Leila Gofti-Laroche

Chapter 18 Intervention Studies 191

Pierre Payment and Paul R. Hunter

Section 1

Surveillance of Waterborne Disease

Pierre Payment

INTRODUCTION

The surveillance of infectious diseases has gained significant attention over the last decade. Many industrialized countries have had in place systems for the surveillance of transmissible diseases for over 100 years. This surveillance was often very minimal. A few countries have invested in surveillance, recognizing that forecasting or rapidly identifying a developing threat would be advantageous. Authorities have been alerted by large outbreaks of waterborne disease, by trans-border outbreaks due to the globalization of food markets, and finally by the rapid dissemination of disease by worldwide travel. The first section of this book focuses on the various aspects of the surveillance of waterborne disease.

Chapter 1 presents the fundamental principles that should guide surveillance systems that will lead to public health interventions. To design a good surveillance system requires well-defined objectives, characteristics, and suitable evaluation processes. The remaining three chapters of this section discuss a number of surveillance systems that are currently operating at local, national, or even international levels. Consideration is also given to the ethical aspects of surveillance systems. The point is made that it is unethical to develop surveillance unless there is likely to be a real benefit to the health of the population under surveillance.

Chapter 2 builds on the principles outlined in Chapter 1 by presenting both a British and an American perspective of local surveillance. For the British perspective, responsibilities, legislative background, and the components of the local surveillance (notifications, laboratory data, and data from other sources) are presented, using cryptosporidiosis as an illustration. The value of active local analysis of local surveillance data, above just data collection and transmission to national surveillance systems, is highlighted. The American perspective focuses on the state level surveillance. Each state has its own local systems and the results are integrated to a higher level at the state level that in turn are transmitted to the national level at the U.S. Centers for Disease Control (USCDC). Paper transmission remains the main format, but the electronic transmission of data is becoming more prevalent, thereby permitting more rapid responses. The deficiencies of the system are again illustrated using cryptosporidiosis. As an appendix to this chapter, a novel cooperative surveillance system between a water utility and public health team in England is presented.

The responsiveness of the surveillance systems at the national level in the U.K., U.S., and Sweden are presented in Chapter 3. Surveillance systems in all three countries appear to have a low level of sensitivity to detect waterborne outbreaks, and reported outbreaks are uncommon. In most cases, this is due to the fact that the local surveillance lacks sensitivity and rarely has adequate information on risk factor exposure. An ideal national surveillance would build on the established reporting of outbreaks and develop more comprehensive local surveillance through education, training, and access to specialists in all fields of water microbiology and engineering.

The final chapter in this section considers a number of international surveillance systems. The point is made that it is only when the local and national surveillance systems are in place that a meaningful international system be fruitful. Many countries, even in the West, do not have adequate national surveillance systems. Within this chapter a number of models for international surveillance systems are presented. The system for cholera surveillance is run by the World Health Organization (WHO) and is a centrally managed surveillance system. The European legionella surveillance system is managed in a more collaborative way between national surveillance centers. Finally the ProMEDmail system is run independent of any national surveillance system, but operates on the basis of e-mail between participants. These systems vary in the quality of their data and the timeliness of reporting.

1 Principles and Components of Surveillance Systems

Paul R. Hunter

CONTENTS

1.1 Introduction....................3
1.2 A Model of Public Health Practice....................4
1.3 Designing a Surveillance System....................5
1.3.1 Agree upon the Objectives of the Surveillance System....................5
1.3.1.1 The Health Problem to be Addressed....................5
1.3.1.2 The Purpose of the Surveillance System....................5
1.3.1.3 The Target Population....................5
1.3.2 Determine the Characteristics of the Surveillance System....................6
1.3.2.1 The Data Set....................6
1.3.2.2 Data Flow....................6
1.3.2.3 Analysis....................7
1.3.2.4 Outputs....................7
1.3.2.5 Outcomes....................8
1.4 Evaluating a Surveillance System....................8
1.4.1 Output Measures....................8
1.4.1.1 Sensitivity....................8
1.4.1.2 Representativeness....................9
1.4.1.3 Predictive Value Positive....................9
1.4.1.4 Timeliness....................9
1.4.2 Process Measures....................9
1.4.2.1 Acceptability....................9
1.4.2.2 Simplicity....................10
1.4.2.3 Flexibility....................10
1.4.2.4 Cost....................10
1.5 Conclusions....................10
References....................10

1.1 INTRODUCTION

Surveillance is an essential part of public health practice and is vital in the control of waterborne disease. Later chapters in this section will discuss in some detail the design and management of surveillance systems for waterborne disease at local and national levels. In this chapter, we will take the opportunity to discuss some of the general principles behind the design of effective surveillance, but before progressing any further we should consider the purpose of surveillance systems. To this author, surveillance systems have value only if they lead directly or indirectly to the improvement of the health of the people surveyed.

0-8493-1259-0/03/$0.00+$1.50

For waterborne disease issues there is further value in developing adequate public health surveillance systems, in that the Third Ministerial Conference on Environment and Health of the Protocol on Water and Health to the 1992 Convention on the Protection and Use of Transboundary Watercourses and International Lakes committed signatory states to a number of actions.[1] In Article 4, signatory states were to take appropriate measures to ensure effective systems for monitoring situations likely to result in outbreaks or incidents of water-related disease and for responding to such outbreaks and incidents and their risks. Under Article 7, parties were required to collect and evaluate data on indicators designed to show how far a process contributed towards preventing, controlling, or reducing water-related disease. Under Article 8, signatories were required to ensure that comprehensive national and/or local surveillance and early-warning systems were established, improved, or maintained which would:

- Identify outbreaks or incidents of water-related disease or significant threats of such outbreaks or incidents, including those resulting from water-pollution incidents or extreme weather events
- Give prompt and clear notification to the relevant public authorities about such outbreaks, incidents, or threats
- In the event of any imminent threat to public health from water-related disease, disseminate to members of the public who may be affected all information that is held by a public authority that could help the public to prevent or mitigate harm.

All these activities require efficient and effective surveillance public health systems. Let us now consider the role of surveillance in a simple model of public health practice before going on to discuss the principles behind the design of effective surveillance systems, and once they have been designed, how best to evaluate them.

1.2 A MODEL OF PUBLIC HEALTH PRACTICE

We can think of public health practice as a negative feedback loop controlling the health of the population in much the same way that a thermostat controls the temperature of a room. Figure 1.1 shows a diagrammatic model of such a thermostat that may control the temperature of a room heated by a single radiator. The black box represents the radiator and the input is hot water from the central heating boiler; the output is heat warming up the room. The sensor is a temperature gauge that continuously measures the room temperature. Information about the room temperature is passed back to the comparator where it is compared with a predetermined ideal temperature. If the room temperature differs from the ideal, information is transmitted to the actuator where the flow of hot water into the radiator is varied until the ideal temperature is reached.

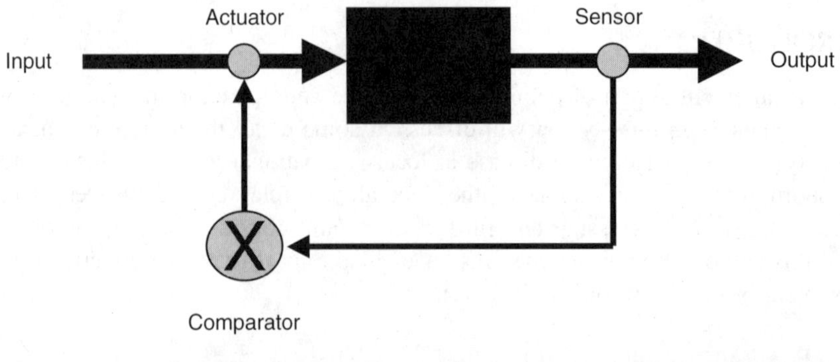

FIGURE 1.1 Basic diagram of a negative feedback control loop such as a simple thermostat.

In the negative feedback loop model of public health practice, the sensor represents the surveillance system that monitors incidence of disease in a community. The incidence of disease (the risk of illness) is then compared with what is considered acceptable. Determining acceptable disease risk is a complex mix of political and public health decision-making. A discussion of the rationale for these decisions is beyond the scope of this chapter but is considered elsewhere.[2] If the risk of illness in a population is unacceptably high (I cannot envisage a public health system that would ever consider that a disease risk was unacceptably low), then the actuator would represent some form of public health intervention. The value of this model is that it emphasizes the link between public health surveillance and public health intervention in order to benefit the health of the population. We shall return to this latter point a number of times in this chapter.

1.3 DESIGNING A SURVEILLANCE SYSTEM

Designing a new surveillance system requires a series of logical steps. The schema used here is derived from one first developed by the United States Centers for Disease Control (CDC).[3]

1.3.1 Agree upon the Objectives of the Surveillance System

This may seem obvious, but it is sometimes forgotten. Unless clear objectives are agreed upon at the outset, it will not be clear whether the surveillance system has met its objectives. The objectives can be described in terms of the health problem to be addressed, the purpose of the surveillance system, and the target population.

1.3.1.1 The Health Problem to be Addressed

The health problem surveyed must be sufficiently important to make the effort required to develop and run a surveillance system worthwhile. Whether a disease is sufficiently important is determined by how common the disease is and the severity of its outcomes. In addition, the disease must be amenable to control or amelioration if detected early enough by an adequate surveillance system. It seems unethical (as well as a waste of money) to develop and run a surveillance system that does not have the potential to benefit the health of the population surveyed.

Also, early on in the development of a system we need to be clear about what disease is being surveyed, and this requires an appropriate case definition. Case definitions can be specific or broad and can be based on clinical syndrome or laboratory-confirmed diagnoses. For example, we may wish to survey cases of self-reported diarrheal disease or we may wish to restrict the surveillance to cases of gastroenteritis from which one of a range of pathogens has been identified by laboratory tests.

1.3.1.2 The Purpose of the Surveillance System

There are a number of possible purposes for which surveillance systems can be developed. They can be designed to identify outbreaks or other adverse events early enough to implement control measures that reduce the number of cases. This is the basis of several national surveillance systems. Surveillance systems may have a longer-term purpose to identify the patterns of disease in order to identify risk factors so that control measures can be implemented. They may also be used to measure the impact of public health interventions by evaluating the impact of prevention and control programs. Finally, they may be used to help managed health care delivery by projecting future health care needs.

1.3.1.3 The Target Population

The target population also needs to be chosen with care. Clearly, the population should be one which will experience the disease under study. There is obviously little value in designing a surveillance system for testicular cancer that includes both men and women. For most infectious diseases, one would wish to include the entire population in the surveillance system. However, such an all-encompassing surveillance system may be too costly to run in some countries. In this case, the surveillance may be focused on certain subgroups within the population. For example, the surveillance system may be focused on preschool children, elderly residents of nursing homes, patients on hospital wards, or people with a pre-existing disease such as patients with AIDS. These subgroups may be chosen because the disease under study usually attacks a certain group in preference to the general population (e.g., pneumocystis pneumonia in AIDS patients). It may also be easier or less costly to study subgroups in order to get a picture of the prevalence of disease in the general population (e.g., surveillance of influenza in elderly persons' residences). Whatever group is chosen for the surveillance system, it should be clear what criteria are to be used to determine whether people belong to such groups and who should or should not be included in any surveillance data.

1.3.2 Determine the Characteristics of the Surveillance System

Once the system objectives are agreed upon, then the attention turns to the design of the system. Several key aspects of the design of any surveillance system will need to be addressed: the data set, the data flow, the analysis, and the outputs and outcomes of the system.

1.3.2.1 The Data Set

The data set is basically the information collected on each case. Choosing what data are to be collected is one of the most difficult issues to resolve in the design of a new surveillance system. On the one hand, most researchers would like to collect as much information as possible. The more information collected, the more one can learn about the disease under investigation. On the other hand, the more information collected per case, the less likely people are to report cases as the effort involved in reporting a case will be correspondingly greater. There is also an ethical issue in that collecting information not related strictly to the primary objectives of the surveillance system is an abuse of an individual's right to privacy.

Consequently, the data set should be the minimum that allows the objectives to be achieved. For infectious diseases, this minimum data set will typically include the diagnosis, some measure of the date of onset (usually the date the specimen was taken or the date the case was reported), the age and sex of the case, and some measure of the geographical location of the case (ideally this would be the post-code of the case's home address, though often this may be the work address of the diagnosing doctor or laboratory). It may be appropriate for some disease surveillance systems to collect data on possible risk factors. The most common potential risk factor to include in routine surveillance is a history of foreign travel. In some systems a wide range of risk factor data may be collected. This is typically done as a form of enhanced surveillance for a particularly important or severe disease such as tuberculosis or meningococcal disease, or after the introduction of a new public health intervention such as a new immunization. Enhanced surveillance systems are more costly to run and are typically short lived.

1.3.2.2 Data Flow

Data flow concerns itself with issues about who collects the data, to whom the data is sent by what routes, and via what intermediaries. These data flows can be quite complex as shown in Figure 1.2. Perhaps the most important link in the chain is the first one. Who makes the first report is vital to any surveillance system. Without someone making that first notification, no surveillance system will work. Unfortunately, the person responsible for making the initial notification, usually a family doctor, frequently has the least interest in the system. A substantial proportion of all surveillance data is lost because the person making the diagnosis does not report his or her findings (hence the

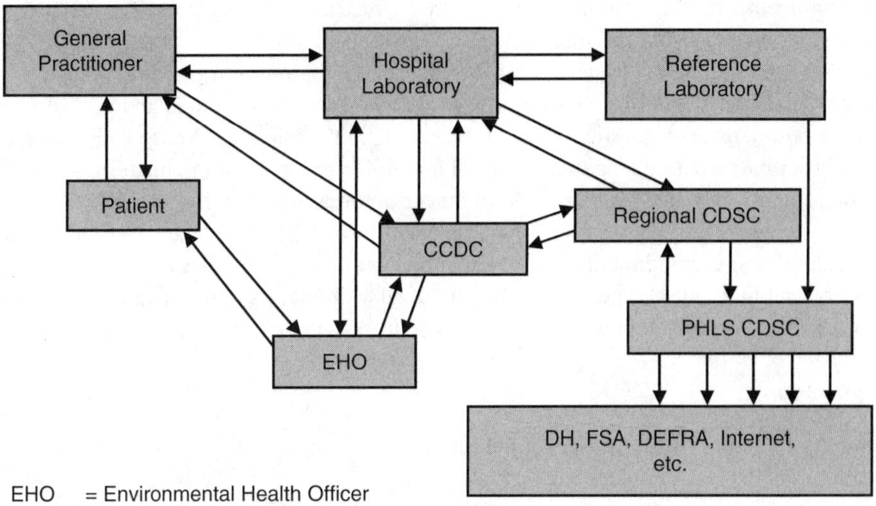

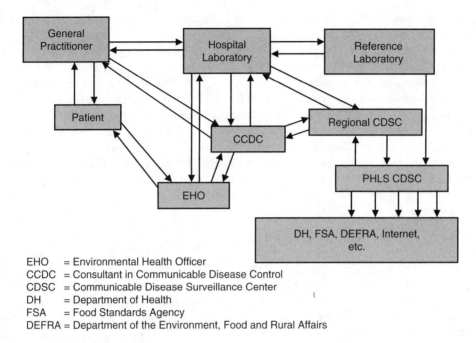

EHO = Environmental Health Officer
CCDC = Consultant in Communicable Disease Control
CDSC = Communicable Disease Surveillance Center
DH = Department of Health
FSA = Food Standards Agency
DEFRA = Department of the Environment, Food and Rural Affairs

FIGURE 1.2 Data flow for *Salmonella* surveillance in England and Wales.

need to make the reporting as simple as possible). As well as determining who is responsible for reporting cases, consideration will have to be given to how the data are recorded and transmitted. The options are paper or electronic records that are either sent by post or over some network. Electronic records are becoming more the norm as such records can be rapidly transmitted and incorporated into a central database. Consideration must be given to the security of the data and what steps have to be taken to prevent unauthorized access.

1.3.2.3 Analysis

Once the data has been collected centrally, it has to be analyzed before any useful information can be derived from the surveillance system. Consideration must be given to what types of analyses are needed and how such analyses will be carried out. For some surveillance systems, it may be sufficient to present the count of reports made over a set time period (weekly, monthly, or even annually). Some simple additional analyses may include breakdown by geographical area or by age and sex. It may be that more sophisticated statistical analyses are appropriate. As will be discussed in a subsequent chapter, geographical information systems have increasing value in the analysis of surveillance data.

1.3.2.4 Outputs

Any surveillance system will serve no purpose unless the results of the analyses are distributed to individuals and organizations that will be able to act on those results. This is the output of the surveillance system. Consideration will therefore need to be given towards what form this output should take and to whom it should be sent. The output of a surveillance system can be circulated in many ways. A weekly or monthly newsletter may summarize the relevant information. Perhaps the best-known examples of this format are the American Morbidity and Mortality Weekly Report (MMWR) and the British Communicable Disease Report (CDR). However, many similar newsletters are produced. The data may also be presented in the form of papers in peer-reviewed journals, particularly if some additional analyses have been done or the data show some especially topical or interesting event. Increasingly the outputs may be restricted to electronic presentation on Web sites that can be accessed via the Internet.

This brings us to consideration of who should receive the output of a surveillance system. As a minimum the output should be sent to individuals who may need to take action as a result. This may include policy makers, public health professionals, or clinicians. Policy makers may need to know the output in order to change national policy on, for example, immunization strategy. Public health professionals may need information to detect outbreaks or modify interventions. Clinicians may need to know so they can modify their diagnostic or therapeutic interventions, as would be the case in an influenza epidemic. Increasingly public health professionals are recognizing the right of the general public to have access to the results of surveillance systems. The increased use of the Internet for presenting surveillance data is one way to provide greater freedom of information.

1.3.2.5 Outcomes

Finally we must consider the outcomes of the surveillance system. This refers back to our discussion of aims and objectives. The outcome of any surveillance system should be enhancement of public health either by identification of disease or its risk factors so that control measures can be put in place, or by alerting clinicians to allow them to change therapy or the range of diagnostic tests. For example, a pediatrician may wish to await laboratory test results before giving antibiotics to a baby with a chest infection if the pediatrician knows that respiratory syncitial virus infection is common at the time. As I have previously stated, in my view it is unethical as well as a waste of resources to run a surveillance system that does not have the potential to improve the health of the population surveyed.

1.4 EVALUATING A SURVEILLANCE SYSTEM

When evaluating a surveillance system a number of key factors need to be considered: the sensitivity of the system, its representativeness, predictive value positive, timeliness, acceptability, simplicity, flexibility, and cost. When deciding whether a surveillance system is achieving its objectives most effectively, each of these factors needs to be considered. The first four factors can be considered measures of the output, and the remaining four measures of the process.

1.4.1 Output Measures

1.4.1.1 Sensitivity

The sensitivity of a system is a measure of its ability to detect events that are under surveillance. An event may be a case of infection or it may be an outbreak. Sensitivity is usually presented as the proportion of cases occurring in the community that are recorded by the system. Unfortunately we have a relatively poor knowledge about the sensitivity of most systems other than knowing that only a minority of cases ever get recorded. Sensitivity is affected by a number of factors, known as the reporting pyramid. Not everyone who is infected will become ill; not everyone who is ill will seek medical attention; not everyone who attends a doctor will have a stool specimen taken; not every stool specimen will be examined for the relevant pathogen; not every time a pathogen is present will the laboratory correctly identify it; not all positive laboratory tests are reported to the surveillance system. The data within any surveillance system represents the tip of the iceberg with the major part of its structure under the water. Unlike real icebergs, however, one cannot easily determine what proportion lies under the water.

One of the best studies to investigate the issue of sensitivity found that the sensitivity of the system for enteric pathogen surveillance varied from as little as 0.06% for Norwalk-like virus to 7.9% for *Campylopbacter* to 31.8% for *Salmonella*.[4] Because of the very poor sensitivity of most surveillance systems, they are of little value in determining disease burden. Their value is in identifying sudden changes in incidence.

One of the biggest problems facing anyone trying to compare disease burden across different countries is that the sensitivity of any surveillance system varies substantially from one country to another. The large variation in reported waterborne disease between European countries is a clear example of this.[5] The surveillance systems of many European countries are incapable of detecting waterborne disease.

1.4.1.2 Representativeness

The fact that only a small proportion of cases are detected by even the best surveillance systems raises the issue of whether the ascertained cases are representative of the typical case in the community. If a surveillance system has high representativeness, then cases ascertained from the surveillance system can be used to make assumptions about the disease in the community; if not, then any assumptions are likely to be systematically biased. For example, if only the relatively affluent can afford a doctor in a particular country, then any surveillance system based on reports from doctors would give a very biased picture of the typical case, suggesting that cases of a particular illness were present only in the wealthy.

1.4.1.3 Predictive Value Positive

In even the best-run surveillance systems, not every case will actually have had the disease. It is not uncommon in medicine for patients to be misdiagnosed. There have even been reports of pseudo-outbreaks resulting from laboratories misdiagnosing artifacts as pathogens.[6] The predictive value positive (PVP) of a surveillance system is the proportion of cases included in the data set who do actually have the disease. As with the sensitivity measure, this is very difficult to estimate exactly and would require significant effort to review patient records. PVP also varies substantially from one surveillance system to another. A system to detect waterborne outbreaks by capturing cases of infectious diarrhea through sales of antidiarrheal medication is likely to have low PVP as changes in medication sales may reflect outbreaks, or it may reflect increased sales because of a television advertisement campaign.

1.4.1.4 Timeliness

Does the surveillance system give information early enough to enable people to take appropriate public health action? Laboratory-based surveillance systems often take some time to provide effective information. Once a patient is infected, it may be a few days before he becomes ill, and once ill he may delay going to the doctor for a day or so. Even when the patient attends his doctor, the doctor may decide not to take a fecal sample on the first visit. Time is also lost during transport of the sample to the laboratory, during specimen processing, and in reporting the result to the surveillance center. Even after the case has been reported, there may be a delay before the data are analyzed and an event recognized. Most outbreaks of food and waterborne disease are detected only after the primary contamination event has passed.

1.4.2 Process Measures

1.4.2.1 Acceptability

For any surveillance system to work well it should be acceptable to the people intended to make it work. The most important are the people who make the initial report. Unless the system is acceptable to them, initial reports will not be made and there will be little information available for analysis. Acceptability for most medical staff equates with ease of use. If doctors are required to complete long questionnaires, it will not be done. Also of vital importance is the acceptability of the system to the people surveyed. An acceptable system does not collect any personal information unless it is absolutely necessary for public health, and any data collected should not traceable back to an individual or, if it is, should be held securely.

1.4.2.2 Simplicity

A simple system is one where the case definition is clear, the data collected are kept to a minimum, lines of reporting are clear, and the analysis is relatively straightforward. Simple systems are likely to be less costly, more robust, and easier to understand and monitor.

1.4.2.3 Flexibility

The public health priorities of a particular surveillance system may change with time. This may be because of a change in the epidemiology of the disease, new evidence of potential risk factors, a change in political priorities, or a change in available information technology. Clearly the best surveillance systems will be able to accommodate these changing events, allowing changes in the design of the system to cope with them. For example, a surveillance system that relies on the presence of a particular information technology in doctors' offices may fail when that technology becomes obsolete. Flexible systems are also likely to be simple systems.

1.4.2.4 Cost

Although not explicitly included in the CDC guidelines,[3] the cost of the system is of high importance. Surveillance systems can be very costly in terms of both financial and human resources. The resources required will be a major factor in deciding whether a particular surveillance system is likely to be implemented. The costs of surveillance systems need to be compared with the potential benefits to public health. The costs and benefits of surveillance will be dependent on the problem addressed, the context, and society's priorities at that time.

1.5 CONCLUSIONS

Surveillance is an extremely important tool of modern health practice. Without surveillance systems we would not be able to design or implement appropriate interventions to improve public health.[7] Even if we did implement public health interventions we would not know whether they had been effective in improving the health of the population. The need for public health surveillance systems is just as important for waterborne disease as for other health problems. Without adequate surveillance systems it will not be possible to identify what burden of disease is due to drinking water, and without this knowledge there will be little impetus for improvement. It is a sad fact that many countries, even in the developed world, have no adequate surveillance system to protect their population from waterborne disease.[5]

REFERENCES

1. United Nations Economic and Social Council, Economic Commission for Europe and World Health Organization's Regional Office for Europe, *Protocol on Water and Health to the 1992 Convention on the Protection and Use of Transboundary Watercourses and International Lakes.*
2. Hunter, P.R. and Fewtrell, L., Acceptable risk, in: *Water Quality: Guidelines, Standards and Health. Risk Assessment and Management for Water-Related Infectious Disease,* Fewtrell, L. and Bartram J., Eds., IWA Publishing, London, 2001, 207.

3. Centers for Disease Control, Guidelines for evaluating surveillance systems, *MMWR,* 37 (Suppl 5), 1, 1988.
4. Wheeler, J. G. et al., Study of infectious intestinal disease in England: rates in the community, presenting to general practice, and reported in national surveillance, *Brit. Med. J.,* 318, 1046, 1999.
5. Anonymous, *Water and Health in Europe*, World Health Organization Regional Office for Europe 1999.
6. Casemore, D.P., A pseudo-outbreak of cryptosporidiosis, *CDR Rev.,* 2, R66, 1992.
7. Eisenberg, J., Bartram, J., and Hunter, P.R., A public health perspective for establishing water-related guidelines and standards, in: *Water Quality: Guidelines, Standards and Health. Risk Assessment and Management for Water-Related Infectious Disease,* Fewtrell, L. and Bartram J., Eds., IWA Publishing, London, 2001, 229.

2 Local Surveillance Systems

Catherine Quigley, James J. Gibson, and Paul R. Hunter

CONTENTS

2.1 Introduction....................13
2.2 Local Surveillance in England and Wales....................14
2.2.1 Components of Local Surveillance....................14
2.2.1.1 Notifications....................14
2.2.1.2 Laboratory Isolates....................14
2.2.1.3 Further Information Collected at the Local Level....................14
2.2.1.4 Dissemination of Local Surveillance Data....................15
2.2.2 Do Local Surveillance Data Pick Up Outbreaks?....................15
2.2.3 Identification of Risk Factors and Trends for Sporadic Disease....................15
2.3 Local Surveillance in the United States....................16
2.3.1 Authorities....................16
2.3.2 Weaknesses....................17
2.3.3 Other Sources of Case Surveillance Data....................18
2.3.4 Sensitivity of Surveillance....................19
2.3.4.1 Innovative Approaches to Increasing Sensitivity in Outbreak Detection....................19
2.4 Conclusions....................19
References....................20
Appendix A: Developing an Integrated System of Health and Technical Data....................21

2.1 INTRODUCTION

The foundation for any surveillance system rests on the quality of those surveillance activities that are closest to the patient. In this chapter we consider two surveillance systems that are undertaken at the local level, one in the U.K. and the other in the U.S.

The functions of local surveillance systems are similar to the functions of all surveillance, as discussed in Chapter 1. However, local surveillance systems have a number of special characteristics and functions.

A key feature of many local systems is that they act as the point of entry for case data that may eventually become part of national or international surveillance systems. Because local surveillance systems are closer to the patient, the results of these systems tend to be more timely than those undertaken at national level. Similarly, local surveillance must be more closely linked to intervention. On the other hand, local surveillance tends to be based on relatively small populations and so the power to detect uncommon occurrences is low. It is also unlikely that local surveillance systems would have the resources to adequately monitor a broad range of different infections; consequently attention should be given to full surveillance of key problems. We will now turn our attention to the two examples.

0-8493-1259-0/03/$0.00+$1.50

2.2 LOCAL SURVEILLANCE IN ENGLAND AND WALES

In England and Wales, health authorities are required to have arrangements in place for the surveillance and control of communicable diseases. At present a typical district health authority covers a population of about 450,000. The legislation governing the control of communicable disease (including the requirement to notify certain diseases) rests with local authorities who usually appoint consultants in communicable disease control (CCDCs) for that function. CCDCs act as "proper officers" for purposes of the legislation.

2.2.1 Components of Local Surveillance

The main components of local surveillance in England and Wales are:

- Notifications to the proper officer by doctors attending patients suspected of having certain specified infectious diseases
- Reports of isolates from public health laboratories and hospital laboratories to the CCDC

Other sources of data relevant to waterborne infection include:

- Outbreaks from settings such as schools, nursing homes, and residential homes are reported to the CCDC or to local authority environmental health departments
- Incidents that might lead to illness are reported by water companies to the CCDC and to local authority environmental health departments

2.2.1.1 Notifications

Doctors attending patients suspected of having certain specified infectious diseases have a legal duty to notify the proper officer of the local authority using a standard form which includes name, address, age, and date of onset of illness. Doctors are paid a small fee for each notification. One of the notifiable diseases, food poisoning, refers to waterborne disease: "any disease of an infectious or toxic nature caused by or thought to be caused by the consumption of food or water."

This system has serious problems; many doctors are not aware of their legal duty to notify, and the list of notifiable diseases is out of date. There are particular problems relating to foodborne and waterborne diseases because the clinical diagnosis of food poisoning (including waterborne infections) is extremely difficult. In general a patient presents with diarrhea, the cause of which (food poisoning or person-to-person spread) may not be obvious.

2.2.1.2 Laboratory Isolates

Reports of laboratory isolates are the mainstay of local surveillance of waterborne disease in the U.K. General practitioners are encouraged to send fecal specimens to the laboratory for patients who present with suspected gastrointestinal infection. Testing is provided free of charge to patients as part of National Health Service general medical services. While reporting is voluntary, the majority of laboratories do report to the CCDC. However, this system also underestimates disease occurrence because many patients with gastrointestinal illness do not present to a doctor and of those who do, not all are tested.[1] In addition, testing policies vary between laboratories (for example, some laboratories have age-related policies with regard to testing for certain organisms).[2]

2.2.1.3 Further Information Collected at the Local Level

As indicated above, the information provided on patients with suspected or proven waterborne disease via the notification and laboratory reporting systems is very limited. The extent to which further information on apparently sporadic cases is ascertained varies throughout the country. However, there are exceptions. For example, as *Cryptosporidium* is the most commonly reported organism in outbreaks associated with drinking water in the U.K., particular attention is given to monitoring and investigating sporadic cases of cryptosporidiosis. In the Cheshire and Wirral Communicable Disease Unit, which provides a communicable disease control service on behalf of three health authorities in the North West of England, standard information is collected on all cases of cryptosporidiosis by environmental health officers. A standard questionnaire recommended by a national group of experts is used and the information collected includes: occupation, date of onset of illness, details of others ill in the household, source of drinking water, and details of risk factors such as travel, contact with animals, and exposure to recreational water.[3] A more detailed questionnaire is used in the event of an outbreak.

When informed by a water company that cryptosporidial oocysts have been detected in treated water, a pro forma is used to collect information that contributes to a health risk assessment. This information includes details regarding the water sample, the number of oocysts detected, the source and treatment of the affected water supply, the distribution area, and any recent problems or changes in the source or treatment.[4]

2.2.1.4 Dissemination of Local Surveillance Data

Local surveillance data are fed back to laboratories, environmental health departments, and general practitioners. Information from the statutory notification system is submitted weekly to the Communicable Disease Surveillance Center. Laboratories report isolates to the regional epidemiologist at the same time that they report to the CCDC, and surveillance data at the regional level are fed back in regular bulletins to CCDCs, laboratories, and environmental health departments.

2.2.2 Do Local Surveillance Data Pick Up Outbreaks?

Local surveillance should be able to:

- Monitor background rates of disease that could be transmitted by drinking water
- Allow recognition of outbreaks

Does local surveillance meet these goals?

In the Cheshire and Wirral Communicable Disease Unit, surveillance data are scrutinized daily and tabulated weekly. In 1996, local surveillance data analysis uncovered an outbreak of cryptosporidiosis that affected a community in Wirral and Ellesmere Port (in South Cheshire). During April of that year, 22 laboratory isolates of cryptosporidiosis were reported in Wirral and Ellesmere Port compared with fewer than 5 cases per month previously. Twelve of the 22 cases were reported during week 17, and this prompted an outbreak investigation, which began at the end of that week (Figure 2.1). By the end of the investigation, 52 cases of cryptosporidiosis were identified and it was concluded that the outbreak was probably associated with drinking water. Local surveillance systems had quickly identified outbreaks by comparing the observed increase with expected levels.

Since 1996, less dramatic increases were similarly identified and reported which resulted in meetings with local environmental health officers where data were reviewed and common source outbreaks ruled out (Figure 2.2). However, a recent study reported from the North West of England has suggested that many outbreaks of waterborne disease may go undetected.[5]

2.2.3 Identification of Risk Factors and Trends for Sporadic Disease

Local surveillance, as mentioned, has the potential to identify risk factors and trends with regard to sporadic cases of waterborne disease. However, gathering data on sporadic cases can be time consuming and may not be considered worthwhile. Risk factors for cases of cryptosporidiosis in

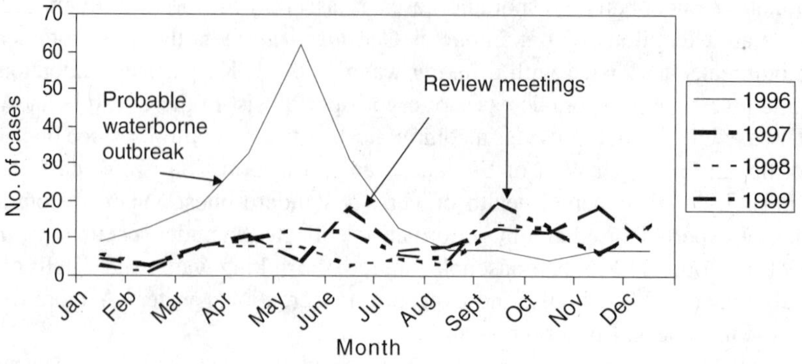

FIGURE 2.1 Laboratory reports of cryptosporidiosis in Cheshire and Wirral, by month, 1996–1999.

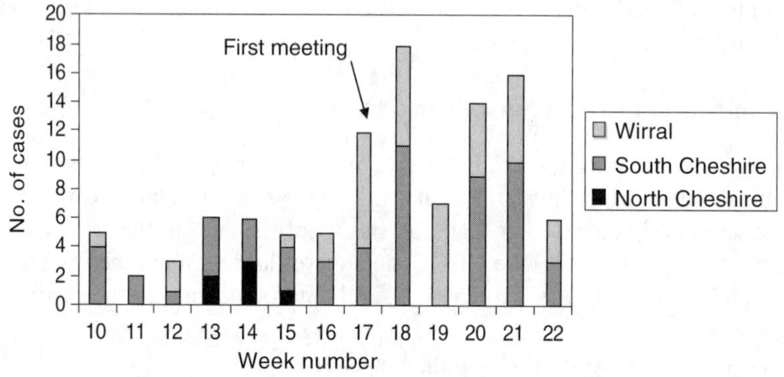

FIGURE 2.2 Probable waterborne outbreak in Wirral and Ellesmere Port, April 1996. Cases by week of report.

Cheshire and Wirral during 1999 were identified in only 39% of cases (41 of 105). However, even though incomplete, this information was considered worthwhile as it identified that contact with farm animals (reported by 14 of the 41) may be an important factor for prevention.

2.3 LOCAL SURVEILLANCE IN THE UNITED STATES

2.3.1 Authorities

Surveillance and response for acute public health diseases is conducted by a three-level system in the United States (Figure 2.3). While this system varies from state to state, the following essential elements are similar in all states. Initial reports (notifications) are usually sent by physicians and clinical laboratories on a standard reporting card or called in by phone to the local county or city health department or multi-county health district, which may serve a jurisdiction from under 5000 to over 8 million persons. This report is reviewed briefly to determine if it fits a standard case definition,[6] if an investigation is needed, or if a preventive response is indicated. It is then forwarded by mail or courier to the second level of the system, the state health department. There the report is again reviewed, usually daily, for conformity to a case definition or need for further clinical or risk factor data, for indication for an immediate preventive response, or for indications of a possible cluster of similar cases that may cross local jurisdictional boundaries. Reported cases are tentatively classified as "suspect, probable, or confirmed" according to standard definitions determined by the U.S. Centers for Disease Control and Prevention (CDC) and the Council of State and Territorial Epidemiologists.[6] A standard case investigation form, usually that specified by the CDC, may be sent back to the local department or directly to the reporting health provider to gather further clinical and epidemiologic

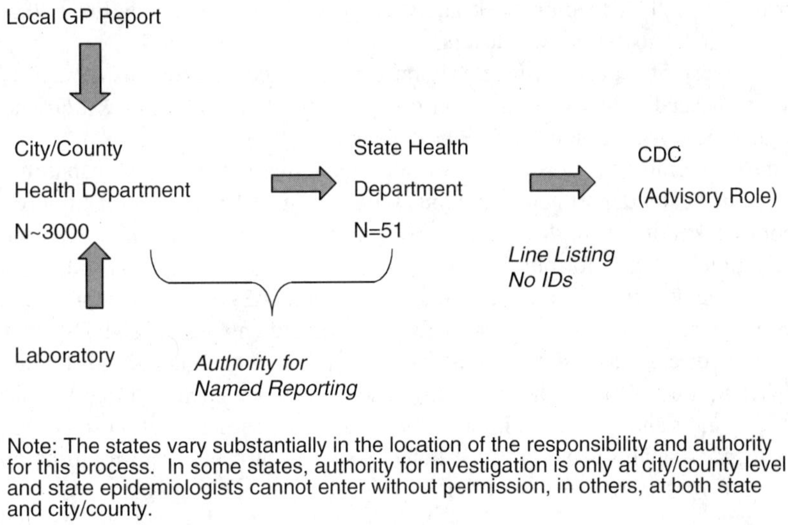

FIGURE 2.3 Communicable disease case reporting in the U.S.: a three-tiered system.

data. The report is then entered into the state's National Electronic Telecommunications Surveillance System (NETSS) database, into which are also entered similar reports from clinical laboratories (usually computer printouts), and results of more detailed laboratory characterization of some agents or subtyping data from the state public health laboratory. At the end of each week provider and laboratory reports are compared and merged, and duplicate reports are deleted. The week's reported cases are classified for level of diagnostic certainty (suspect, probable, or confirmed), stripped of identifiers, and sent in line-listed form by e-mail to the third level of the system, the CDC.

Statutory authority to require reporting, investigation, and preventive response by public health authorities lies at the state and large-city levels. Thus, with some rare exceptions such as investigation of a potential bioterrorist incident, outbreak investigations always begin at the state or local level and federal participation happens only at the invitation of the state health department. Likewise, the list of reportable conditions and manner of reporting is specified by state law and varies somewhat from state to state. A general principle is that a condition should be reportable only if a public health preventive action might reasonably follow that report.

2.3.2 Weaknesses

This system has a number of flaws in most jurisdictions. These originate primarily from lack of staff at the local level to investigate or give a preventive response to all the reports from clinicians and laboratories, as well as a lack of modern communication systems.[7] These flaws include:

1. Timeliness: because most notifications are sent on paper, and laboratories (the most complete sources of reports) report cases only in batches, delays of days to months can intervene from the date of onset to the time a public health response is begun.
2. Completeness: the system is based on submission of reports of clinical conditions by clinical laboratories and health care providers, mostly primary care physicians and hospital infection control practitioners. Clinician reporting is essential for a number of conditions such as AIDS, most of the vaccine-preventable diseases, and meningococcal infections, since they are clinical diagnoses or would not be reported by laboratories in time to allow effective public health action. However, with the exception of a few high-profile conditions, reportable diseases are incompletely reported by health care providers, even though they are required to do so by law. No positive reinforcement is given for

reporting other than feeding back analyzed surveillance data. This limits the system's sensitivity for detecting case clusters.

3. Paper delivery of reports: clinical laboratories are excellent sources of reports but currently most send batches of cases on computer printouts or hand-written cards which must then be re-keyed into NETSS at the state level.
4. Routine gathering of exposure data on reported cases is beyond the capability of most local public health departments, and thus such exposure data is rarely routinely collected, except in cases of severe diseases (e.g., HIV, meningococcal meningitis, typhoid fever) or conditions targeted for elimination such as measles, rubella, or syphilis.
5. Lack of integration of different acute disease surveillance systems: general communicable diseases are reported to one unit at the state level and entered into NETSS, but sexually transmitted diseases are reported to a different unit and maintained in a different database. HIV/AIDS, tuberculosis, lead poisoning, and cancers are each reported to still different state-level units and databases. Each of these databases uses a different software platform, and integrated analyses can only be done as special projects requiring time-consuming merging of files using case identifiers.

In addition, reporting of most waterborne pathogens suffers from the difficulty that the clinical syndrome they cause is usually not specific for any particular pathogen. To compound this problem, most cases of gastroenteritis do not have a specimen submitted for diagnostic microbiology, particularly in recent years as the incentives for medical cost reduction mount. These facts reduce probability of detection of clusters of potentially waterborne agents such as *Cryptosporidium*, *Giardia*, or Norwalk-like virus (or even milder cases of Shiga-toxin producing *Escherichia coli*). The result is low completeness of detection of infections with waterborne pathogens and low frequency of detection of waterborne outbreaks.[8]

2.3.3 Other Sources of Case Surveillance Data

Three other methods provide valuable data to detect apparent clusters.

1. Telephone reports from hospital emergency departments, nursing homes, and schools: for focal, high-incidence outbreaks of gastroenteritis (for example) emergency department or other institutional staff are one of the commonest sources of notification that "something is going on."
2. Sentinel surveillance for influenza and other respiratory virus isolates: before each influenza season many state health departments provide a number of "sentinel" practices or clinics with respiratory virus specimen collection kits and a method of sending the specimen to the state laboratory for viral isolation as a way of monitoring the range of influenza viral types and subtypes occurring during that season. Health department HIV testing and counseling clinics provide a sentinel surveillance system as well.
3. Routine subtyping of isolates of common bacterial pathogens (e.g., pulsed-field gel electrophoresis [PFGE] of *Campylobacter*, non-enteritidis *Salmonella*, *E. coli* O157:H7) to detect time-space clusters of individual subtypes: these clusters might indicate a common source of infection. Usually foodborne sources are the target. Such subtype clusters must then be investigated using a case-control study in search of an exposure associated with disease. It is unclear how cost effective this approach is for detecting true common source outbreaks, considering the work involved and the number of false-positive clusters that must be investigated. More such subtype clusters need to be studied with this issue in mind. A recent study of effectiveness of investigation of clusters of foodborne bacterial infections of the same subtype suggested that only clusters with at least six cases are worth taking to a case-control study.[9]

2.3.4 Sensitivity of Surveillance

An example of reporting sensitivity from the Milwaukee, WI outbreak of cryptosporidiosis gives some idea of the expected sensitivity for culturing cases of gastroenteritis, and for their reporting.[10] Using a conservative estimate of 285,000 cases of gastroenteritis, there were 17,100 persons who sought medical care, and of them 971 received a stool test for a protozoan cause of their disease (0.3% of cases and 5.7% of those with a medical encounter). Of those, only 41 were diagnosed with *Cryptosporidium*, and only a fraction of those were eventually reported. The outbreak was not detected by the routine communicable disease system in place, but rather by astute clinicians and public health officers who noted the striking increase in sales of antidiarrheal medications.

In another example, in the state of South Carolina (population 4,012,000 in 2000) the total number of cases of *Cryptosporidium* reported in 1996 through 1999 was 61, for a median annual incidence rate of 0.4/100,000. In spite of a special level of sensitization to *Cryptosporidium* in pediatricians in the city of Greenville (population 300,000) because its water supply is from unfiltered surface water, during that entire period only three cases were detected. Routine surveillance data did, however, allow the State Health Department to detect a *Cryptosporidium* outbreak in Charleston County from recreational exposure to a neighborhood swimming pool in 1999.[11] We therefore concluded that the current system may be able to detect larger outbreaks in areas where physicians order appropriate microbiologic tests for gastroenteritis, but that many cases and smaller outbreaks are probably missed.

2.3.4.1 Innovative Approaches to Increasing Sensitivity in Outbreak Detection

One approach is routine sentinel reporting of all gastroenteritis cases from hospital emergency departments ("syndromic surveillance" for gastroenteritis). In this method numbers of cases of gastroenteritis from a fixed set of sentinel clinical settings are followed to detect unusual increases in incidents that are not explained by known environmental or seasonal factors. Such sentinel syndromic surveillance is currently being evaluated in several jurisdictions.

Another approach is routine reporting of sales of over-the-counter antidiarrheal medications to monitor for significant increases above normal utilization. Such a striking increase in sales accompanied the famous waterborne outbreak of cryptosporidiosis in Milwaukee, WI in 1994, but trials of this method of surveillance in New York City discovered that an advertisement for an over-the-counter antidiarrheal during television coverage of the football superbowl resulted in a similar significant increase in sales.[12]

2.4 CONCLUSIONS

The two surveillance systems discussed in this chapter illustrate some of the key features of local surveillance systems. In both, reporting of cases is a legal requirement, but despite that there is evidence of substantial under-reporting by diagnosing physicians. The reasons for this under-reporting include a lack of understanding by physicians of their responsibilities and uncertainty about what should or should not be reported. In the United States at least, additional reasons for incomplete reporting include the increasing cost disincentives for ordering diagnostic laboratory testing for cases of gastroenteritis, and a lack of positive incentives for clinicians to take the time to report.

In both systems, reports are regularly scrutinized to identify possible outbreaks. However, the sensitivity for detection of outbreaks and identification of risk factors is probably poor. These issues are addressed in more detail in later chapters. It would also appear that those responsible for local disease surveillance in both countries are investigating possible alternative ways to identify outbreaks of waterborne disease, though as yet these systems also suffer from substantial weaknesses.

One approach, discussed in the appendix to this chapter, is to link public health and water utility to identify outbreaks in a more timely manner than currently possible.

One issue not discussed by either contributor is that those responsible for the management of local surveillance systems usually have many other responsibilities. For example, in the U.K., the CCDC is also responsible for managing outbreaks, contact tracing, developing policies, monitoring hospital control of infection activities, immunization campaigns, as well as many other things. It is in the wide demands on local people's time that the main weakness of local surveillance rests. Local surveillance systems are frequently under-resourced and supervised by people who may just not have the time to devote to the monitoring and analysis that surveillance systems require to be most effective.

REFERENCES

1. Wheeler, J.G. et al., Study of infectious intestinal disease in England: rates in the community, presenting to general practice, and reported in national surveillance, *Brit. Med. J.*, 318, 1046, 1999.
2. Chalmers, R.M. et al., Laboratory ascertainment of *Cryptosporidium* and local authority public health policies for the investigation of sporadic cases of cryptosporidiosis in two regions of the United Kingdom, submitted.
3. Department of the Environment, Transport and the Regions & Department of Health, *Cryptosporidium* in Water Supplies, Third Report of the Group of Experts, 1998.
4. Hunter, P.R., Advice on the response from public and environmental health to the detection of cryptosporidial oocysts in treated drinking water, *Comm. Dis. Public Health*, 3, 24, 2000.
5. Hunter, P.R., Syed, Q., and Naumova, E.N., Possible undetected outbreaks of cryptosporidiosis in areas of the North West of England supplied by an unfiltered surface water source, *Comm. Dis. Public Health*, 4, 136, 2001.
6. CDC, Case definitions for infectious conditions under public health surveillance, *MMWR*, 46, RR10, 1, 1997
7. Parrish II, R.G. and McDonnell, S.M., Sources of health-related information, in *Principles and Practice of Public Health Surveillance*, Teutsch, S.M. and Churchill, R.E. (Eds), Oxford Univ. Press, 2000, 30.
8. Levy, D.A. et al., Surveillance for waterborne-disease outbreaks — United States, 1995–1996, *MMWR*, 47 (No. SS-5), 1, 1998.
9. Osterholm, M., personal communication, 2001.
10. Mackenzie, W.R. et al., A massive outbreak in Milwaukee of *Cryptosporidium* infection transmitted through the public water supply, *New Engl. J. Med.*, 331, 161, 1994.
11. South Carolina Department of Health Communicable Disease Reporting Registry, issues for 1996–1999.
12. Layton, M., personal communication, 2001.

Appendix A: Developing an Integrated System of Health and Technical Data

Alan Thompson

CONTENTS

The water industry has for a long time collected and held information in a number of fields including process/operational and research data, as well as information required in terms of regulatory monitoring. It has, then, a large, complex, comprehensive, and well organized database but one which is under-utilized outside of the strict domain of water supply compliance. In contrast, health data tends to be unstandardized, reactive in nature, and limited in size.

Ideally, the community would be best served by an integrated system of both technical and health data working in as close to "real time" as possible. It would be necessary to distinguish the needs at national and local levels, the former allowing identification of trends by using very large data sets, probably over a considerable period of time, whereas at a local level the need is for a prompt and appropriate reaction to a particular event.

A.1 CURRENT SITUATION

The data from both the public health and water utility departments are inextricably linked. Efficient exchange of information between these two is required to answer two fundamental questions:

- If there is evidence of noncompliance in the water supply, whether bacteriological, chemical, or physical, is there evidence of illness in the community?
- If there is evidence of an emerging outbreak in the community, is there reason to believe that the water supply is implicated?

The problem with such a concept is the timeliness of data acquisition and interpretation. Classical water quality testing is of a known standard and duration (e.g., 18 h for coliform analysis). However, increasingly water utilities are challenging this basic approach. An increased awareness of risk has led utilities to consider the treatment process as a whole and hence the overall process risk, incorporating resource quality and process efficiency as well as final water quality.

In terms of analysis, genetic techniques are increasingly able to identify distinct pathogenic organisms rather than simply "indicators," and in a greatly reduced analytical period. The devel-

0-8493-1259-0/03/$0.00+$1.50

opment of the "DNA chip" by Ondeo Services (formerly Lyonnaise des Eaux) is a good example of this approach whereby selected pathogenic organisms will be extracted and positively identified from water samples in approximately 4 h. Overall, then, the trend is for greatly reduced analytical timescales with many tests becoming available on-line.

Health surveillance has traditionally relied upon both clinical notification by family doctors and a "gold standard" of laboratory isolates of pathogenic organisms from people who are ill. Typically the time from exposure to confirmed isolate is a week or more. As the clinical notification system is very weak, the problem remains that hard evidence becomes available long after the health crisis has occurred.

A.2 THE WAY AHEAD

The key, then, is the early detection of emerging foci of infection. Current surveillance systems do not do this well, as they are geared to meeting national analysis of trends. Outbreak detection demands prompt information, which is of necessity incomplete and provisional. Trend analysis, by comparison, needs precise information, which inevitably means it will be delayed. As an interim until hard data becomes available, increases in the number of symptomatic people can be used as early warning markers. Such markers include school absenteeism, pharmaceutical sales, NHS Direct help-line enquiries, and, of course, water utility complaints. These can be collected daily allowing a very fast (early) response. Clearly, they have a higher degree of inherent uncertainty than a laboratory isolate. They can, however, trigger an active case search, particularly with family doctors, to confirm the likelihood of excess community illness. An increase in any single early warning marker may be random, but concurrent increases in several "soft" markers should generate an alarm.

A.2.1 Episys

A project between the North of Tyne Communicable Disease Control Unit and Northumbrian Water Limited currently running in the North East of England aims to satisfy many of these requirements. The early warning marker surveillance and active case search have been established for three years. Supporting these has required a radical redesign of computer support to store dissimilar data, quantify the levels of uncertainty, and analyze for space–time clustering on a daily basis. The immediate objectives are to:

- Produce comparative infection rates for an irregular polygon (corresponding to whatever area water has been supplied)
- Compare rates of infection in the same area at different times
- Produce a probabilistic model which takes into account the patterns of all the previous illness data in an area (the "accrued wisdom")

Episys is person-based rather than case-based and is sufficiently eclectic to allow syndromic surveillance as determined by changing hypotheses. These systems have shown themselves capable of:

- Detecting traditional episodes (salmonella in schoolchildren)
- Tracking non-notifiable illness (viral community outbreaks, which were subsequently laboratory confirmed)
- Detection of episodes where no laboratory data exists (viral illness, data from multiple sources)

Human resources are required to maintain data input and remove anomalies, but these are modest in comparison to the benefits. There are also, of course, major advantages for the water utility. The ability to predict with some certainty the outcome of a particular level of hazard (nonconformity) will allow the preparation of detailed and appropriate response plans by both utility and local authority, to be implemented in "real time."

A.3 CONCLUSIONS

In the role of public health, both the water industry and local authorities have different but complementary skills in the realm of data acquisition storage and interpretation. The technical challenges are relatively well understood, and so it remains a question of coordination, capacity, leadership, and cooperation, as well as resources; however, the benefits of early detection and appropriate response to community infection are clearly of enormous value.

3 National Surveillance Systems

Rosalind Stanwell-Smith, Yvonne Andersson, and Deborah A. Levy

CONTENTS

3.1 Introduction....25
3.2 Surveillance in the United Kingdom....25
3.2.1 Detected Waterborne Outbreaks in England and Wales....27
3.3 Surveillance in the United States....28
3.3.1 Characteristics of the Surveillance System....29
3.3.1.1 Sources and Types of Data....29
3.3.1.2 Methods....30
3.3.1.3 Classification of Outbreaks....30
3.3.1.4 Representativeness and Usefulness of the Surveillance System....31
3.3.1.5 Sensitivity of the Surveillance System....32
3.3.2 Strengths and Weaknesses of the Surveillance System....32
3.4 Surveillance in Sweden....32
3.4.1 Organization of the Surveillance of Communicable Diseases....33
3.4.1.1 Detection of Waterborne Outbreaks by the Surveillance System....33
3.4.1.2 Alternative Ways of Recognizing Waterborne Outbreaks....35
3.4.2 Reported Waterborne Outbreaks....36
3.5 Limitations with National Surveillance Systems....37
3.6 National Surveillance Systems of the Future....38
References....39

3.1 INTRODUCTION

This chapter builds on the previous one by broadening the focus of attention to national surveillance systems of waterborne disease. Three national surveillance systems are described: the ones in the U.K., the U.S., and Sweden. In many ways these three nations are relatively uncommon, even in the developed world, in having adequate disease surveillance systems in place that are able to detect and record outbreaks of waterborne disease.[1] In Europe, for example, most of the member states of the European Union currently have no adequate disease surveillance systems for waterborne disease. The situation in the developing world is even more problematic. Most national surveillance systems rely heavily on local surveillance for primary data collection. Local surveillance for the U.K. and U.S. was discussed in detail in Chapter 2, and that discussion will not be repeated here.

3.2 SURVEILLANCE IN THE UNITED KINGDOM

Detailed records of water-related outbreaks of infectious disease in the U.K. date back to the 1850s and were collated nationally from reports by Medical Officers of Health, supplemented from the 1940s on by reports from the Public Health Laboratory Service (PHLS) in England

0-8493-1259-0/03/$0.00+$1.50

and Wales, and from the Communicable Disease Surveillance Center (CDSC) after 1978.[2–5] The current U.K. surveillance system was established in the early 1990s to supplement the previous outbreak-based surveillance and to provide regular summaries of reported outbreaks. Scotland has a separate system for the surveillance of water-related disease: outbreak reports and incidents of chemical contamination are collated by the Scottish Center for Infection and Environmental Health (SCIEH).[6] No formal surveillance system currently exists for non-infectious waterborne disease. The four main sources of information in the surveillance system in England and Wales are:

1. Reports of suspected outbreaks received from consultants in communicable disease control in each health district, environmental health officers in local authorities, microbiologists in the PHLS and other relevant centers, regional epidemiologists, and occasionally other sources (e.g., school medical officer reports, primary care physician reporting system, the press and other media)
2. The national surveillance of routine laboratory reports used to monitor trends in water-related organisms, such as *Campylobacter* spp., *Cryptosporidium* spp., *Giardia lamblia,* and *Salmonella typhi*
3. Surveys of water quality and environmental sampling
4. Reports from the Drinking Water Inspectorate on incidents of suspected or established water contamination

The main change introduced in the last decade was grading reported outbreaks by strength of association with the putative water cause (Table 3.1).[7–10] This change was introduced as an acknowledgment of the difficulty of attributing cause in water-related disease. Attribution of a strong association usually requires microbiological confirmation of the organism in human cases and in the suspected water source. Evidence of water quality failure and a statistical association with illness in an analytical epidemiological study is now included in the criteria for a strong association with water.

Reported outbreaks are investigated with a standard pro forma followed up by additional enquiries for further details. In the U.K. the outbreaks are collated and reported in the PHLS publication *Communicable Disease Weekly* at 6-month intervals. The information is checked with those people who reported the outbreaks, updated case numbers, and the results of any further investigations noted when the 6-month reports are compiled. District reports on large outbreaks are also collated nationally and regionally.

TABLE 3.1
Criteria for the Strength of Association of Water with Human Infectious Disease and How They Are Applied in the National Surveillance for Water-Related Disease in England and Wales

	Criteria
	(a) The pathogen found in human case samples was also found in water samples
	(b) Documented water quality failure or water treatment failure
	(c) Significant result from analytical epidemiological study (a case control or cohort study)
	(d) Suggestive evidence of association from a descriptive epidemiological study
Strength of Association	
Strong	a + c, a + d, or b + c
Probable	b + d, (c) only, or (a) only
Possible	(b) + (d)

3.2.1 Detected Waterborne Outbreaks in England and Wales

As discussed above, the current surveillance system has only been operational since the early 1990s, although reports of waterborne outbreaks go back for over a century.[3]

Figure 3.1 shows the number of reported outbreaks associated with mains water-related outbreaks and the number of people affected by them. Figure 3.2 shows the same data for private water supplies. Table 3.2 shows the etiological causes of these outbreaks. It can be seen that mains water-related outbreaks in the UK have been almost exclusively due to cryptosporidiosis in the past 2 decades. In part, this represents the fact that *Cryptosporidium* is an emerging pathogen, and many water supply systems were not designed to cope with it. Outbreaks associated with private supplies, though less common, are due to a wider range of pathogens, especially *Campylobacter*. The presence of *Campylobacter* in reports of outbreaks associated with small private supplies reflects the general lack of treatment for these supplies and the lack of chlorination.

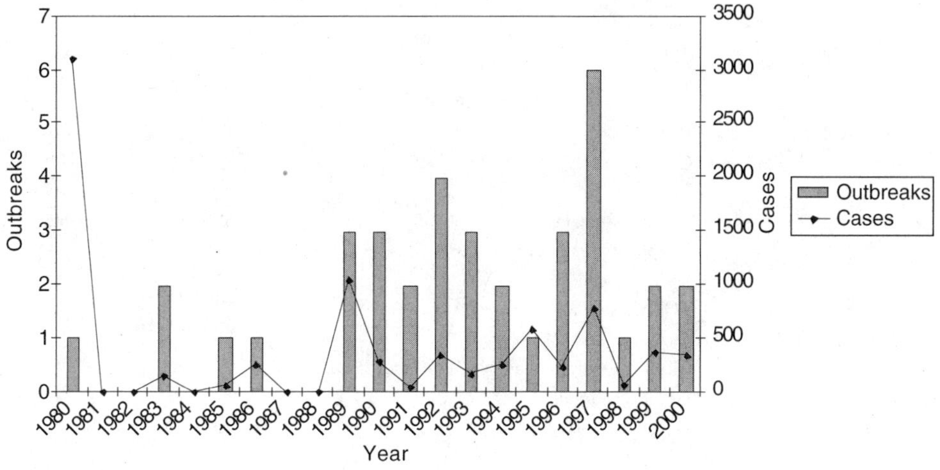

FIGURE 3.1 Outbreaks of waterborne disease associated with public water supplies in England and Wales from 1980–2000.

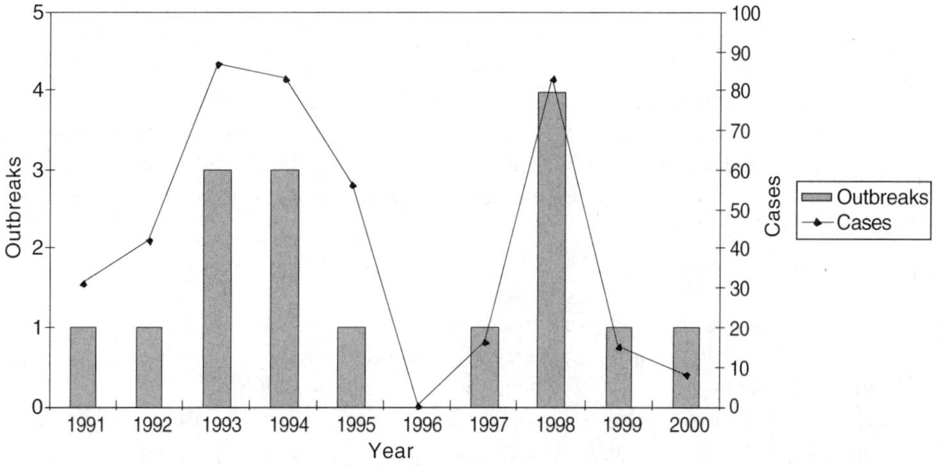

FIGURE 3.2 Outbreaks of waterborne disease associated with private water supplies in England and Wales from 1991–2000.

TABLE 3.2
Causes of Outbreaks of Waterborne Disease in England and Wales.

Decade	Cause	No. Outbreaks	No. Cases
	Public Supplies		
1971 to 1980	Gastroenteritis	2	3114
	Giardia	1	60
	TOTAL	3	322
1981 to 1990	*Cryptosporidium*	7	1157
	Campylobacter	3	629
	Gastroenteritis	3	310
	TOTAL	13	2096
1991 to 2000	*Cryptosporidium*	23	2837
	Campylobacter	1	281
	Gastroenteritis	1	229
	TOTAL	25	3347
	Private Supplies		
1971 to 1980	Paratyphoid	1	6
	Gastroenteritis	1	160
	TOTAL	2	166
1981 to 1990	*Campylobacter*	3	520
	Streptobacillary fever	1	304
	Gastroenteritis	1	56
	TOTAL	5	962
1991 to 2000	*Campylobacter*	8	178
	Mixed *Campylobacter* and *Cryptosporidium*	1	43
	Cryptosporidium	3	74
	Gastroenteritis	2	81
	Giardia	1	31
	E. coli O157	1	14
	TOTAL		421

3.3 SURVEILLANCE IN THE UNITED STATES

In the United States, national statistics on outbreaks associated with drinking water have been available since 1920.[11] The Centers for Disease Control and Prevention (CDC), the U.S. Environmental Protection Agency (EPA), and the Council of State and Territorial Epidemiologists have maintained a collaborative surveillance system of the occurrences and causes of waterborne disease outbreaks (WBDOs) since 1971.[12–16] This surveillance system collects and reports data regarding outbreaks associated with drinking water and recreational water. The objectives of the surveillance efforts at the federal level are to:

- Characterize the epidemiology of WBDOs
- Identify the etiologic agents that caused the outbreaks
- Determine the reasons for the occurrence of the outbreaks
- Train public health personnel to detect and investigate WBDOs
- Collaborate with local, state, federal, and international agencies on initiatives and programs to prevent waterborne diseases

The public health actions that have been taken as a result of this surveillance system include joint efforts by the EPA and CDC to estimate the national prevalence of waterborne disease attributable to consumption of municipal drinking water and to study emerging waterborne pathogens that might require regulatory consideration by the EPA, meetings with the recreational water industry, focus groups to educate parents on prevention of waterborne disease transmission in recreational water settings, and publications with guidelines for parents and swimming pool operators.

3.3.1 Characteristics of the Surveillance System

3.3.1.1 Sources and Types of Data

State, territorial, and local public health agencies have the primary responsibility for detecting and investigating WBDOs. Reporting the outbreaks to the CDC on a standard form is voluntary, and the surveillance system is passive. The CDC annually requests reports from state and territorial epidemiologists or from persons designated as WBDO surveillance coordinators, and the data are analyzed, summarized, and published every 2 years. Data collected on the completed report form include:

- Type of exposure (i.e., drinking water or recreational water)
- Location and date of outbreak
- Actual or estimated number of persons exposed, ill, and hospitalized, and number of fatalities
- Symptoms, incubation period, and duration of illness
- Etiologic agent
- Epidemiologic data (e.g., attack rate, relative risk, or odds ratio)
- Clinical laboratory data (e.g., results of fecal and blood tests)
- Type of water system (i.e., community, non-community, or individual system for drinking water; swimming pool, hot tub, water park, lake, etc. for recreational water)
- Environmental data (e.g., results of water tests)
- Factors contributing to contamination of the water

Additional information regarding water source, supply, quality, and treatment is obtained from the state's drinking water agency if needed. Data are summarized and presented in the CDC bi-annual surveillance report in various formats, including, for example, by etiologic agent and water system for drinking water (Figures 3.3 and 3.4). See Chapter 10 for a more detailed discussion of recent outbreaks of waterborne disease in the U.S.

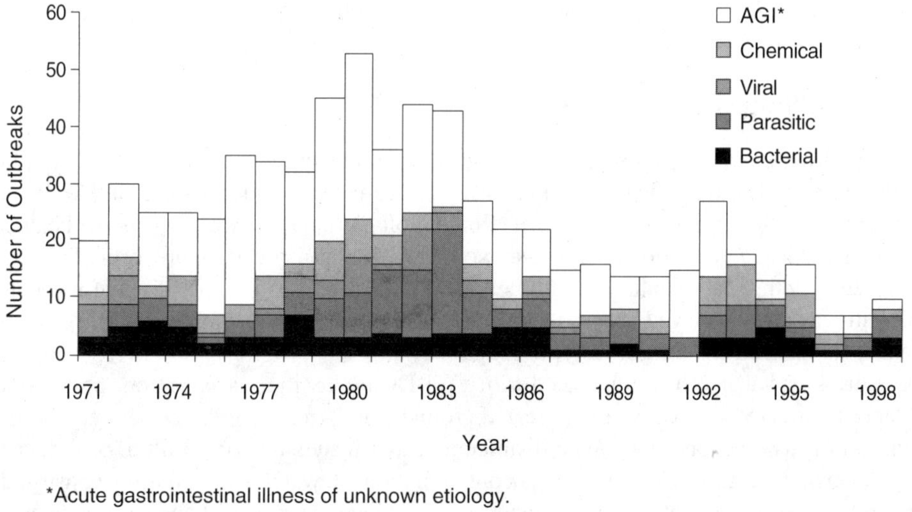

FIGURE 3.3 Waterborne disease outbreaks associated with drinking water by year and etiologic agent, United States 1971–1998 (N = 689).

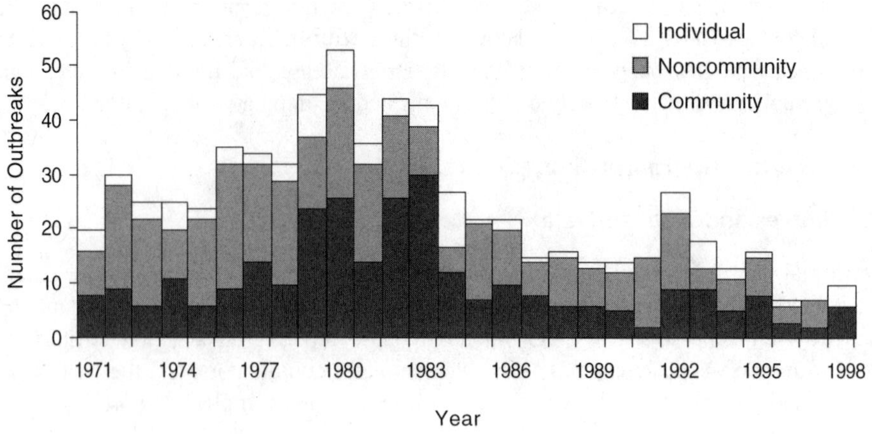

FIGURE 3.4 Waterborne disease outbreaks associated with drinking water by year and type of water system, United States 1971–1998 (N = 689).

3.3.1.2 Methods

The unit of analysis for the waterborne disease outbreak surveillance system is an outbreak rather than an individual case of a disease. Two criteria must be met for an event to be defined as a WBDO. First, at least two persons must have experienced a similar illness after ingestion of drinking water or exposure to recreational water, with the exceptions of single cases of laboratory-confirmed primary amoebic meningoencephalitis and single cases of chemical poisoning if water quality data indicate contamination by the chemical. Second, epidemiologic data must implicate water as the probable source of illness. Outbreaks caused by contamination of water or ice at the point of use (e.g., a contaminated water faucet or ice bucket) are noted but not classified as WBDOs.

If primary-case patients (e.g., persons exposed to contaminated water) and secondary-case patients (e.g., persons who became ill after contact with primary-case patients) are distinguished on the report form, only primary-case patients are included in the total number of cases. If both actual and estimated case counts are provided in the report, the estimated count is used if it was calculated using attack rates or was obtained from a randomly sampled study population.

3.3.1.3 Classification of Outbreaks

Waterborne disease outbreaks are classified according to the strength of the evidence implicating water (Table 3.3). The classification numbers are based on the epidemiologic and water quality data provided on the outbreak report form. Epidemiologic data are weighted more heavily than water quality data, and reports without supporting epidemiologic data are excluded from the surveillance system. Classifications II through IV do not necessarily imply that the investigations of the outbreaks were flawed, because the circumstances of each outbreak differ and not all outbreaks can or need to be rigorously investigated.

Each drinking water system associated with a WBDO is classified as having one of the following deficiencies: untreated surface water, untreated ground water, treatment deficiency (e.g., temporary interruption of disinfection, inadequate disinfection, and inadequate or no filtration), distribution system deficiency (e.g., cross-connection, contamination of water mains during construction or repair, and contamination of a storage facility), or unknown or miscellaneous deficiency (e.g., contamination of bottled water). If more than one deficiency is reported on the form, the deficiency that was most likely to have caused the outbreak is noted.

TABLE 3.3
Classification of Investigations of Waterborne Disease Outbreaks in the United States[a]

Class[b]	Epidemiologic data	Water-quality data
I	Adequate[c] a) Data were provided about exposed and unexposed persons b) The relative risk or odds ratio was ≥2, or the p-value was <0.05	Provided and adequate Could be historical information or laboratory data (e.g., the history that a chlorinator malfunctioned or a water main broke, no detectable free-chlorine residual, or the presence of coliforms in the water)
II	Adequate	Not provided or inadequate (e.g., stating that a lake was overcrowded)
III	Provided, but limited Epidemiologic data were provided that did not meet the criteria for Class I The claim was made that ill persons had no exposures in common besides water, but no data were provided	Provided and adequate
IV	Provided, but limited	Not provided or inadequate

[a] The following types of waterborne disease outbreaks are not classified according to this scheme: outbreaks of *Pseudomonas* and other water-related dermatitis; single cases of primary amoebic meningoencephalitis; and single cases of chemical poisoning.
[b] Based on the epidemiologic and water-quality data that were provided on the form (CDC form 52.12).
[c] Adequate data were provided to implicate water as the source of the outbreak.

3.3.1.4 Representativeness and Usefulness of the Surveillance System

The passive and voluntary characteristics of the WBDO surveillance system lead to questions about the representativeness of WBDOs that are reported to the CDC. Several factors affect the recognition and investigation of WBDOs, including:

- Size of the outbreak — the larger the outbreak the more likely it will be detected.
- Severity of the illness caused by the outbreak — the more severe the illness (e.g., bloody diarrhea caused by *Escherichia coli* O157:H7) the more likely the outbreak will be detected.
- Public awareness that an outbreak might be occurring — a person who is aware is more likely to call the health department to report an illness.
- Clinician's interest in the etiologic agent — heightened interest is more likely to lead to a request for laboratory testing to identify the specific agent.
- Resources available to the local and state health departments — local and state health departments have limited budgets and allocate resources according to perceived health risks.
- Routine laboratory testing practices for pathogens in clinical specimens — state reference laboratories and private laboratories vary in the types of tests that are included in routine examinations of specimens (e.g., a test for *Cryptosporidium parvum* may or may not be included in a request for routine ova and parasite testing of a fecal specimen).

Despite the fact that certain types of WBDOs are much more likely to be detected while others are more likely to be missed, the data gathered through this surveillance system are useful for identifying major deficiencies in providing safe drinking and recreational water. The data are used to determine or update the biology and epidemiology of etiologic agents and to determine epidemiologic trends in the occurrence of WBDOs. Surveillance information also influences research priorities and can lead to improved water quality regulations.

3.3.1.5 Sensitivity of the Surveillance System

The sensitivity of the waterborne disease outbreak surveillance system is unknown because it is not possible to determine how many outbreaks actually occur. However, the sensitivity is assumed to be low, and the primary cause of under-reporting of outbreaks is under-recognition.

Many obstacles to reporting cases of illness to the local and state health departments exist. Certain steps need to occur for a case patient to be recognized and counted, and at each step additional potential cases go unrecognized and thus are lost to the surveillance system. The steps that need to occur for cases to be recognized and a waterborne disease outbreak to be detected include the following:

- An infected person must become ill.
- A person who is ill must seek medical care (less than 8% of persons with gastrointestinal illness seek medical care).
- The physician must order a laboratory test.
- The laboratory test requested must be the appropriate test.
- The patient must provide the specimen.
- The laboratory must perform the test.
- The test result must be positive.
- The laboratory or physician must report the positive result to the health department.
- The health department must review and analyze the reports in a timely manner and conclude that an outbreak might be occurring.
- The epidemiologic investigation must implicate water as the most likely source of the outbreak, even in the absence of an identified etiologic agent.

In addition, standardized laboratory methods that are both sensitive and specific are lacking for many viruses, and routine testing for parasites is not always done. Therefore, outbreaks caused by viruses and parasites are more likely to be missed than those caused by bacteria. Finally, the incubation period for parasitic diseases such as cryptosporidiosis averages 7 days and can be as long as 14 days, thus making the association between illness and water much more difficult and less likely.

3.3.2 Strengths and Weaknesses of the Surveillance System

The primary strength of the waterborne disease outbreak surveillance system includes its ability to capture many types of waterborne outbreaks including: (1) outbreaks of unknown etiology; (2) outbreaks associated with both infectious and chemical agents; (3) outbreaks associated with gastrointestinal illnesses as well as those associated with respiratory illnesses and dermatitis; and (4) outbreaks that are very small (e.g., N = 2). The surveillance system can also easily accommodate new or emerging pathogens, and the type of data collected can be expanded or modified with minimal effort.

The weaknesses of the surveillance system include: (1) its low sensitivity; (2) its inability to capture sporadic cases of illness associated with waterborne transmission; (3) its lack of uniformity in hard data collected (i.e., not all outbreaks are confirmed by laboratory positive results); and (4) its inconsistency in the quality and completeness of the outbreak reports received.

3.4 SURVEILLANCE IN SWEDEN

In the northern part of Europe, it is common for people to drink tap water, although use of bottled water has increased in the last decade. Most parts of Sweden have a sufficient amount of high quality mains drinking water. Approximately 85% of the population has access to tap water from community water supply systems; the other 15% use private wells. Surface water is used in about 50% of the community water supply systems, and groundwater or artificially recharged groundwater supplies the other half. A Swedish survey revealed that although most people drink tap water daily, 44% also drink bottled water on a daily basis. However, 4% do not drink tap water at all.[17] In Sweden, the use of bottled water probably has more to do with food habits than with fear of becoming ill from drinking tap water.

3.4.1 Organization of the Surveillance of Communicable Diseases

In 1875, Sweden enacted legislation with a view to avoiding the spread of serious infectious diseases in humans. County medical officers, who deal with communicable diseases at the county council level, have the main responsibility in this area. They are charged with monitoring and coordinating the control of communicable diseases in their respective regions. Local doctors are responsible for investigating the epidemiology of communicable diseases and giving advice on hygiene. They must notify all cases of notifiable communicable diseases to the appropriate county medical officer and to the Swedish Institute for Infectious Disease Control (SMI). Some diseases also require notification to the municipality's Environmental and Public Health Committee.

In each community, the Environmental and Public Health Committee is responsible for investigating infections from environmental sources (food, water, ventilation systems). Environmental and public health officers are responsible for routine water analysis and for taking corrective action. All water treatment plants in Sweden must also have an "in-house control program" designed in accordance with the Hazard Analysis Critical Control Points (HACCP).

The SMI is responsible for the overall surveillance of communicable diseases in Sweden and for providing advice in outbreak situations. In large outbreaks or unusual situations, personnel from the SMI may also be involved in microbiological sampling, epidemiological studies, or technical inspection of the water treatment plant. A sudden increase in reported cases of a communicable disease may launch a thorough investigation (see Chapter 5). The SMI may also coordinate outbreaks involving several counties and participate in investigations of international outbreaks.

A suspected outbreak triggers an epidemiological investigation, which usually requires cooperation between the county medical officer and the municipality's Environmental and Public Health Committee. The county medical officer is responsible for overall coordination of the investigation and focuses on those who have contracted the disease. The environmental and public health inspector is responsible for investigating the suspected source of infection.

Although reporting waterborne outbreaks in Sweden is not mandatory, the environmental and public health inspector or the county medical officer usually reports any outbreaks to the National Food Administration and/or the SMI. All waterborne outbreaks are covered by the SMI. They are thoroughly examined for deficiencies in the water system. The results are then communicated to the responsible personnel at the water treatment plants or the Environmental Health Protection Board. When particular deficiencies are identified frequently, regulations are changed. In Sweden, water regulations are covered under the Food Act. The National Food Administration issues regulations and guidelines based on European directives and Swedish laws, including regulations on water for human consumption.[18] Figure 3.5 shows the different bodies that may be involved in the investigation of a food- or waterborne outbreak.

3.4.1.1 Detection of Waterborne Outbreaks by the Surveillance System

In Sweden, there are three systems of surveillance of communicable diseases:

1. Compulsory reporting of notifiable diseases by doctors
2. Compulsory reporting of positive findings from laboratories
3. Voluntary reporting by laboratories

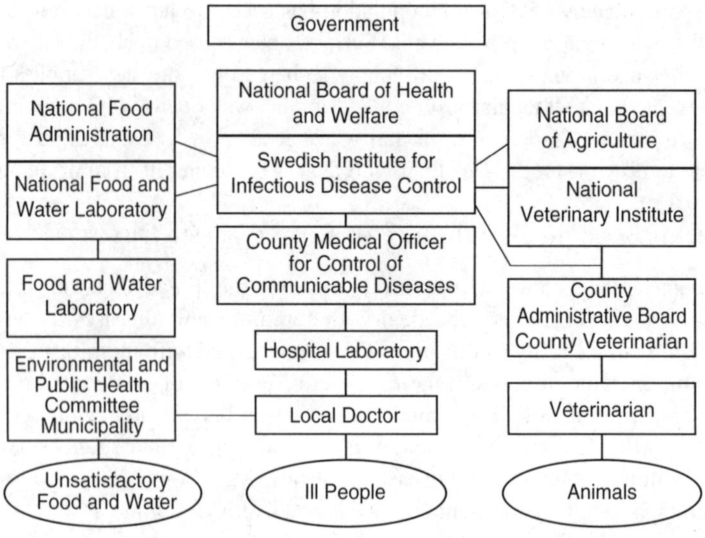

FIGURE 3.5 Organization of the epidemic surveillance in Sweden in case of food and waterborne outbreaks.

The same diseases are compulsorily reported both by doctors and laboratories. Diseases that may be waterborne include: amoebiasis, campylobacteriosis, cholera, infection with enterohaemorrhagic *E. coli* O157, giardiasis, hepatitis A, paratyphoid fever, salmonellosis, shigellosis, typhoid fever, and yersiniosis. Diseases that are reported voluntarily by laboratories are: infection with calicivirus, *Cyclospora* diarrhea, cryptosporidiosis, infection with enterohaemorrhagic *E. coli* other than O157, and rotaviral enteritis.

Waterborne pathogens usually give rise to mild symptoms including diarrhea, abdominal pain, and vomiting. Duration is normally only a few days, although some individuals may be ill for a longer period. In waterborne outbreaks, people may be ill enough to be absent from work but not sufficiently ill to consult a doctor. There have been waterborne outbreaks that have affected several hundred or a thousand people but were discovered more or less accidentally. When those who are ill see a doctor (clinical surveillance), the doctor takes a fecal sample, which may show the presence of a pathogenic microorganism (laboratory surveillance) (Figure 3.6).

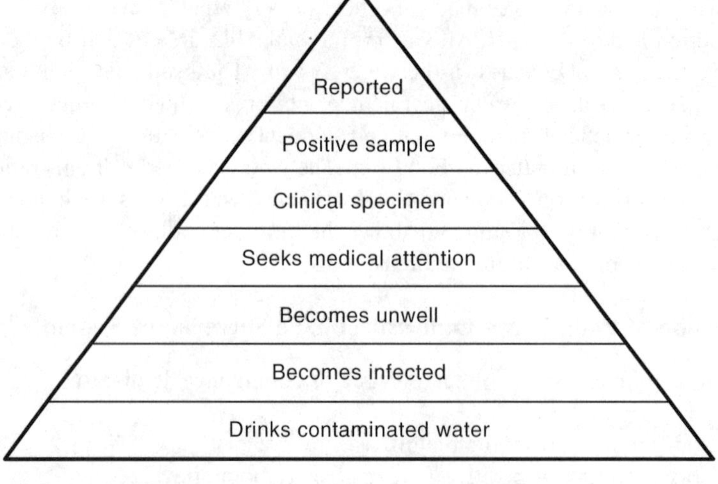

FIGURE 3.6 Conditions for a pathogenic microorganism to be diagnosed and reported in a waterborne outbreak.

Waterborne outbreaks may be recognized by an increase in:

- Acute gastrointestinal illness (AGI) in general practice or in hospitals (clinical surveillance)
- Positive laboratory results from possible waterborne agents (laboratory surveillance)
- AGI in the community or part of the community, although most people are not sick enough to visit a doctor (community surveillance)

Because of delays (from sampling to microbiological investigation and reporting), it normally takes 1 to 2 weeks before the surveillance system recognizes an increase in cases of waterborne disease. Usually, the surveillance system only identifies the tip of the iceberg (Figure 3.6). In a large outbreak, hundreds of sick people (community surveillance) may be the sign of a breakdown in the water system.

In fact, clinical and laboratory surveillance systems seldom reveal waterborne outbreaks. Most Swedish outbreaks are recognized as a result of the increased numbers of sick people and not by the surveillance system. For example, an increase in reported cases of giardiasis over a few months in one community revealed that tap water may have been the source. In another case, the medical laboratory reported seven cases of campylobacteriosis to the county medical officer. In fact, this revealed a waterborne outbreak involving 2500 people. Except for family outbreaks, the surveillance system has difficulty recognizing small waterborne outbreaks and sporadic cases.

3.4.1.2 Alternative Ways of Recognizing Waterborne Outbreaks

The prompt discovery of an outbreak and its source usually involves several participants. The capacity for detection depends on the knowledge and resources available. It is important to interpret what may have happened and start an investigation quickly.

Apart from laboratory, clinical, and community surveillance of communicable diseases, other phenomena to be monitored include:

- Non-potable water found by routine sampling
- Complaints about water quality (color, taste, smell)
- Accident or incident at the water treatment plant
- High turbidity in source water or an unusually large amount of microorganisms in source water
- Increase in sales of antidiarrheic treatments

Non-potable water found by routine sampling can seldom prevent an outbreak but may reveal weak points in the water system. Waterborne outbreaks have sometimes been identified in this way.

One outbreak started with complaints about the smell and taste of the water. The lines were flushed, but complaints about water quality continued to come in. A few days later, reports of illness followed.

Accidents or errors occur now and then at water treatment plants. One of the most common mistakes is failure to disinfect, normally by chlorination. The largest reported waterborne outbreak in Sweden was due to the absence of chlorination. During the installation of a computer control system, the chlorination and the associated alarm were out of order.[19]

Different types of connections between community water systems and surface or sewer systems have been the reason for several waterborne outbreaks. In one instance, about 3600 people (attack rate 90%) contracted gastroenteritis (giardiasis and amoebiasis). The drinking water reservoir had been constructed with a spillway overflow connected to the sewer system.[20] A blockage in the latter caused sewage to backflow into the drinking-water reservoir.

A conventional method of recognizing waterborne outbreaks is unusually high sales of antidiarrheic treatments. In one case, this triggered the beginning of an outbreak investigation which revealed a waterborne outbreak involving about 1000 people at a ski resort. An additional indication was that almost no one skied because of illness. The tap water was judged potable when investigated using common indicator microorganisms and was therefore difficult to incriminate as the source of the outbreak. A cohort study later revealed that the water was in fact the source of the outbreak.

The National Food Administration records sales of devices used for boiling water in order to gain information about possible water incidents or suspected waterborne outbreaks.

3.4.2 Reported Waterborne Outbreaks

An improved system for reporting outbreaks of waterborne disease was established in 1980. It included directions for epidemiological investigation of large outbreaks. Because of its greater effectiveness, the number of reported outbreaks has increased. During the period 1980 to 1999, 116 outbreaks of waterborne diseases were reported.[17] They affected about 58,000 people, and two deaths were reported (Figure 3.7). About 70% of the outbreaks were due to unknown agents causing AGI (Figure 3.8). In the 100-year period between 1880 and 1979, by contrast, 77 waterborne outbreaks occurred, with 26,867 recorded cases and 789 deaths. Most of the outbreaks (88%) during that period were due to known agents, and the diseases most commonly reported were typhoid

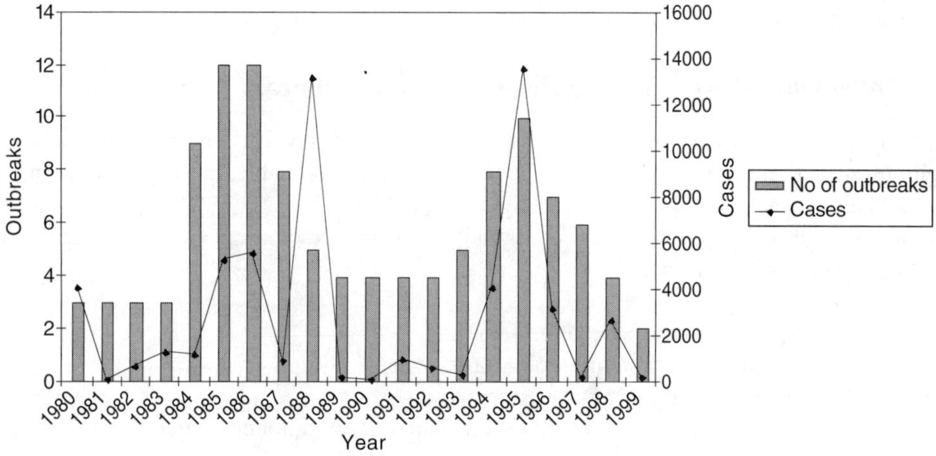

FIGURE 3.7 Outbreaks and cases of waterborne disease in Sweden, 1980–1999.

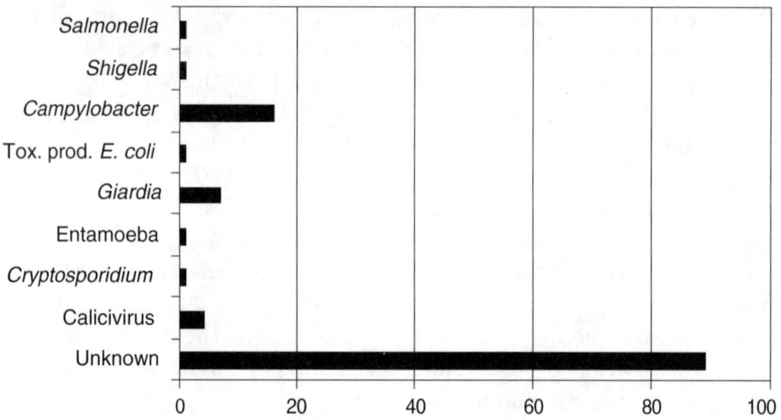

FIGURE 3.8 Microbial agents associated with waterborne outbreaks in Sweden, 1980–1999.

fever, hepatitis, and shigellosis.[21] During these 100 years only serious waterborne disease outbreaks, mostly involving known agents, were reported.

The change is attributable to the more systematic investigation of large waterborne outbreaks, using a standardized questionnaire and sampling of sick people and polluted water. The most commonly identified agent involved in waterborne outbreaks in Sweden is *Campylobacter.* On the other hand, waterborne outbreaks due to *Cryptosporidium*, which are more common in the U.S. and the U.K., have been reported only once in Sweden (Figure 3.8).

The strength of the Swedish reporting system is the close cooperation between different bodies. It is important that the laws are enforced quickly when the surveillance system reveals deficiencies in water systems. Some years ago, several waterborne outbreaks were due to the backflow of surface water or sewage into a low-water reservoir. The National Food Administration acted promptly and took appropriate action.

The surveillance system for waterborne outbreaks could be made more efficient if the reporting of such outbreaks was compulsory.

The Swedish surveillance system provides less information about private and family wells. Such information normally only comes to the knowledge of the authorities accidentally. It is the owner's responsibility to take action if a private well is polluted. Sporadic cases of infection due to tap water containing a small amount of pathogens or to occasional contamination will not usually be detected by any surveillance system.

Better knowledge at community level of water microbiology, methods for investigating outbreaks, and epidemiology should increase the quality of the outbreak investigations. Teams specially trained to investigate water- and foodborne outbreaks are available in most counties in Sweden. These teams are seldom used, but strengthening their role could be a way to investigate outbreaks more quickly and effectively.

Rapid and reliable information about waterborne outbreaks is essential in order to improve surveillance methods. Our experience in Sweden is that more information and education at local and county levels can increase the number of reports and the attention given to waterborne outbreaks when they occur.

The following actions should improve the surveillance system of waterborne outbreaks:

- Feedback to all parties involved in the investigation of waterborne outbreaks
- Support (telephone and/or on the spot) during the outbreak investigation
- Use of effective investigations as examples for other authorities in the public health sector
- Compulsory reporting of outbreaks

3.5 LIMITATIONS WITH NATIONAL SURVEILLANCE SYSTEMS

The strong historical influence of descriptive epidemiology has had and still has a significant influence on all three waterborne disease surveillance systems described in this chapter. Waterborne disease surveillance in all three countries has been shaped largely as an outbreak-driven system. There is, however, growing recognition of the need for a more innovative approach to waterborne disease surveillance to respond to new influences such as:

- The development of a "risk management" culture
- The threat of newly emerging diseases related to water
- A greater understanding of the importance of multiple exposures to pathogens and host factors increasing susceptibility to infection
- The possibility of bioterrorism
- The effects of climate change on disease patterns, such as temperature changes influencing breeding cycles of microorganisms, increased flooding, and changing patterns of precipitation

A number of barriers must be overcome in order to establish an improved national system, including:

- Attributing cause — analytical epidemiological studies are needed to provide evidence of strength of association between illness and water, but these are costly and time consuming. The majority of reported outbreaks are still investigated by descriptive epidemiological and environmental studies.
- Statutory notification system — although notification of certain infectious diseases is compulsory in all three countries, distinguishing waterborne illness from other causes such as food poisoning is problematic. For example, in the U.K. waterborne diseases are included within food poisoning. Furthermore, several important diseases caused by waterborne pathogens may not be statutorily notifiable in their own rights (i.e., giardiasis, campylobacteriosis, cryptosporidiosis, legionellosis, and some viral pathogens). In some situations, the national laboratory-based surveillance systems can be used to ascertain these infections, but reporting may still be voluntary and a suspected association with water may not be reported.
- Resources — it has become more difficult to justify surveillance and secure the necessary funding when overall numbers of outbreaks are decreasing. In recent years in the U.K., only a few drinking outbreaks have been reported annually, including those with only a probable or possible association with water.
- Confidentiality and access to patient-identifiable data — there is increasing public concern about confidentiality of patient data. Within the European Union there have been changes in human rights legislation that have changed what is considered acceptable use of patient-identifiable data. This has implications for local and possibly national surveillance.
- Environmental factors — unlike other disease surveillance systems, a waterborne disease system has to take environmental factors into account. This requires an integrated approach with other agencies and disciplines, for example in hydrogeology and water engineering.
- Training and specialized experience — in most countries, detected waterborne outbreaks are uncommon, so there are fewer opportunities to gain experience and expertise in their investigation and management. Incidents are often managed at the local level with little or no input from regional or national centers unless the outbreak develops into a major incident. Some countries have made recent attempts to standardize the approach, for example, a detailed appendix on epidemiological investigation of outbreaks in the recent U.K. report on *Cryptosporidium* in water supplies.[22]

3.6 NATIONAL SURVEILLANCE SYSTEMS OF THE FUTURE

The ideal national surveillance for waterborne disease would build on the established reporting of outbreaks, where this is already in place, and develop more comprehensive surveillance of clusters, sporadic cases, and reported episodes of water quality failure. Because of the need for particular expertise across a broad range of disciplines, many countries could not expect to provide the full range of expertise at the local level and need to rely on national experts to assist in outbreak investigation (see Chapter 9 for a description of the involvement of a national resource in local outbreak management).

There may be an argument in some countries for setting up a high profile national unit with multidisciplinary membership and clear leadership in regard to waterborne disease management. This unit would have access to a wide range of databases including geographical information systems (GIS), water supply areas, disease data, and behavioral data on water consumption patterns and trends. In England and Wales, responsibility for the surveillance of infectious and chemical illness related to drinking water is managed by separate agencies. Economy of scale could be achieved by bringing the responsibilities for these two types of disease together.

Education and training are essential components of the ideal national system; in addition to knowledge of microbiology and epidemiology, specialists in water surveillance need also to understand the principles of water engineering and domestic plumbing. Any lead organization for waterborne disease surveillance should have the provision of education and training as a key objective.

Finally, any national surveillance system for waterborne disease must feed into appropriate international surveillance. This is particularly important for European countries, which have many shared water resources. Links with international surveillance systems are also becoming more important as travel-related waterborne infections seem to be on the rise. International surveillance systems will be discussed in the next chapter.

REFERENCES

1. Anonymous, *Water and Health in Europe*, World Health Organization Regional Office for Europe, 1999.
2. Galbraith, N.S., Historical review of microbial disease spread by water in England and Wales, in *Water and Public Health,* Golding, A.M.B., Noah, N., and Stanwell-Smith, R., Eds., Smith-Gordon, London, 1994, ch. 2.
3. Galbraith, N.S., Barrett, N.J., and Stanwell-Smith, R., Water and disease after Croydon: a review of water-borne and water-associated disease in the UK 1937–86, *J. Inst. Water Environm. Managt.*, 1, 7, 1987.
4. Stanwell-Smith, R., Water and public health in the United Kingdom. Recent trends in the epidemiology of water borne disease, in *Water and Public Health,* Golding, A.M.B., Noah, N., and Stanwell-Smith, R., Eds., Smith-Gordon, London, 1994, ch. 3.
5. Furtado, C. et al., Outbreaks of waterborne infectious intestinal disease in England and Wales, 1992–5. *Epidemiol. Infect.,* 121, 109, 1998.
6. Benton, C. et al., The incidence of water-borne and water-associated disease in Scotland from 1945 to 1987. *Water Sci. Technol.,* 21, 125, 1989.
7. Nazareth, B. et al., Surveillance of waterborne disease in England and Wales. *Comm. Dis. Report Rev.*, 4, R93, 1994.
8. Communicable Disease Surveillance Center. Strength of association between human illness and water: revised definitions for use in outbreak investigation. *Comm. Dis. Weekly,* 6, 65, 1996.
9. Tillett, H.E., de Louvois, J., and Wall, P.G., Surveillance of outbreaks of waterborne disease: categorizing levels of evidence, *Epidemiol. Infect.,* 120, 37, 1998.
10. Stanwell-Smith, R., Waterborne disease surveillance, *Public Health Med.,* 2, 53, 1999.
11. Craun, G.F., Ed., *Waterborne Diseases in the United States*, CRC Press, Inc., Boca Raton, FL, 1986.
12. Barwick, R.S. et al., Surveillance for waterborne disease outbreaks — United States, 1997–1998, *MMWR*, 49, SS4, 1, 2000.
13. Levy, D.A. et al., Surveillance for waterborne disease outbreaks — United States, 1995–1996, *MMWR*, 47, SS5, 1, 1998.
14. Kramer, M.H. et al., Surveillance for waterborne disease outbreaks — United States, 1993–1994, *MMWR*, 45, SS1, 1, 1996.
15. Moore, A.C. et al., Surveillance for waterborne disease outbreaks — United States, 1991–1992, *MMWR*, 42, SS5, 1, 1993.
16. Herwaldt, B.L. et al., Surveillance for waterborne disease outbreaks — United States, 1989–1990, *MMWR*, 40, SS3, 1, 1991.
17. Anonymous, *Environmental Health Report 2001* (Miljöhälsorapport 2001, in Swedish), Socialstyrelsen, 2001.
18. Anonymous, The Swedish Food Administration Ordinance on Drinking Water (in Swedish), 1993 SLV FS 1993:35.
19. Andersson, Y., A waterborne disease outbreak, *Water Sci. Technol.*, 24, 13, 1991.

20. Andersson, Y. and de Jong, B., An outbreak of giardiasis and amoebiasis at a ski resort in Sweden, *Water Sci. Technol.*, 21, 143, 1989.
21. Andersson, Y., Outbreaks of waterborne disease in Sweden in a historical, hygienic and technical perspective (in Swedish), Master of Public Health, Nordic School of Public Health, Gothenburg Sweden, 1992.
22. Department of the Environment, Transport and the Regions (DETR), Cryptosporidium *in Water Supplies: Third Report of the Group of Experts to: DETR and Department of Health*, London: DETR, 1998.

4 International Surveillance

Paul R. Hunter

CONTENTS

4.1 Introduction....41
4.2 Principles of Collaboration....42
4.3 Examples of International Surveillance....43
4.3.1 WHO Surveillance of Cholera....43
4.3.2 EWGLI Surveillance Network for Travel-Associated Legionnaires' Disease....44
4.3.3 ProMEDmail....45
4.4 Conclusions....46
References....46

4.1 INTRODUCTION

So far we have considered a number of surveillance systems set at local and national levels. In this chapter we shall consider the value of international surveillance and look at some international surveillance systems.

To be worthwhile, international surveillance systems need to bring value to public health over and above that provided by national or local surveillance systems. International surveillance systems provide additional value to national surveillance in a number of situations.

Perhaps the most obvious situation is when infection affects people from more than one country, and where the number of cases in a single country may not be sufficient to enable adequate investigation. Typically, this would apply to the situation of a foodborne outbreak where there is a low attack rate, but the food is sold into several countries. In this context, the surveillance system is most likely to be effective at detecting outbreaks of strains that were previously uncommon. There have been a number of incidences of such foodborne outbreaks.[1–3] However, given that most drinking water is distributed over relatively short distances for consumption, it is unlikely that small numbers of people in several countries will be affected.

The second reason for developing international surveillance systems is to detect outbreaks of illness that affect travellers who are likely to receive a diagnosis only after they return home. This group includes people who may only become unwell after their return home and travellers to countries where medical systems are insufficient to give a full etiological diagnosis in most cases. Perhaps the best example of this is in the surveillance of Legionnaire's disease, which is discussed in more detail below.[4] Another example of the value of international surveillance is the recent identification of an outbreak of cryptosporidiosis associated with a hotel swimming pool on a Mediterranean island, which was only identified following investigation of people after they had returned to the U.K.[5] As discussed below, such systems work best when they also act as a means of helping the countries where the initial infection occurs to improve their technical ability to diagnose the infections and investigate and control outbreaks.

The third major reason for developing international surveillance systems is when an outbreak or epidemic in one country has the potential to spread to neighboring countries. Classic examples

0-8493-1259-0/03/$0.00+$1.50

of such international surveillance systems are the ones organized by the World Health Organization for influenza and cholera.[6] The value of these systems is that they alert countries early to impending epidemics of disease so that appropriate preventative action can be taken. Such action may include the stockpiling of vaccines, developing health education programs, or building up health care facilities to enable them to cope with the increased need.

The remaining reason for conducting international surveillance is the ability to detect other emerging problems that have the potential for adversely impacting on human health. These may represent sentinel events that are likely to be uncommon and difficult to predict in advance. Indeed, it can be difficult to know what pathogens or diseases will arise that can threaten public health. The ProMEDmail surveillance system has been developed as a way of communicating rapidly about emerging issues (see below).[7]

4.2 PRINCIPLES OF COLLABORATION

Given the potential for misunderstanding and confusion inherent in all international endeavors, it is important that the principles of any surveillance system are clearly agreed upon by all participants at the outset. The principles associated with one international surveillance network, the European Enter-Net System, were recently set out in print.[8] These principles include:

- Commitment to rapid exchange of data
- Access to the database
- Confidentiality
- Data protection requirements
- Legal liability
- Wider dissemination of data

For any surveillance system to meet its objective of improving public health, its results must be available in a sufficiently timely fashion to enable implementation of appropriate control measures. Any international surveillance network runs a greater risk of delay than that inherent in national surveillance systems. For international surveillance networks to work, participants should have access to adequate electronic communications and be committed to report appropriate events without delay. Ideally the timeliness of reporting from participants should be monitored so that sources of delay can be identified and resolved.

The problem inherent in all surveillance systems of balancing need for access with right to privacy is even more difficult for international surveillance networks. This issue is especially important when the countries involved have differing laws on confidentiality. Within the European Union, a directive prohibits the processing and transmission of health data, except for the purpose of preventative medicine.[9] Even so, an individual's rights of access to data varies from one country to another. The Enter-Net System resolves this issue by referring all enquiries about data generated by an individual country to that country.

Despite concerns about confidentiality, participants need access to the data or else the surveillance system will not make any contributions to public health. The key is to be able to identify the minimum data set that enables participants to do their jobs with the minimum encroachment on civil liberties. All key participants should have full access to the data, but this list of individuals should be restricted to professional people responsible for their countries' own surveillance systems. Ideally such people should have on-line access.

During the analysis and interpretation of surveillance data, various draft and speculative reports may have to be shared with participants. It is essential that confidentiality levels of the reports are clearly documented and understood.

Another confidentiality issue concerns legal liability around the naming of foods or products that may be implicated in disease outbreaks. Participants must exercise due care in drafting reports.

Nevertheless, there are times when suspect products have to be named. Despite the potential for claims of libel, the Enter-Net management's legal opinion is that there is no reason why such product detail should not be included. It is up to individual participant countries to determine what they do with the data.

It is likely that data within any international surveillance system will need to be shared with other institutions and surveillance systems that are not part of the key team. Should these other institutions need access to a particular data set, they will need to formally agree to abide by the same principle as the key participants. Wider access to the data set should not be allowed. However, many countries have freedom of information laws, and participants in any surveillance network should be prepared to produce regular reports on the outputs of the network. These reports should be available to both the public health community and the public. Similarly, should a surveillance network identify an adverse event such as an outbreak, this information (once verified) should be made available to the public.

4.3 EXAMPLES OF INTERNATIONAL SURVEILLANCE

International surveillance systems will vary in their designs. The main differences relate to the degree of centralization of control of the data. The three examples of international surveillance discussed below reflect increasing decentralization of data control. The centrist model is similar to the national surveillance systems described in Chapters 4 through 6. In this model there is an international communicable disease center which receives information for participant countries, analyzes the data, and produces regular reports and alerts, as with the WHO system for cholera. The next example is more of a hub-and-spoke system with a coordinating center, but all participants have equal access to the data and can use the information as appropriate. In the final example, there is very loose control of data, though such systems are moderated to prevent misuse. As central control reduces, the timeliness usually increases, though the reliability and consistency of the data may be reduced.

In Europe there has been some serious debate about whether the surveillance systems should be based around a single center or should follow a network model.[10,11] Giesecke and Weinberg argue that effective public health action is facilitated more by enabling coordination and collaboration than by bricks and mortar.[11] Although this is probably right in the European setting, the structure of each surveillance system must be designed to best operate in its context. Networks work better when the partners have or can acquire the skills and resources needed to support their own surveillance. Adequately resourced centers should have the staff available to manage the surveillance system as a whole and to support local people when outbreaks and other adverse events occur. On the other hand, network systems are probably better at building local competence, though they may struggle to find the resources to assist local agencies directly in outbreak investigation. For example, the WHO cholera surveillance system probably has the most appropriate design, considering that many of the participant countries are reticent about reporting disease and may not have their own resources to deal with outbreaks.[6] The network structure is likely to be more appropriate in the European setting, where partners should have the skills and resources to manage their own national surveillance.

4.3.1 WHO Surveillance of Cholera

Cholera is one of the three diseases currently reportable under the International Health Regulations.[6] Under these regulations, signature states must report the first cases of cholera in their territories to the WHO within 24 hours of becoming aware of a case. Reports of cholera cases and deaths are published each week in the *Weekly Epidemiological Record*. Annual summaries are also published, as are summaries of outbreaks. Figure 4.1 shows the cases reported to the WHO from 1950 to 1998.

Despite the fact that reporting under this scheme is mandatory, reporting is still not complete. Many countries are reluctant to report cases of cholera, as they fear the economic and political

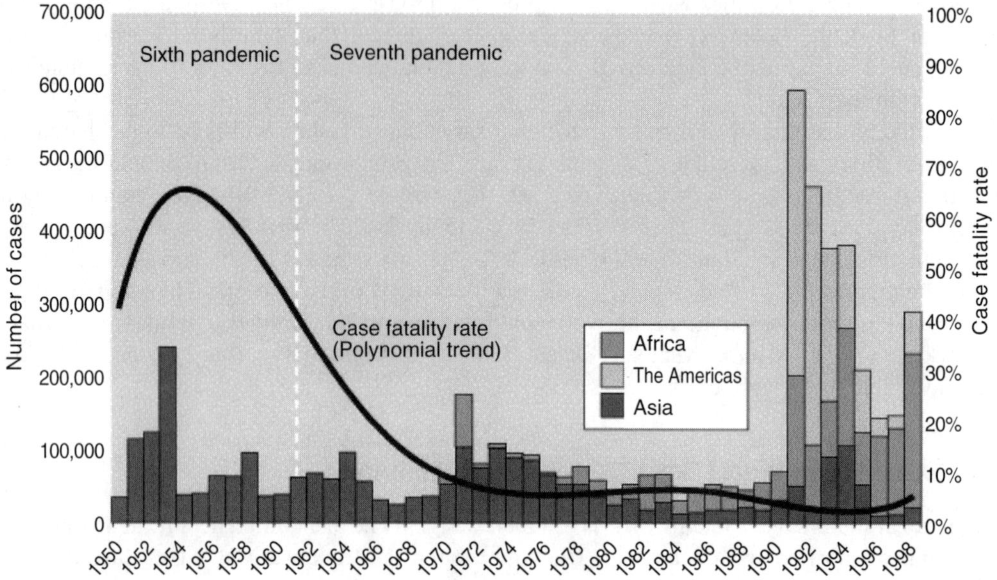

FIGURE 4.1 Cholera, reported number of cases and case fatality rates, 1950 to 1998.

fallout that may ensue. This is a particular problem in those countries that rely on tourism as a major source of income. Even when eventually reported, there may be considerable delay by the time the official report is made. Another problem is that some countries may report watery diarrhea in order to avoid the stigma.

4.3.2 EWGLI Surveillance Network for Travel-Associated Legionnaires' Disease

One of the most effective and earliest European surveillance systems was set up by the European Working Group for *Legionella* Infections (EWGLI). This network was set up in 1986 to investigate Legionnaires' disease in travellers. The network was initially coordinated by the National Bacteriology Laboratory in Stockholm, and in 1993 the responsibility for coordination was transferred to the U.K. Public Health Laboratory Service (PHLS) Communicable Disease Surveillance Centre (CDSC). The EWGLI surveillance system is described in more detail elsewhere.[4] Regular summaries are also published in the scientific literature.[12–14] In 1999, 31 countries and 38 collaborating centers were participating in the network.

Each country has at least one collaborator, usually the microbiologist in charge of the national *Legionella* reference laboratory. It is this person's responsibility to report on each travel-associated case diagnosed in his or her country. Collaborators are notified in turn by fax of all cases of *Legionella* infection satisfying the case definition in their country. If a case is part of a cluster (two or more cases diagnosed within 6 months who shared the same accommodation), then all collaborators and the WHO are informed.

From its inception in 1987 up to 1999, 1886 cases of travel-associated Legionnaires' disease have been reported to the EWGLI network (Figure 4.2). There were also 183 clusters identified in the same period. The pattern of notification varies substantially from one country to another, and this pattern does not reflect only the propensity of a country's citizens to travel abroad (Table 4.1). At least part of the explanation for the difference in reporting between countries reflects the competence of national diagnostic and surveillance services.

One of the other benefits of the surveillance network has been the provision of support for the investigation of outbreaks of Legionnaires' disease to countries that have not had the necessary

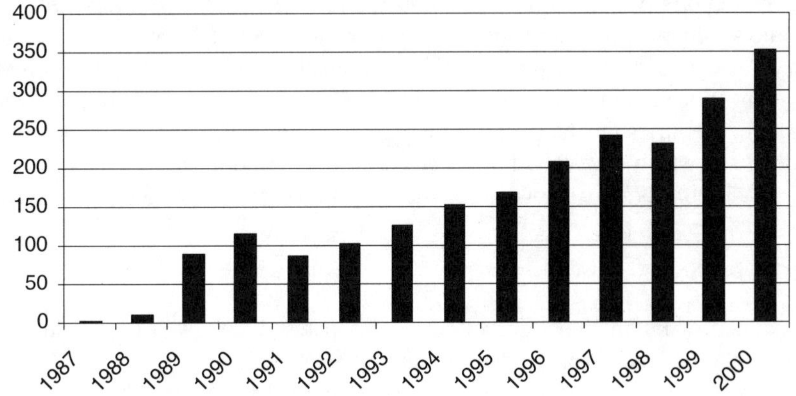

FIGURE 4.2 Reports made to European Working Group on *Legionella* infection surveillance scheme for travel-associated *Legionella*.

expertise to investigate such outbreaks. The network has also acted as a focus and driving force to develop and improve research programs in the diagnosis and prevention of this infection. For example, an external quality assurance scheme for *Legionella* diagnosis has been developed which has led to marked improvements in diagnostic methods in Europe. The network has also been involved in improving methods for the typing of *Legionella*.

4.3.3 ProMEDmail

The ProMEDmail surveillance network is an entirely new type of surveillance network that was set up by the Federation of American Scientists in 1994. As of November 2000, ProMEDmail had some 21,000 individual and institutional subscribers in 150 countries.[7] Reports are submitted by e-mail from any subscriber and then e-mailed to all subscribers. The system is free of charge to subscribers. It is moderated by infectious disease specialists. Some reports are generated by diagnosing clinicians; others relate items that have appeared in the media.

Typically, ProMEDmail is faster than other international surveillance systems and information is often published several days before the WHO has permission from the involved state to report. On the other hand, there have been concerns raised about the accuracy of some ProMEDmail

TABLE 4.1
Countries Reporting Cases to EWGLI in 1999

Country Making Report	Number of Reports
England and Wales	69
Netherlands	66
Italy	31
France	28
Scotland	27
Sweden	22
Denmark	18
Austria	12
Spain, Switzerland, Ireland	3 each
Finland, Slovenia	2 each
Germany, Norway, U.S.	1 each
Belgium, Croatia, Czech Republic, Greece, Malta, Portugal, Turkey	None

postings. Of 351 reports posted during a 7-month period, 15 (4.3%) were retracted, though 6 of those were official reports that were subsequently retracted. Only 6 (2.6%) were due to incorrect reports from contributors. To this author this is an acceptably low error rate, given the benefits of rapid notification. When compared with the formal WHO surveillance system, the WHO reported cholera from three countries that had not been identified on ProMED, and the latter identified three other countries from which the WHO had received no official notification.

One thing that ProMEDmail cannot do is provide data for year to year or geographical comparisons.

4.4 CONCLUSIONS

The picture painted of international surveillance so far may have given the reader a fairly rosy view. However, international cooperation and surveillance of infectious disease is still far from perfect. A recent review of the management of five outbreaks affecting more than one country highlighted a number of weaknesses:[15]

- Failure to identify and report cases within countries
- Failure to inform other countries
- Inadequate preparedness planning
- Inadequate funding arrangements
- Failure to link information to action
- Failure to provide the capacity for international outbreak investigation
- Failure to share lessons

Several of these weaknesses relate to surveillance. As discussed in Chapter 1, not all occurrences of an infectious disease are reported to national surveillance systems.[16] The proportion of cases reported varies from one infection to another, even in those countries with the best surveillance systems. The problem is that many countries, even within Europe, have very poor surveillance systems in place and will not be able to adequately contribute to international surveillance networks.[17]

Even when countries become aware of infectious disease, there may be considerable reticence about letting other countries know of these problems. The desire to resist informing other countries may be most strong in nations that rely heavily on tourist income.

As discussed in Chapter 1, surveillance systems only have value if they lead to action that improves public health either now or in the future. All too often it would appear that appropriate action was not taken, despite the surveillance system identifying the problem.

The role of international surveillance systems will increase in future years as intercountry trade and travel increase. International surveillance systems are only as good as the component national surveillance. If we are to develop effective international surveillance, then considerable efforts will have to be invested into bringing many national surveillance systems up to an acceptable minimum standard. One vision of the future of surveillance is the Public Health Intelligence Network run by Health Canada.[18] This surveillance system works by systematically and automatically monitoring the internet for information on target diseases. This system relies not on reports from clinicians and laboratories, but on reports by news agencies and other grey sources. To date, this system has identified several important outbreaks that had not been officially reported to the WHO.[18]

REFERENCES

1. Tauxe, R.V. and Hughes, J.M., International investigation of outbreaks of foodborne disease. *Brit. Med. J.*, 313, 1093, 1996.
2. Killalea, D. et al., An outbreak of *Salmonella agona* infection caused by a ready to eat savoury snack. I. England and the United States, *Brit. Med. J.*, 313, 1105, 1996.

3. Mahon, B. et al., An international outbreak of salmonella infections caused by alfalfa sprouts grown from contaminated seed, in *Abstracts of the 36th Interscience Conference on Antimicrobial Agents and Chemotherapy*, American Society for Microbiology, New Orleans, 258, 1996.
4. Hutchinson, E.J., Joseph, C.A., and Bartlett, C.L.R., EWGLI: a European surveillance scheme for travelassociated Legionnaires' disease, *Eurosurveillance*, 1, 37, 1996.
5. Anonymous, British tourists return from Majorca with cryptosporidiosis, *CDR Weekly,* 10, 285, 2000.
6. World Health Organization, *WHO Report on Global Surveillance of Epidemic-Prone Infectious Diseases*, WHO/CDS/CSR/ISR/2000.1, WHO, Geneva, 2001.
7. Woodall, J.P., Global surveillance of emerging diseases: the ProMEDmail perspective, *Cad. Saude Publica, Rio de Janeiro*, 17 (Suppl), 147, 2001.
8. Fisher, I.S.T. and Gill, O.N., International surveillance networks and principles of collaboration, *Eurosurveillance*, 6, 17, 2001.
9. EC directive 95/46/EC (3) on the protection of individuals with regard to the processing of data and on the free movement of such data, October 1995, *Official J. European Communities*, L281, 31, 1995.
10. Tibayrene, M., European centres for disease control, *Nature,* 389, 433, 1997.
11. Giesecke, J. and Weinberg, J., A European centre for infectious disease?, *Lancet*, 352, 1308, 1998.
12. Lane, C.R., Joseph, C.A., and Bartlett, C.L.R., Travel-associated Legionnaires' disease in Europe in 1996, *Eurosurveillance*, 3, 6, 1998.
13. Slaymayer, E., Joseph, C.A., and Bartlett, C.L.R., Travel-associated Legionnaires' disease in Europe: 1997 and 1998, *Eurosurveillance*, 4, 120, 1999.
14. Lever, F. and Joseph, C.A., Travel-associated Legionnaires' disease in Europe in 1999, *Eurosurveillance*, 6, 53, 2001.
15. MacLehose, L. et al., Communicable disease outbreaks involving more than one country: systems approach to evaluating the response, *Brit. Med. J.*, 323, 861, 2001.
16. Wheeler, J.G. et al., Study of infectious intestinal disease in England: rates in the community, presenting to general practice, and reported in national surveillance, *Brit. Med. J.,* 318, 1046, 1999.
17. Anonymous, *Water and Health in Europe*, World Health Organization Regional Office for Europe, 1999.
18. Health Canada, Detecting emerging health risks around the world, http://www.hc-sc.gc.ca/hpb/transitn/gphin_e.pdf.

Section 2

Investigation of Outbreaks of Waterborne Disease

Will Robertson and Al Dufour

INTRODUCTION

This section of the book covers two of the sessions of the expert group meeting. The first of these two sessions concerned itself with a discussion of best practice in outbreak investigation, and the second with the value of data held by water utilities.

In this section of the book, recognized experts representing various disciplines describe their perspectives and contributions to the detection, characterization, and control of infectious waterborne disease outbreaks.

Chapter 5 provides an overview of outbreak detection and investigation. Successful outbreak investigations follow a systematic approach. The importance of preparing for outbreaks is stressed, as is the development of a learning culture whereby lessons learned from an outbreak are implemented and fed into the preparations for future outbreaks. Once an outbreak has been confirmed, it is essential to identify the source of the pathogen and to quickly control its spread to minimize human suffering and negative economic impacts. This requires a coordinated effort by an established, functional multi-disciplinary team of key participants (public health physicians, epidemiologists, clinical and environmental microbiologists, media spokespersons, and in the case of waterborne outbreaks, drinking water purveyors). Epidemiological studies to link illness and exposure route can be simply descriptive (i.e., collection of case information and generation of an epidemic curve) or based on a case-control approach (i.e., comparison of the incidence of illness in exposed and non-exposed populations). There is some concern among epidemiologists that case-control studies may suffer from various biases leading to the misclassification of data and may not possess sufficient statistical power to link illness and exposure source. The presence of acquired immunity within the exposed population can also affect the power of the study.

The detection of infectious outbreaks has traditionally relied upon clinical laboratory-based surveillance methods. While these methods can detect outbreaks affecting many people, smaller outbreaks are often missed due to the under-reporting of cases. In addition, because of delays in reporting, outbreaks may be detected only after the fact. These unrecognized and missed outbreaks can have significant public health and economic consequences. Earlier detection of disease clusters and possible outbreaks, based upon indirect evidence such as the increased sale of antidiarrheal drugs, has been demonstrated. Other means, such as physician requests for fecal analyses hold some promise. Computer-assisted technologies used in conjunction with these early indicators could be used to quickly detect outbreaks or possibly even predict outbreaks. Chapter 6 discusses a number of approaches for improving the early detection of outbreaks.

If the epidemiological study identifies a public drinking water supply as the most likely source of an outbreak, environmental and engineering studies must be initiated quickly to maximize the chances of finding the responsible infectious agent in the drinking water and to determine how it was able to breach the treatment or distribution system in sufficient quantities to cause a detectable outbreak. At the same time clinical and environmental microbiology investigations are essential to characterize the responsible pathogen and to link confirmed cases to the suspected drinking water. In many instances, the contaminated water has passed through the distribution system rendering it impossible to isolate the suspected organism from the water. In these instances the pathogen may be isolated from sewage. Increasingly, molecular techniques such as polymerase chain reaction and pulse field gel electophoresis are being used to match human and drinking water isolates and thus confirm that contaminated water was the source of the outbreak. Chapters 7 and 8 describe in more detail the impact of microbiological methods on the investigation of waterborne outbreaks, using enteric viruses and *Cryptosporidium* as examples.

The three remaining chapters in this section of the book switch their focus away from public health action and data to water utility data. The most obvious data held by water utilities are the results of routine coliform testing. Coliform monitoring of drinking water is usually performed to determine if the water meets some predetermined level of quality that is protective for public health. There is very little evidence, however, that coliform monitoring is predictive of disease associated with drinking water. Studies that have been conducted in an attempt to show a relationship between outbreaks of disease and previous detection of non-compliant levels of coliforms have not been able to show a significant association between these two events. This inability to forecast risk using coliforms as an indicator of water quality has led some authorities to consider other approaches to monitoring the quality of drinking water.

Chapter 9 is a discussion of the value of engineering investigations in confirming an association between disease and drinking water. The author describes his role as an engineer in investigating a number of outbreaks where standard water quality data, such as coliform counts, did not provide the outbreak investigation team with the answers they needed.

Although the value of the information provided by indicator bacteria has been questioned, the information provided by careful investigation of outbreaks of disease associated with drinking water has been shown to be very useful. Outbreak information that describes the risk factors associated with disease linked to drinking water has been a key driving force for improving water treatment technologies, source water protection, and water protection regulations. Only by careful and systematic review of the results of a number of outbreak investigations can appropriate general lessons be drawn. Chapter 10 is one such review of the causes of outbreaks of waterborne disease that have occurred in recent years in the U.S.

Chapter 11 is a review of the United Kingdom's experience of dealing with a recurrent problem, cryptosporidiosis. This chapter is a good example of how outbreak investigation can have a significant impact on the management of waterborne outbreaks by impacting on legislation. Following a legal ruling that epidemiological data was not admissible evidence, the U.K. took significant steps to remedy the shortcomings of coliform bacteria by legislating a treatment standard based on the detection of oocysts from the protozoan pathogen *Cryptosporidium*. The daily standard is based on a continuous sampling procedure that examines water filtered at a rate of at least 40 liters per hour. The sample should not contain more than an average of one oocyst per 10 liters. This approach is a radical departure from traditional practices used around the world and will provide useful data that may show a relationship between water-linked cryptosporidiosis and oocysts in water.

The approaches described above will be treated in greater detail in the following discussions. Their use will undoubtedly lead to improvements in the quality of drinking water, and they may provide an early warning for potential outbreaks of waterborne disease. The use of oocysts of *Cryptosporidium* as a treatment standard should provide some interesting results regarding the relationship between pathogens in drinking water and their linkage to disease in exposed populations. This approach may also provide an answer to the frequently posed question: can one pathogen, when used as an indicator, provide safe drinking water with regard to other potential pathogens? The need for visionary new approaches to providing high quality drinking water is well established. Improving the way we collect and use data, especially waterborne disease surveillance data and routine monitoring data, is a sensible way to begin fulfilling that need. Ultimately, however, we should aspire to setting goals for a system that will be able to forecast, rather than monitor, risks. A predictive system will not prevent outbreaks of disease associated with drinking water, nor will monitoring. We must continue to look for variables in the treatment process and distribution system that will tell us that something is going to happen and not that something has already happened.

5 A Systems Approach to the Investigation and Control of Waterborne Outbreaks

Catherine Quigley and Paul R. Hunter

CONTENTS

5.1 Introduction....53
5.2 The Stages in Outbreak Investigation....54
5.2.1 Preparation for an Outbreak....55
5.2.2 Outbreak Detection....55
5.2.3 Outbreak Confirmation....56
5.2.4 Outbreak Declaration....56
5.2.5 Outbreak Description....57
5.2.6 Hypothesis Formulation....59
5.2.7 Remedial Control Measures....60
5.2.7.1 Options for Intervention....60
5.2.7.2 Making Intervention Decisions with Inadequate Data....61
5.2.8 Hypothesis Testing....61
5.2.8.1 Analytic Epidemiological Investigations....61
5.2.8.1.1 Selection of Cases and Controls....62
5.2.8.1.2 Sample Size and Power....62
5.2.8.1.3 Bias....63
5.2.9 Control Measures....63
5.2.10 Formal Report....64
5.3 Conclusions....64
References....64

5.1 INTRODUCTION

In this chapter we shall describe a general approach to outbreak investigation and discuss some of the limitations and pitfalls inherent in the process. As should be clear from the introduction to Section 2, many aspects of outbreak investigation are dealt with in more detail in subsequent chapters. Further discussion of the epidemiological approaches important to waterborne outbreak investigation can be found elsewhere.[1–5]

The approach suggested here is a systems approach to outbreak investigation.[1] This approach considers the whole system and follows a logical sequence of actions in the investigation that will be broadly similar in each case. In outbreaks of waterborne disease, the whole system includes the water extraction, treatment, and distribution system, the population affected and relevant health care system responsible for the diagnosis, and management prevention of infectious disease (Figure 5.1). The

0-8493-1259-0/03/$0.00+$1.50

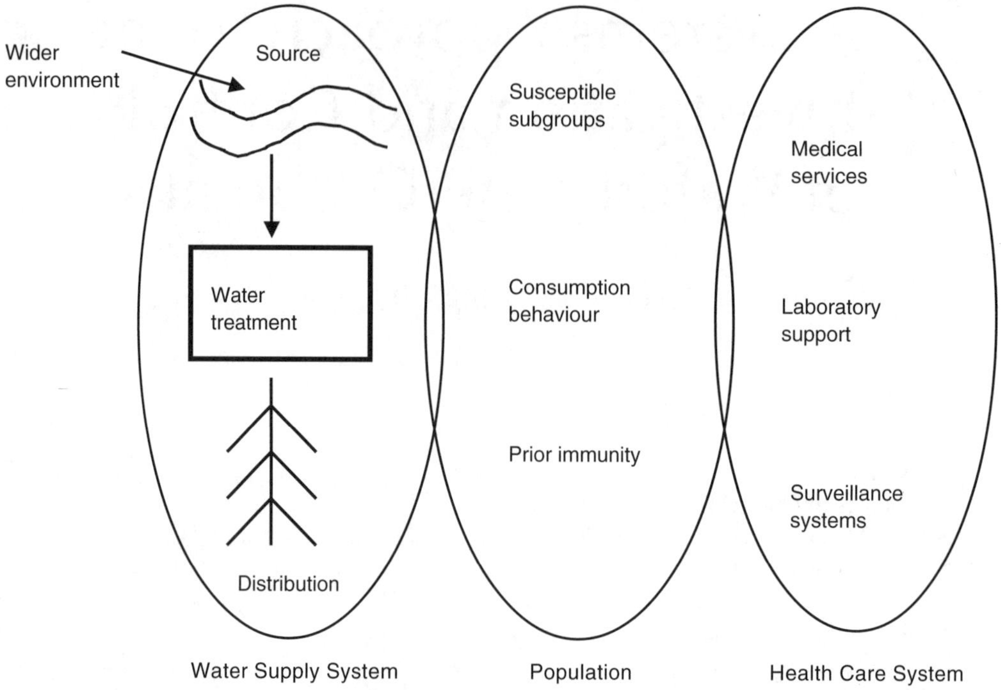

FIGURE 5.1 A systems map of an outbreak of waterborne disease.

outbreak team must be aware of each of the areas identified in the system map and systematically consider how these may contribute to the outbreak or its investigation.

The stages of an outbreak investigation are listed below:[1]

1. Planning
2. Outbreak detection
3. Confirmation that an outbreak is occurring
4. Declaration of outbreak and calling the outbreak committee together
5. Description of the outbreak
6. Generation of a hypothesis as to the cause of the outbreak
7. Implementation of an initial control measure
8. Testing the validity of the hypothesis
9. Implementation of further control measures
10. Learning the lessons for the future

Although the process is generally sequential, more than one stage can be undertaken at a time; however, it is definitely not a good idea to be doing step 1 (preparation) while an outbreak is under way. Furthermore, a good outbreak investigation will continue to iterate back to earlier steps to check its previous conclusions and hypotheses (Figure 5.2). Finally, as also shown in Figure 5.2, all outbreak investigations should be circular in that lessons learned should feed into preparation and planning for the next outbreak.

5.2 THE STAGES IN OUTBREAK INVESTIGATION

We will now discuss the stages in outbreak investigation following the sequential list given in the introduction.

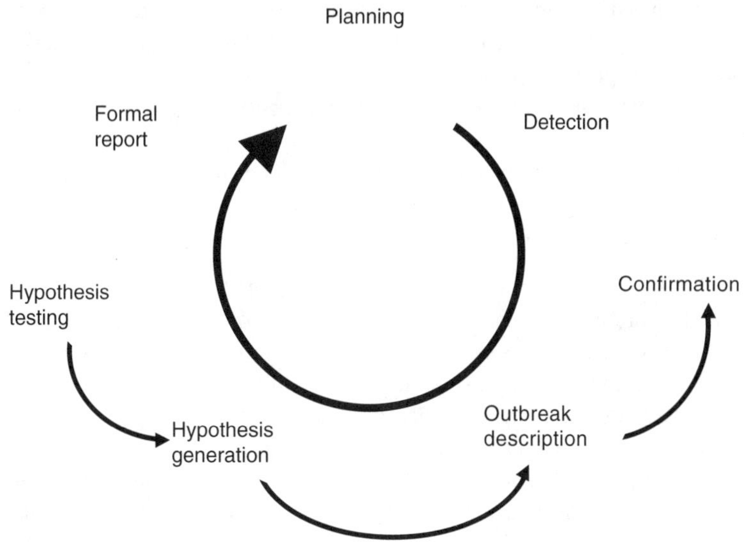

FIGURE 5.2 The learning curve for outbreak investigations, showing important iterations.

5.2.1 Preparation for an Outbreak

The investigation of any outbreak is a complex activity that calls on the skills and experience of individuals from a variety of organizations and professional backgrounds. One of the keys to successful outbreak management is planning. Such planning will need to address issues such as who should be involved and what their roles and responsibilities will be. Planning will also ensure that everyone can agree in advance on the terms of reference for the outbreak control team, what the key steps in the outbreak investigation will be, and how and to whom the work of the team will be communicated. The outbreak plan must also be explicit about who will manage the outbreak team

Although most public health practitioners working in communicable disease control will have regular experience of outbreak management, few will have managed an outbreak of waterborne disease. Furthermore, the team brought together for a waterborne outbreak is likely to differ from the team that investigates outbreaks of, say, meningococcal disease. It is also important that people who are likely to work together under potentially difficult conditions should meet regularly and build up trust. A useful activity for any prospective outbreak team is to have occasional exercises to test outbreak plans and enable colleagues to get to know each other.

Once an outbreak is under way and the local press is outside the door, it is too late to resolve potentially difficult issues such as who will be the lead investigator and which organization will take the lead in press relations.

5.2.2 Outbreak Detection

Most waterborne disease outbreaks are detected because of an increase in the number of cases of a particular infection being reported through the local or national surveillance system. The chain of events leading to notification of a case and the falloff in number of cases reported to a particular surveillance system are discussed in Chapters 1 to 4.

Surveillance systems at local, regional, and national levels should be sufficiently robust to allow recognition of outbreaks. A sudden increase in laboratory isolates locally should prompt an enquiry regarding any changes in laboratory testing policies. Assuming the increase is real, experience and scrutiny of weekly rates will usually indicate the level at which an outbreak should be suspected and a meeting should be called to investigate further. Agreed-upon threshold levels for investigation may be useful; these are calculated on the assumption that baseline weekly numbers of cases follow a Poisson distribution.[5] An outbreak may also be recognized following a report of a treatment failure from a water company; it is therefore very important that such reports involve the recording of appropriate information to enable health risk assessment.[6]

The issue of outbreak detection is discussed in more detail in Chapter 6.

5.2.3 Outbreak Confirmation

Before acting on the diagnosis of an outbreak it is important to think whether the outbreak is real or an artifact. There is often quite marked variation in the reported incidence of some infections from one week to the next and it is possible that an apparent outbreak simply reflects normal random variation. Even if the magnitude of an increase is unlikely to have arisen by chance, it may be that laboratory methods have changed or clinicians have suddenly become aware of their responsibility for notifying particular infections. Pseudo-outbreaks as a result of laboratory error have been detected on more than one occasion.[7] A small amount of double checking of data can lead to big savings in embarrassment that would accompany any announcement that the apparent outbreak was a false alarm.

5.2.4 Outbreak Declaration

Once the outbreak is confirmed then the appropriate person should declare that an outbreak is occurring. This declaration activates the various outbreak plans, and the investigation proper begins with the calling together of the outbreak team. The membership of the outbreak control team will be governed by the outbreak plan. The core membership of the outbreak control team will vary from country to country depending on existing public health practice and structures. However, it should include:

- The public health professional responsible for communicable disease control in the area affected by the outbreak; this person should be the lead and chair the outbreak control team meetings
- An environmental health specialist from the local area who should be sufficiently senior to make decisions and allocate resources
- A microbiologist from the local hospital or Public Health Laboratory who would be responsible for examining stool samples from affected cases
- A press officer

In these authors' views, it is also important that a senior representative of the implicated water utility should also be a member. This person would be able to present the outbreak committee with data from the water utility which would enable the implementation of appropriate control measures.

In addition to these core team members, there are a number of other people who may be asked to attend. These include:

- An epidemiologist, who may or may not be part of the local authority, to advise on adequate design and analysis of epidemiological investigations
- A public health microbiologist to advise on microbiological sampling and interpretation
- Water supply engineers
- A representative of the national environment agency, if one exists
- A representative of the local agriculture ministry
- Physicians
- Infection control or public health nurses

At its first meeting the outbreak team should agree on terms of reference. The example terms of reference listed here, from a 1990 U.K. expert committee report, are still valid today:[8]

- To review the evidence for an outbreak by examination of the epidemiological, microbiological, and other data
- To identify the population at risk in order to institute additional measures required for gathering further relevant information
- To decide on measures of controlling the outbreak and protecting other members of the community at risk
- To make arrangements for the commitment of personnel and resources considered necessary
- To monitor the implementation and effectiveness of the measures taken
- To make arrangements for informing the public and media
- To decide on the point at which the outbreak can be considered of no further significance
- To prepare a report as soon as it is practicable on the outbreak and make recommendations for further action

Also at its first meeting, and each subsequent meeting, the outbreak committee will review all new information about the outbreak, plan further investigations, and decide whether any control measures can be put in place. The outbreak control committee will also decide what information about the outbreak should be made public.

Before progressing to consideration of the outbreak investigation in more detail we must also consider some of the resource implications in outbreak management. The following must be easily available to enable high quality epidemiological investigation of outbreaks of waterborne illness:

- Relevant information including maps of water distribution and supply zones (provided by water companies) and population data for the area affected
- Staff with appropriate skills including epidemiological, statistical, data handling, interviewing, leadership, and organizational
- Facilities, including an "incident room"

The setting up of an incident room has been described by Mitchell.[9] The functions of the incident room are to provide a headquarters where the work of the investigating team may be coordinated, to act as a communications control center, and to facilitate the collation of all data.

5.2.5 Outbreak Description

Outbreak description is the use of descriptive epidemiological techniques to describe and summarize certain key information about the people affected and their illness. It is the most important stage in the investigation of any waterborne outbreak and may even be sufficient epidemiology.[10] The key information that we are primarily concerned about in descriptive epidemiology is often abbreviated to time, person and place, or who, when, and where — the person related to key demographic data on cases (age and sex), the time to when the illness developed, and the place where the person lives. These simple sets of data when collected over a sufficient number of cases will often provide most of the information required to judge whether or not an outbreak is likely to be waterborne. In order to be able to do descriptive epidemiology, however, one needs to know whether an ill individual should be included as a case in the study. To know this requires a case definition.

Case definitions are usually phrased in terms of the illness, geographical location, and date of onset. Illness may be defined by clinical symptoms (e.g., presence or absence of diarrhea) or by laboratory results (e.g., stool positive for *Cryptosporidium*). Often cases are called "possible" based on clinical features and "confirmed" once laboratory results are available. For many pathogens, there can also be two levels of confirmation based on further typing (i.e., knowing that a particular infection is due to the calf genotype of *Cryptosporidium*). The case definition should also state the time period for dates of onset that the outbreak team is interested in (e.g., diarrhea with a date of onset after April 1st). The case definition should also include some geographical locator as well (i.e., residence in particular city). There is a certain art to getting useful case definitions. If the case definition is drawn too narrowly (say, residence within too narrow a geographical area), then actual cases will be excluded from analysis and potentially vital information will be lost. On the other hand, if case definitions are drawn too widely then much time could be wasted investigating cases that are extremely unlikely to be part of the outbreak. The inclusion of too many cases that are not part of the outbreak under investigation would also impair the power of any analytical study.[11] Case definitions should be revisited regularly during the investigation and possibly changed as more information becomes available.

In practice, the data collected on individual cases are broader than suggested by the time, person, and place suggested above. A basic set of data will be collected on every individual who satisfies the case definitions. At a minimum, this will include name, address, age, sex, date of onset, the results of microbiological examination, and sufficient clinical information to prove that the individual satisfies the case definition. It is also usual to record place of work or school, a basic food or contact history, and any travel history. Example questionnaires for the investigation of potentially waterborne *Cryptosporidium* outbreaks are given elsewhere.[5]

The results of the descriptive epidemiology are then collated and presented in tabular or graphical form. The epidemic curve (a histogram showing the distribution of dates of onset) is probably the most useful descriptive technique in any outbreak investigation (Figure 5.3). The epidemic curve is the clearest indication of how the outbreak is progressing and whether control measures have been effective. Another valuable data presentation technique is geographical mapping, which shows how cases are distributed. This allows the investigators to see whether cases are clustered around particular water supply areas (Figure 5.4).

An outbreak of cryptosporidiosis in Wirral and Ellesmere Port in the North West of England in 1996 illustrates the value of descriptive epidemiology, especially when supported by a significant association between illness and residence in a particular water supply area, and by microbiological results. The investigation has been described elsewhere.[12] In summary, in April 1996 an outbreak investigation followed an increase in the number of cases of cryptosporidiosis among residents of Wirral and Ellesmere Port supplied by a single water treatment plant. Fifty-two laboratory-confirmed cases of cryptosporidiosis satisfied the case definition employed in the investigation.

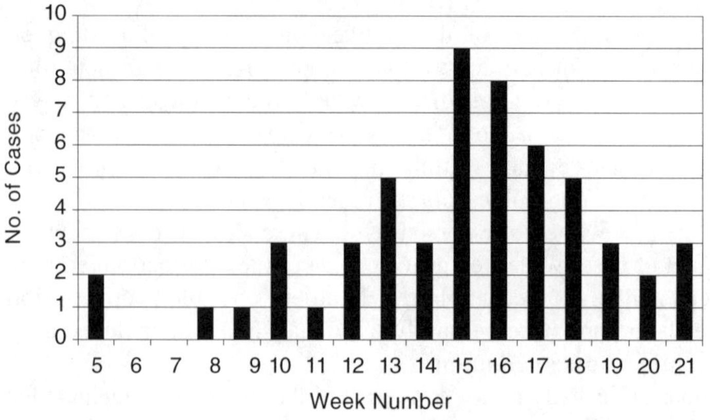

FIGURE 5.3 Outbreak of cryptosporidiosis, Wirral and Ellesmere Port, 1996: cases by week of onset (n = 51).

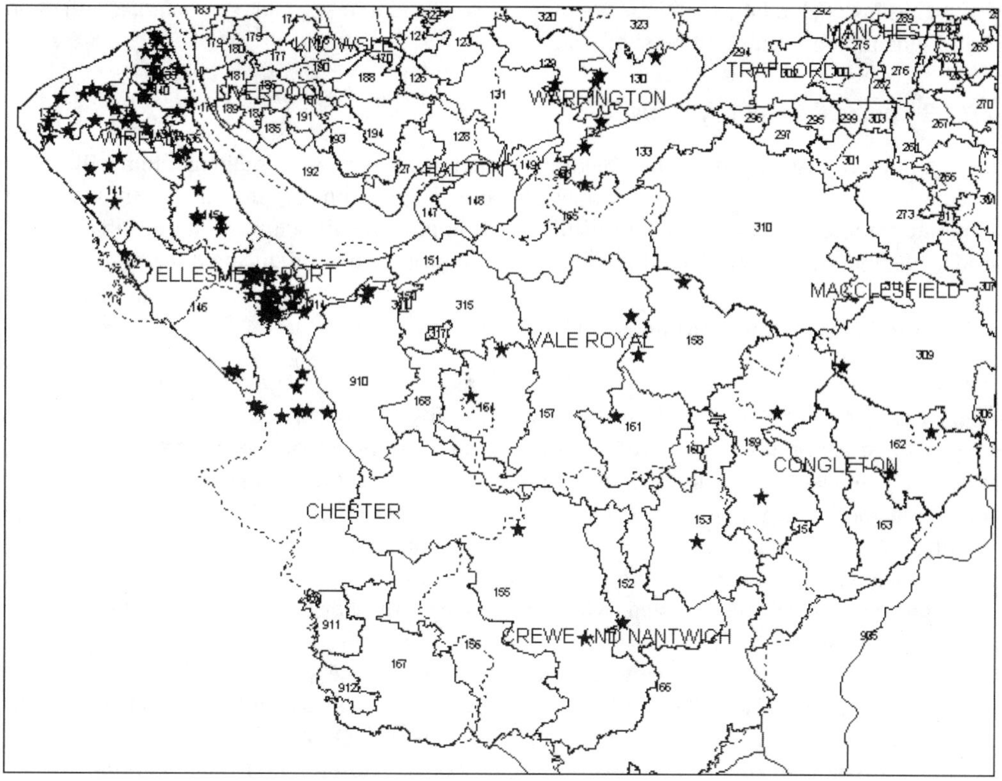

FIGURE 5.4 Outbreak of cryptosporidiosis, Wirral and Ellesmere Port, 1996: geographical distribution.

The epidemic curve (Figure 5.3) and the geographical distribution of cases (Figure 5.4) suggested a common source outbreak. In addition, no other common risk factor that would explain the outbreak was identified when cases were interviewed. The attack rate among those whose water was supplied solely from the plant was 1.42 per 10,000 compared with 0.42 per 10,000 among those having some, but less than 50%, of their water supplied from the plant ($p = 0.045$; relative risk 3.40, 95% confidence interval: 1.06 – 10.9). On four occasions in April, May, and June a single oocyst was recovered from treated water, though there was no "event" or problem identified with the water treatment process that could explain the outbreak. The results of the descriptive epidemiology together with the difference in attack rates among the population and the detection of oocysts indicated that the outbreak was strongly associated with drinking water.

5.2.6 Hypothesis Formulation

As the initial outbreak data are being collected and analyzed, it is important to keep asking what these data suggest about the possible cause of the outbreak. This is known as hypothesis generation. Indeed, at some point during the investigation a hypothesis as to the cause of the outbreak should be clearly stated. The formal statement of the hypothesis is important for a number of reasons. If analytical studies (see below) are being considered, they will be designed to test one or more hypotheses. Any control measures that are being considered will presume a particular hypothesis as to the cause of the outbreak (whether or not the outbreak is waterborne).

In deciding the hypotheses as to the cause of the outbreak, the outbreak team will rely on the descriptive epidemiology, initial environmental investigations, knowledge of the epidemiology or microbiology of the causative agent, and their experience of similar outbreaks. Although prior experience is invaluable in generating hypotheses it is essential to keep an open mind, as infectious disease epidemiology can often be surprising.

5.2.7 Remedial Control Measures

If consumption of drinking water has been implicated as a cause of an outbreak, this will lead to consideration of what can be done to prevent more people from getting ill. Control measures appropriate for waterborne disease will be discussed in more detail below. In this section we shall consider possible options available to the outbreak control team for reducing risk.

5.2.7.1 Options for Intervention

Early in the investigation of an outbreak there are relatively few interventions that can reduce a presumed risk to public health. Basically, a water utility can either take action to improve the quality of the water or advise consumers to avoid drinking unboiled tap water. Options to improve water quality are also limited and will depend in part on the technical cause of the failure in water quality. Some of the causes of failure are discussed in more detail in Chapters 9 through 11. If the cause of the failure is known, say, a failure in chlorination, it may have already been rectified. If not, then water treatment failure can be corrected.

In many cases, the cause of failure will be more long term. For example, a groundwater source that is subject to surface-water intrusion may not have a filtration system. The immediate options available to the water utility in such circumstances depend on the size of the supply and whether alternate sources are readily available. If the source is relatively small and an adequate alternate supply is available, then it may be relatively simple to switch sources. On the other hand, if the source is large then it may not be possible to access sufficient water from elsewhere. Even if there are alternate sources, it may not be prudent to switch to a source that has not been used recently and does not have adequate water quality data available. Similarly, if switching source to another water treatment facility would put undue stress on that facility, then improved water quality could not be guaranteed.

If steps cannot be taken to enhance water quality, then consideration must be given to advising consumers to boil all water before drinking. Issuing of "boil water notices" or "boil water advisories" is one of the more common responses to risk reduction in the outbreak setting. However, recent opinion has highlighted concerns about the potential benefits and adverse health effects of advice to boil water.[13,14] There is now some good evidence that boil water advice is frequently ignored by the consumer who may be confused.[15–17] Consequently many people continue to drink unboiled tap water during boil water notices. Even with 100% compliance, it is doubtful that many boil water notices reduce risk to health. By the time the outbreak is detected and the notice is delivered to consumers, it is likely that any contaminated water has long since left the distribution system.[14]

On the negative side, boil water notices may also be associated with very real negative health effects. There has been very little published research on the benefits and disadvantages to health associated with boil water notices. The potential risks to health from boil water notices were first raised in the 1980s.[13] Boil water notices cause inconvenience and some cost, especially if people start buying bottled water. In a recent study, 13 of 675 (1.9%) hospital employees responding to a questionnaire claimed that they or a member of their family had suffered a burn or scald following a boil water notice.[17] The psychological effects in terms of anxiety and loss of confidence in the water supply have not been properly studied. However, in one study it was noted that 10% of respondents did not revert to normal tap water consumption after a boil water notice in North London.[17] Whatever the adverse health effects of boil water notices, it is likely that the elderly will have more difficulties. As far as we are aware, there have been no studies of the impact of boil water notices on this vulnerable group.

In conclusion, with the current state of knowledge it is not known whether there would be any health gain from issuing a boil water notice following the detection of *Cryptosporidium* oocysts in drinking water. Indeed, it is possible that the issue of such a notice may have a negative health effect. Nevertheless, where the risk assessment does indicate the need for issuing a boil water notice, public health personnel should ensure that the notice is issued as quickly and effectively as possible.

Given that boil water notices may have negative as well as positive effects on public health, one should always be cautious about advocating their use. This caution is particularly valid early in an outbreak investigation when there may be considerable uncertainty as to the cause. We will now consider the difficulties associated with intervention decisions in more detail.

5.2.7.2 Making Intervention Decisions with Inadequate Data

At this stage of outbreak investigation the outbreak control team has rarely proven the source of the outbreak. Even if the outbreak team is reasonably confident that water is the source, it may not be known whether any contamination event was a short-lived or continuing problem.

In our experience, this is probably the most difficult decision in outbreak investigation. If decisions are delayed, more people are likely to become ill. On the other hand, as discussed above, control interventions may have their own problems for public health and can also be very costly for the water utility to implement. Decisions to introduce control measures for erroneously presumed waterborne outbreaks are also potentially very embarrassing for the outbreak team. We do not have any magic formulae to help outbreak control teams make these decisions. After all, making difficult decisions is what public health doctors are paid to do. Nevertheless we would suggest that outbreak committees should ask themselves three questions before implementing control measures.

- How confident are we that the cause of this outbreak is drinking water?
- What would likely be the worst effect of not introducing a particular control measure?
- What would likely be the worst effect of introducing a particular control measure?

5.2.8 Hypothesis Testing

Once the outbreak control team has generated one or more hypotheses as to the cause of the outbreak, the next stage is to attempt to prove these hypotheses in a more rigorous fashion. In Chapter 3, we were presented with two schemes for assessing the strength of association between water and outbreaks of disease. These are based on a combination of epidemiological and microbiological evidence as well as on information about the operation of the water distribution system. Thus there are three complementary approaches to proving hypotheses as to the cause of potentially waterborne outbreaks: further microbiological, epidemiological, or environmental/engineering investigations.

Microbiological proof rests, at best, on identifying the causative agent in the water supply or demonstrating microbiological evidence of treatment failure such as coliforms. However, the further microbiological examination of patients and contacts also provides considerable additional proof. Chapters 7 and 8 describe in more detail the potential value of microbiological investigations in outbreak investigation.

Environmental evidence comes from a full study of the water supply and distribution system, looking for potential causes of failure. This study will include a review of the supply records as well as a thorough inspection of the system. These investigations will aim to identify possible breakdowns in the integrity of the system or in the application of standard procedures. The engineering/environmental investigations of possible waterborne outbreaks are discussed in more detail in Chapter 9.

5.2.8.1 Analytic Epidemiological Investigations

The most common analytical epidemiological investigation of potential waterborne outbreaks is the case–control study. For outbreaks affecting water supplies to small communities, a retrospective cohort may also be used. The conduct of both these types of study are discussed in more detail elsewhere.[1,2]

A cohort study is a study of a group of individuals for whom exposure data are known. Typically for outbreaks, retrospective cohort studies are done where all people are potentially exposed to a single risk factor (say, supplied by water from a single well). By contrast, case–control studies are retrospective studies of events that preceded the onset of disease in a group of individuals. In a case–control study, hypotheses are tested by comparing the incidence of a preceding event in those with disease (cases) with a group of individuals who do not appear to have disease (controls). For outbreaks, cases are those people who satisfy the agreed case definition. Case–control studies have the advantage of being relatively quick and inexpensive compared to other some other designs of epidemiological study, and they can also be used to examine several hypotheses simultaneously.

However, case–control studies potentially suffer from a number of problems that can bias their conclusions. For example, a case–control study was undertaken during the investigation of the Wirral and Ellesmere Port outbreak described above. Detailed data were collected for the 52 cases that met the case definition and 106 controls (15 of whom were excluded because of gastrointestinal illness). Cases and controls were matched for age within 5-year age bands. The results of the study were inconclusive in that there was no statistically significant association between regular drinking of tap water and risk of illness. The potential problems associated with case–control studies in outbreak investigation will be discussed next. Case–control studies, albeit in the context of sporadic disease, are discussed further in Chapter 17.

5.2.8.1.1 Selection of Cases and Controls

Ideally, cases used to identify a risk factor and generate a hypothesis in the descriptive epidemiological study should be excluded from a case–control study used to test that hypothesis. However, the power of the study may be compromised by too few cases, and the size of the outbreak may not be apparent when deciding to carry out a case–control study. A pragmatic approach is to ensure at the outset that data collected from cases for the descriptive study, especially with regard to risk factors, are appropriate for a case–control study. In the Wirral and Ellesmere Port outbreak, cases interviewed early in the investigation were included in the case–control study; however, this is not thought to have introduced bias because the same detailed questionnaire was used throughout the investigation, so early cases did not have to be re-interviewed.

Could the selection of controls have led to overmatching and thus underestimating the true effect of exposure to drinking water? Controls were selected from a computerized list of patients registered with general practitioners, held by the Health Authority. They should therefore have been representative of the general population. A more convenient method of obtaining controls is to ask each case to nominate a friend of similar age who lives in the same community. The advantage of this method is that friends may be more willing to cooperate with a study than members of the general population, and they may also offer a degree of control of important confounding factors, e.g., socioeconomic status.[2] However, this method is more likely to lead to overmatching because controls may be too similar to the cases in relation to exposure of interest.

5.2.8.1.2 Sample Size and Power

The most likely explanation for the inconclusive results of the case–control study in Wirral and Ellesmere Port is that the study did not have sufficient statistical power. The power (the probability that a variable with a true association with illness will be statistically significant) of a case–control study is increased by:

- Increased sample size
- Increased magnitude of effect (measured by odds ratio in a case–control study)
- The number of controls per case (though there is little to be gained beyond 4 controls per case)
- Increased immunity in cases
- Reduced exposure among controls

For example, if 90% of cases drink tap water and 80% of controls drink tap water, 219 cases and 219 controls would be needed to demonstrate that this 10% difference in exposure to tap water is unlikely to be caused by chance alone (confidence level: 95%, power: 80%). (Andrews, N., personal communication, 1996). While one can influence sample size by increasing the number of controls per case, the effect of immunity cannot be altered, and it does have an important effect. Taking the Wirral and Ellesmere Port outbreak, a power calculation suggested that a study with 50 cases and 100 controls, with 70% of controls drinking tap water, would have 80% power to detect an odds ratio of 4, assuming no immunity among controls. However, if 20% of controls were immune, the true odds ratio would have to be 7 for a study of this size to show a statistically significant association between drinking water and illness. It is possible that the population in Wirral and Ellesmere Port, where 85% of the water is abstracted from river water, was repeatedly exposed to *Cryptosporidium* oocysts and thus developed sufficient immunity to affect the power of the study.[12]

5.2.8.1.3 Bias

Bias is a particularly important issue in case–control studies. Selection bias can occur if response rates are unequal among cases and controls; this was not the case in the investigation described here. Interviewer bias is almost impossible to eliminate since the interviewer is usually part of the outbreak investigation. This, however, would be more likely to lead to an exaggeration of the difference in exposure between cases and controls rather than an underestimated effect. The other important bias that is particularly difficult to control for in an outbreak is recall bias. Cases are likely to think about exposure histories more than controls; again this is more likely to lead to an overestimate rather than an underestimate of the true odds ratio.

Publicity about an outbreak can have an important effect on controls as well as cases. A community-based survey in Lancashire, North West England, following a large outbreak of cryptosporidiosis that generated a lot of media publicity, found that the prevalence of self-reported diarrheal disease was higher in the control towns than in the outbreak towns.[18] Moreover, there was a strong association between self-reported diarrhea and drinking water in both control and outbreak areas.[19] It was unlikely that infection in the region at the time could have accounted for these results; rather, it was thought that widespread publicity led to recall bias that affected controls as much as cases. The imposition of a boil water notice during an outbreak could have the same effect and would make interpretation of the results of a case–control study difficult.

The factors that have been discussed here should not lead to the conclusion that case–control studies are never worthwhile in the investigation of an outbreak where drinking water is suspected. Several studies have shown an association between drinking water and illness, and in some large outbreaks a significant "dose response" relationship has been found between the quantity of water consumed and illness.[12, 20–24] However, one should be aware of the factors that may lead to misclassification of results — usually an underestimate of the true odds ratio. The power of the study may not be sufficient and the effects of immunity, particularly in populations that normally drink surface water, are often overlooked.[12] The influence of recall bias due to publicity or the imposition of a boil water notice may make interpretation of results very difficult. The value of descriptive epidemiology should not be underestimated.

5.2.9 Control Measures

If an outbreak has been shown to be waterborne or, as discussed above, the degree of evidence is sufficient, control measures may be implemented. We have already discussed control measures that could be implemented early in an investigation. More longer term control measures could be taken by the utility or the appropriate regulator. The exact control measures depend on the cause of the failure that led to an outbreak. If the failure was due to a process failure, new controls and procedures may be implemented. If failure was due to poor plant design, new capital works may need to be commissioned or the works abandoned, provided suitable alternatives are available.

The regulator may also choose to implement changes in its recommendations for best practice and inspection procedures. Very occasionally, the agency may bring in new legislation, as was the case in the U.K. following a large outbreak of cryptosporidiosis (Chapter 11).

5.2.10 Formal Report

For most outbreaks of waterborne disease, the cause of the outbreak has passed before the public health has become aware of the increase in cases. In such a situation, one may be tempted to think that the outbreak report is only of historic interest. However, many different organizations and individuals will have an interest in reports of the outbreak and its investigation. Going back to the introduction to this chapter, a major reason for any outbreak investigation is to learn the lessons so that future outbreaks can be prevented or better managed.

The formal outbreak report enables the participating agencies to review their own contributions and determine whether there are any areas where they could have contributed better. The water utility, in particular, will want to know what went wrong so that measures can be taken to prevent similar problems in the future. The formal outbreak report is also becoming of considerable interest to lawyers who may bring claims for damages against the water company. Chapter 11 discusses in more detail how the investigation of one outbreak impacted on the legal system and how new legislation was passed as a result.

The wider public health, scientific, and industry communities may also have a legitimate interest in a particular outbreak. It is always better to learn from other people's mistakes than from your own. Where there are important lessons to be learned from an outbreak, the investigators have a duty to publish aspects of their work in the scientific press.

5.3 CONCLUSIONS

Outbreak investigation is one of the most stressful and yet most rewarding aspects of the work of public health practitioners. It is stressful because of making decisions that have potentially large effects on people and industry, making decisions within the full glare of the media spotlight, and making decisions on incomplete and uncertain data. On the other hand, good outbreak investigation can have very real benefits in protecting people's health in the short and long term. Short-term health protection arises from identifying and stopping the source of an outbreak, thus preventing illness in people who would otherwise have been exposed to the infection. Longer-term health protection comes from the power of outbreak reports to influence policy and law on the local, national, and international level. Indeed, few people can expect to have as much influence on public health as the authors of outbreak reports.

Many of the causes of stress during outbreak investigation can also be controlled provided that the investigation is based on adequate planning and preparation and follows a logical process as described in this and subsequent chapters. Subsequent chapters discuss in more detail certain aspects of outbreak investigation.

REFERENCES

1. Hunter, P.R., *Water-borne Disease: Epidemiology and Ecology*, Wiley, Chichester, 1997.
2. Hennekens, C.H. and Buring, J. E., *Epidemiology in Medicine*, Little, Brown and Co., Boston, 1987.
3. Andersson, Y. and Bohan, P., Disease surveillance and waterborne outbreaks, in: *Water Quality: Guidelines, Standards and Health. Risk Assessment and Management for Water-Related Infectious Disease,* Fewtrell, L. and Bartram J., Eds., IWA Publishing, London, 2001, 115.
4. Blumenthal, U.J. et al., Epidemiology: a tool for the assessment of risk, in: *Water Quality: Guidelines, Standards and Health. Risk Assessment and Management for Water-Related Infectious Disease,* Fewtrell, L. and Bartram J., Eds., IWA Publishing, London, 2001, 135.

5. Department of the Environment, Transport and the Regions & Department of Health, Cryptosporidium *in Water Supplies, Third Report of the Group of Experts*, HMSO, London, 1998.
6. Hunter, P.R., Advice on the response from public and environmental health to the detection of cryptosporidial oocysts in treated drinking water, *Comm. Dis. Public Health,* 3, 24, 2000.
7. Casemore, D.P., A pseudo-outbreak of cryptosporidiosis, *Comm. Dis. Rep. Rev.,* 2, R66, 1992.
8. Badenoch, J., Cryptosporidium *in Water Supplies, Report of the Group of Experts*, Department of the Environment, Department of Health, HMSO, London, 1990.
9. Mitchell, E. Setting up an incident room, in *Communicable Disease Epidemiology and Control*, Noah, N. and O'Mahony, M., Eds., John Wiley & Sons, Chichester, 1998, ch. 8.
10. Palmer, S.R., Epidemiology in search of infectious diseases: methods in outbreak investigation, *J. Epidemiol. Community Health,* 43, 311, 1989.
11. Hunter, P.R., Modelling the impact of prior immunity, case misclassification and bias on case–control studies in the investigation of outbreaks of cryptosporidiosis, *Epidemiol. Infect.,* 125, 713, 2000.
12. Hunter, P.R. and Quigley, C., Investigation of an outbreak of cryptosporidiosis associated with treated surface water finds limits to the value of case control studies, *Comm. Dis. Public Health*, 4, 234, 1998.
13. Mayon-White, R.T. and Frankenberg, R.A., Boil the water, *Lancet,* 2, 216, 1989.
14. Hunter, P.R., Advice on the response to reports from public and environmental health to the detection of cryptosporidial oocysts in treated drinking water, *Comm. Dis. Public Health,* 3, 24, 2000.
15. O' Donnell, M., Platt, C., and Aston, R., Effect of a boil water notice on behaviour in the management of a water contamination incident, *Comm. Dis. Public Health*, 3, 56, 2000.
16. Angulo, F.J. et al., A community waterborne outbreak of salmonellosis and the effectiveness of a boil water order, *Am. J. Public Health,* 87, 580, 1997.
17. Willocks, L.J. et al., Compliance with advice to boil drinking water during and outbreak of cryptosporidiosis, *Comm. Dis. Public Health*, 3, 137, 2000.
18. Hunter, P.R. and Syed, Q., Community surveys of self-reported diarrhoea can dramatically overestimate the size of outbreaks of waterborne cryptosporidiosis, *Water Sci. Technol.,* 43, 27, 2001.
19. Hunter, P.R. and Syed, Q., A community-based survey of self-reported gastroenteritis undertaken during a waterborne outbreak of cryptosporidiosis, *Epidemiology,* 11, 442, 2000.
20. Tillett, H.E., de Louvois, J., and Wall, P.G., Surveillance of outbreaks of waterborne infectious disease: categorizing levels of evidence, *Epidemiol. Infect.*, 120, 37, 1998.
21. Willocks, L. et al., A large outbreak of cryptosporidiosis associated with a public water supply from a deep chalk borehole, *Comm. Dis. Public Health*, 4, 239, 1998.
22. Furtado, C. et al., Outbreaks of waterborne infectious intestinal disease in England and Wales 1992–1995, *Epidemiol Infect.*, 121, 109, 1998.
23. Maguire, H.C. et al. An outbreak of cryptosporidiosis in South London: what value the p value, *Epidemiol Infect.*, 115, 279, 1995.
24. Bridgman, S.A. et al., Outbreak of cryptosporidiosis associated with a disinfected groundwater supply, *Epidemiol Infect.*, 115, 555, 1995.

6 Early Detection of Water-Related Disease Outbreaks

Jim Black and Christopher K. Fairley

CONTENTS

6.1 Introduction.....67
6.2 Choice of Measures of Illness.....68
6.3 Statistical Techniques for Outbreak Detection.....69
6.3.1. Cluster Detection and Action Thresholds.....69
6.3.1.1 Action Thresholds.....69
6.3.1.2 The Scan Statistic and Related Approaches.....71
6.3.1.3 The Cumulative Sum Chart (CUSUM).....71
6.3.2 Forecasting.....72
6.3.2.1 Auto-Regressive, Moving Average, and Auto-Regressive Integrated Moving Average (ARIMA) Modelling.....73
6.4 Artificial Neural Networks.....73
6.4.1 Origins and Function.....74
6.4.2 Drawbacks.....75
6.4.3 Forecasting.....76
6.4.4 In Practice.....76
References.....76

6.1 INTRODUCTION

Large-scale disease outbreaks are not instantaneous disasters like earthquakes or plane crashes. Contamination often continues for days or weeks, incubation periods vary, and there may be secondary transmission of the disease organism from primary cases by means other than water. Water-related outbreaks generally evolve slowly enough that early detection of the increasing number of cases would allow the application of useful preventive and curative measures. Prompt investigation and correction of treatment plant problems, the early introduction of a general "boil water" alert to consumers, or alerting physicians to the presence of an outbreak could all help reduce case numbers by hundreds or even thousands, with corresponding reductions in mortality. The earlier the outbreak is detected, the smaller the eventual total case numbers and the smaller the number of deaths. To this end, government health departments and public health laboratories around the world undertake surveillance of key organisms with outbreak potential. Astute epidemiologists and laboratory technicians perusing tabulations of recent laboratory isolates have often been the first to spot evolving outbreaks as clusters of isolates in time and/or space.

0-8493-1259-0/03/$0.00+$1.50

Despite these successes, smaller outbreaks probably go undetected quite often. Even at their best, laboratory-based surveillance systems may only detect increasing cases weeks, rather than days, after the initial contamination event.

There are several problems that prevent the early detection of outbreaks, such as the large number of organisms with outbreak potential and the large numbers of geographic areas that need to be monitored. There is also a need for robust statistical techniques that will allow reliable detection of an outbreak as close to its onset as possible

A typical laboratory-based system might recognize several thousand different organisms (counting all the various serotypes, etc), with a considerable range of frequencies and public health importance. The large numbers of data points and the need for more sophisticated statistical tools make it increasingly difficult for a human observer to scrutinize and analyze them all. If we are to improve the quality of water-related disease surveillance, it is increasingly obvious that computers and sophisticated analytical algorithms will be needed to flag unusual events and supplement human judgement. It may also be useful to reconsider the choice of measures to be regularly collected and analyzed, going beyond the traditional dependence on laboratory isolates.

6.2 CHOICE OF MEASURES OF ILLNESS

Key considerations in the choice of surveillance measures are their sensitivity and specificity, ease of collection, and (most importantly in relation to waterborne disease) timeliness in relation to contamination events. The ideal measure should be highly sensitive so that it rarely misses an outbreak, however small or localized. It should also be highly specific for water-related outbreaks, and thus rarely lead to a false alarm (which can be extremely costly and damaging to the water companies and health departments, as well as disturbing to the water consumers). Ideally the information should be very easy to collect, or already collected for other reasons, so that the surveillance system incurs little extra cost to the community. To allow the maximum time for intervention, the measure should rise as quickly as possible after a contamination event. Even better, the measure should be capable of forecasting, so that outbreaks might be foreseen days before they happen, when case numbers are still small.

Unfortunately, individual measures of illness tend to be at opposite ends of the spectrum for these different criteria. Laboratory isolation of organisms from disease sufferers, which is the measure most commonly used by health departments, is highly specific, but weeks can pass between a contamination event and the reporting of increasing isolates. The contaminated water must first be distributed to the consumers (often several days for the most peripheral areas of a large city), then there is a time lag (the incubation period for the given disease, measured in hours to days) between ingesting the water and the appearance of symptoms. The patients must then recognize the need for medical assistance and seek care — often another day or more. Then their medical attendants must decide that testing is necessary and order the test. The testing procedure commonly takes one or two days, sometimes longer. Finally, the results must be communicated to the health department and analyzed. Epidemiologists have at times been embarrassed to find media reports of disease clusters occurring days before their detection by routine surveillance systems.

Several measures have been suggested that are further "upstream" in this process and that have been shown to rise early in past outbreaks. These include absenteeism from work or schools, pharmacy sales of antidiarrheal medications, attendance at hospital casualty departments, and receipt of requests for fecal analysis (rather than positive results). None of these candidate measures has so far proved ideal — they are difficult to measure, or are not specific to diarrheal disease outbreaks, or at least not specific to water-related disease. Nevertheless, as each day's delay in the early stages of a city-wide outbreak may mean hundreds or even thousands more cases, the search continues for more useful measures of disease incidence. It is also likely that some of the candidate measures that are currently difficult to obtain will become easier in the future. For example, it is possible that even small retail pharmacies will change to a computerized stock control and inventory system in the next few years. The fact that useful data for outbreak detection (such as the daily sales of oral rehydration salts or antidiarrheal medicines) would then be routinely collected for other reasons would make acquisition of the same data by surveillance systems much simpler. See Chapter 2 for a further discussion of these issues.

6.3 STATISTICAL TECHNIQUES FOR OUTBREAK DETECTION

Any statistical approach to outbreak detection (and by extension any computer-based algorithm) faces several distinct difficulties. One is the day-to-day random variation inherent in any surveillance measure. A second problem is the tendency of many diseases, and thus also their proxy measures, to seasonal variation. Some measures also exhibit a secular trend — a longer-term tendency to rise or fall over several years. An even more difficult problem, where the surveillance database includes previous outbreaks, is creating an algorithm that can take account of those earlier outbreaks and not tend to include the inflated numbers from outbreak years in its assessment of the "normal" disease rate. Although a human observer can often spot all these different variations and "see through" them to the underlying pattern, they all pose difficulties, and sometimes insurmountable limitations, to statistical algorithms. The underlying processes we attempt to model are highly complex, and models that can accurately reconstruct past data sequences are commonly very poor predictors of the future of the same series.

Although there is a certain amount of overlap, there are currently two main approaches to the question of machine-assisted detection of outbreaks in time series data such as disease surveillance databases. The first approach, more commonly used in current practice, seeks to answer the question, "Are there more cases today than we would expect given our previous experience of the disease in question?" (or, "Has an outbreak begun?"). The other approach asks a different, though related, question, "How many cases are coming in the near future?" In other words, "Is there an outbreak coming, and how big will it be?"

6.3.1. Cluster Detection and Action Thresholds

There are a number of techniques and algorithms that take the first approach of asking whether there are there more cases being reported than would be expected, given previous experience.

6.3.1.1 Action Thresholds

Simple approaches are intrinsically appealing. The simplest approach is to define a certain number of cases as an action threshold above which further investigation or direct action will be taken.[1] This is easy where the disease is rare, and the appearance of one or a small number of cases warrants immediate action (such as poliomyelitis). It is difficult where the disease is relatively rare, but some sporadic cases can occur without signifying an outbreak. It is also very difficult to define an action threshold where case numbers are higher but day-to-day variation is large; a low action threshold will mean many false alarms, but a high action threshold will lead to outbreaks being detected too late for useful action. However, algorithms based on this basic idea are currently among the best in day-to-day use.

The *Morbidity and Mortality Weekly Review* (*MMWR*)[2] is a publication of the Centers for Disease Control and Prevention (CDC) of the United States (Figure 6.1). Each week the *MMWR* includes a graphical presentation of the reports of a short list of notifiable disease for the entire United States.[3] The graph compares the reports for the 4-week period just ended with a baseline number calculated from previous years. The baseline number for each disease is the mean of fifteen earlier 4-week periods: the comparable 4-week period in each of the preceding 5 years as well as the 4-week periods immediately before and after. The calculation is made for a 4-week period so that much of the random week-to-week variation will be smoothed out. The *MMWR* baseline figure

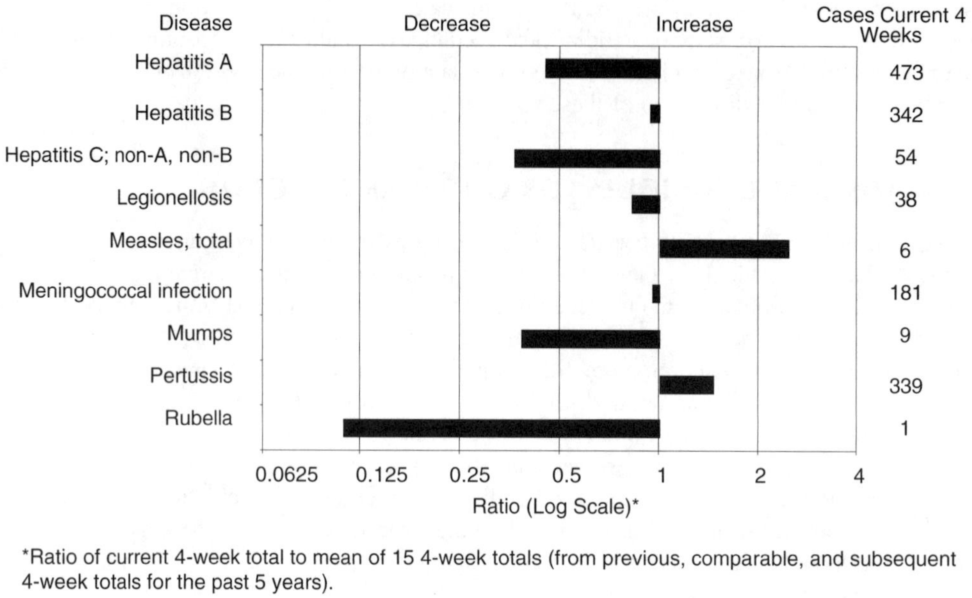

FIGURE 6.1 The MMWR method. (Source: *MWWR*, 50, 10, March 16, 2001.)

should take account of seasonal variation (by comparing with the same season in previous years) and lessen the effect of previous outbreaks (by including 3 months' data from each of 5 previous years). The results are presented as ratios, with a ratio of 1.0 indicating no difference between the period just ended and the baseline. Ratios greater than 1.0 indicate an increase against the baseline. (Ratios beyond historical limits are also flagged.)

The *MMWR* graph is a useful summary, but because it relies on 4-week periods to make it more robust, it is not timely. Although the effect of previous outbreaks is diluted in the baseline, it is still present and still has some influence. Because the summary applies to national data, localized outbreaks such as those associated with drinking water may be missed.

In England and Wales the Communicable Disease Surveillance Center (CDSC) of the Public Health Laboratory Service (PHLS) uses a similar approach, calculating a baseline for comparison with a given week, based on the 6 nearest weeks in the 5 preceding years. However, the PHLS/CDSC goes further, including using the computer algorithm to scan large numbers of reports of individual organisms isolated in the various public health laboratories. The PHLS algorithm also adjusts the baseline to allow for long-term trends by fitting a log–linear trend line to the data set.[4,5] The algorithm reduces the effect of previous outbreaks in the baseline by weighting down the influence of baseline values from previous years that are more than one standard deviation above the general mean. Although the same algorithm is applicable to many different organisms with different weekly frequencies, the action thresholds and confidence intervals are adjusted so that the specificity is similar over a broad range of organisms. Finally, a high threshold was chosen (a 99% confidence coefficient) in order to minimize the number of events flagged each week (i.e., only the events most likely to be real outbreaks are flagged, to make most efficient use of the human resources involved in further investigation).

The PHLS algorithm is undoubtedly useful, but it is still difficult to apply where the baseline mean varies from year to year, and it still uses the final step in the chain (the isolation of specific organisms in clinical specimens) so it is still not as timely as we might wish for the detection of water-related outbreaks. Similarly, the reliance on laboratory reports of specific pathogens will not allow the detection of outbreaks where no pathogen has been detected.

6.3.1.2 The Scan Statistic and Related Approaches

A conceptually related but statistically different approach is to ask, "Are there more disease events in the last time interval than one would expect due to chance?" (or, "Is there unusual clustering of disease in time or space in the latest time period?"). There are a number of conventional (i.e., parametric) statistical techniques that address this question. One of the best known is the scan statistic (which takes various forms).[6–9] Calculation of the scan statistic begins with the null hypothesis that the events will be distributed in each time interval according to a defined probability distribution. In the simplest case the assumption is that the events will be evenly distributed over time. If we define a time interval window of a fixed length shorter than the total time series, then the number of events in each of the possible windows should be approximately equal. The number of events in a given window will vary according to the random day-to-day variation noted above — the scan statistic is a measure of the probability that a given number of events seen in a given window could have occurred by chance. If a large number of events occur in the latest available time window and it is unlikely that number could have occurred by chance, then an outbreak is flagged.

There are variants of the scan statistic, or relatives such as Tango's index,[10,11] that can account for different probability distributions for the disease measure over time, and also variants that can take into account the distribution of cases in space as well as time. They are all susceptible to the influence of previous outbreaks, and the operator adjustments needed to allow for that make automation difficult.

6.3.1.3 The Cumulative Sum Chart (CUSUM)

Proponents of the cumulative sum chart (CUSUM) suggest that rather than setting a threshold for investigation or action and waiting until that threshold is crossed, it should be possible to detect deviations from the background disease incidence that show the measure is approaching the threshold some time before the alert threshold is actually reached.

The CUSUM plots the accumulated diversions of a process away from a preset baseline over time (Figure 6.2). It has its origins in the quality control of industrial manufacturing processes.[12,13]

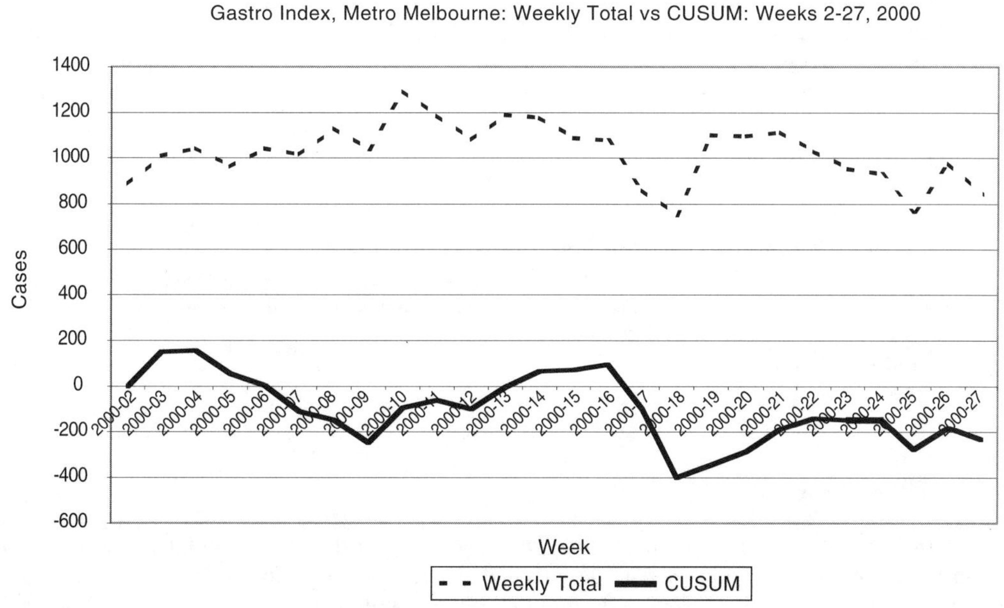

FIGURE 6.2 An example of a CUSUM chart.

A production line may be manufacturing a certain component with clearly defined upper and lower size limits. While the line is functioning normally, the measured size of its outputs should vary in a normally-distributed way around the mean. However, as the machinery begins to wear, for example, the size of the component might begin to slowly drift away from the mean until eventually the production line begins to produce unusable objects. The CUSUM chart is based on periodic sampling of the line's output, and plots the accumulated diversions from the mean over time. As long as the sizes vary in the usual way, the CUSUM value hovers around zero. As soon as the process begins to deviate, the CUSUM (representing the accumulation of small errors) deviates rapidly. The slope of the CUSUM chart can thus indicate a small drift and allow corrective action long before the line's production becomes unusable.

In disease surveillance, a suitable CUSUM measurement might allow the detection of an outbreak long before the defined epidemic threshold is reached, and even before the upward trend can be discerned by eye among the random day-to-day variation.[14–16] Once an outbreak is established, the same CUSUM chart might indicate more rapidly the high point and the beginning of the downward phase.

Unlike a production line, a CUSUM for disease surveillance does not have a simple baseline from which to start. The same problems apply as to other algorithms — day-to-day variation, seasonality and secular trends, and the effect of previous outbreaks. The CUSUM chart will only be as useful as the baseline calculation. Similar approaches have been suggested for this calculation, such as using a baseline calculated from the same time in previous years. The CUSUM then sums up the difference between each day's incidence and the baseline for that day calculated from the same and surrounding days in preceding years.

Disease incidence is a continuous process, so it is also necessary to reset the CUSUM chart to zero from time to time. However, the optimum interval for this is not necessarily clear and will thus be difficult to automate, especially where large numbers of organisms (and thus large numbers of charts) are involved.

Figure 6.2 illustrates a CUSUM chart for the total number of fecal analysis requests outside public hospitals in Melbourne, Australia from weeks 2 to 27, 2000. The total numbers are overplotted for comparison. Note that the rise in numbers in the first quarter is shown by the CUSUM plot to actually be less than expected when compared with the 3 preceding years. This graph illustrates one difficulty with CUSUM charts: the drops in week 17 and 18 are artifacts due to the coincidence of Easter and a local public holiday (ANZAC Day), and the CUSUM chart should possibly be reset to zero from week 19. But what if an outbreak process had begun in week 16 or 17? Even without that possibility, it is clear that the resetting of the baseline would need human intervention and judgement, adversely affecting the CUSUM's suitability as a machine-assisted algorithm in day-to-day use.

Action Threshold Detection Algorithms vs. the Ideal

	Timely	Unaffected by Previous Outbreaks	No Operator Intervention Required
MMWR method	XX	✓	✓✓
PHLS (CDSC) method	X	✓✓	✓✓
Scan statistic	✓	X	✓
CUSUM	✓✓	X	X

6.3.2 Forecasting

The second, or forecasting, approach is less well developed for disease surveillance, but is worthy of further attention. This approach is based on the perception that the development of disease outbreaks, and the pattern of endemic disease in a given population, is essentially deterministic — that there is some underlying mathematical process that can be used to describe it. Once the appropriate mathematical formula linking current disease rates to past ones has been elucidated, it should be possible to predict future disease incidence, at least into the near future. There are two ways that this might be useful. If the beginning of outbreaks proves to be predictable, then the model could give prior warning of the onset of a new outbreak in time to avoid it altogether. If an outbreak turns out to be beyond the predictive power of such a model, then the model should at least give the best possible estimate of the background rate expected, and allow rapid identification of the onset of the unforeseen epidemic. Potentially, at least, these techniques might turn the bugbear of baseline calculation — the presence of past outbreaks in the time series — into an asset.

These techniques all make one basic assumption — that the factors determining current disease distribution will continue to be important into the future. Of course this is the basic assumption of all forms of prediction, but it is worth remembering that it does not always hold true.

Experience with forecasting techniques in routine disease surveillance data sets is so far limited, and results have been mixed, but the potential benefits make them worthy of further study.

6.3.2.1 Auto-Regressive, Moving Average, and Auto-Regressive Integrated Moving Average (ARIMA) Modelling

It might seem tempting to use conventional linear regression techniques to map the association between previous and future disease numbers, but conventional linear regression modelling techniques assume that each of the "independent" input variables is just that — independent from all the others. Linear regression also makes assumptions about the frequency distribution of each input, generally assuming that they are normally distributed. The first assumption is almost never applicable to time series data related to disease incidence. Today's case numbers are usually closely related to yesterday's, yesterday's to the day before, and so on.

There is, however, a class of statistical model that not only takes account of the correlation between adjacent elements of a disease time series but actually uses it to make its predictions more accurate. Using two basic processes — AutoRegressive (AR) and Moving Average (MA) filters — a time series can be generated that uses the preceding events in the series to determine future values.[17] The exact shape of the series depends on the values of a number of internal coefficients, and the technique aims to find the values for these coefficients that best replicate the observed series. The two processes are often used together to create so-called ARMA models.

The process of estimating the coefficients, however, depends on certain assumptions about the original time series. The most important is that the series itself must be stationary (in the statistical sense, meaning that both the mean and the variance of the time series values should not change over time). This condition is commonly not satisfied, but it is often possible to create a new series which is stationary by calculating the difference between the values at successive time points. It is sometimes even necessary to calculate second-order differences — the difference between the differences. ARMA techniques can then be used to model these "differenced" series, and then the final results added together (integrated) to produce a powerful technique called Auto-Regressive Integrated Moving Average (ARIMA) modelling.

Although these are potentially useful tools in disease surveillance, they are very much dependent on being able to achieve stationarity, either in the original data set or in the differenced series derived from it.[18–21] In real life, too, the background environment in which disease events happen may change too quickly for any model to capture — a model that describes the past 2 years very accurately may suddenly fail tomorrow. (Doubters should ask any investors in the NASDAQ "new-economy" share market, who saw their whole paradigm change in early 2000.)

6.4 ARTIFICIAL NEURAL NETWORKS

Many different entities can be described as artificial neural networks.[22–24] The most common, known as feed-forward networks (or sometimes "perceptrons"), are computer software programs in which individual memory objects called neurons or nodes do the processing. Unlike conventional statistical models, they are created ("trained") by a non-linear process known as back-propagation of errors.[25] They can detect non-linear relationships between input and output data, and make no assumptions about the frequency distribution of the input data. They can be usefully thought of as non-linear regression techniques, and have been described as universal function approximators. *

6.4.1 Origins and Function

The inspiration for the development of feed-forward networks came from psychology, and they were originally proposed as models for the way that the human brain learns. As in the human brain, each neuron is connected to a number of others in functional layers (see Figures 6.3 and 6.4). The first layer represents inputs from the external world, and there are one or more hidden layers which

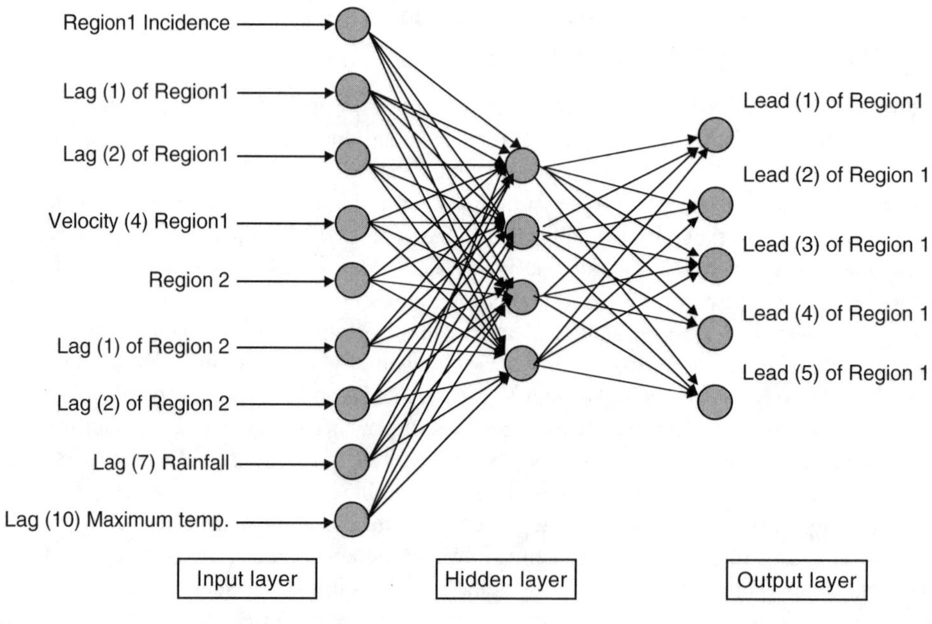

FIGURE 6.3 Structure of a feed-forward neural network.

* Many modelling techniques use a mathematical algorithm to minimize an error function; for example, a linear regression model minimizes the sum of the squared difference between the model fitted line and the actual observations. Neural networks usually minimize the mean squared error — the mean of the squared differences between the network's outputs and the observed output values in the training set. A useful concept in understanding how they do this is the "error surface." If we plot a graph of the model error against the values of one of the model's internal parameters, such as a correlation coefficient in a regression model or a neuron connection weight in a neural network, we see that there are certain values of the parameter that correspond to low errors and others that correspond to high errors. There are commonly several dips in this error line, some deeper than others, corresponding to good or poor solutions. The lowest point on this error graph (the global minimum) corresponds to the best solution, while other dips (local minima) are less good solutions. If we now imagine adding a second parameter to the graph, on the z axis, the combined effects of the two parameters create a three-dimensional surface, now with ridges and valleys corresponding to the local and global minima. It is possible to imagine (but not to draw) a much more complex graph in which each parameter adds one more dimension to the graph, and for n dimensions an n-dimensional "error surface" must be explored and the global minimum found. Conventional statistical techniques find the global minimum quickly because they make assumptions about the shape of the error surface, but if those assumptions are not met by the data, the calculated "optimum" values of the various coefficients can be quite wrong. Neural networks need make no such assumptions because they effectively explore regions of the error surface step by step. Training is slow compared to conventional models, but much less "attractive" data can be used.

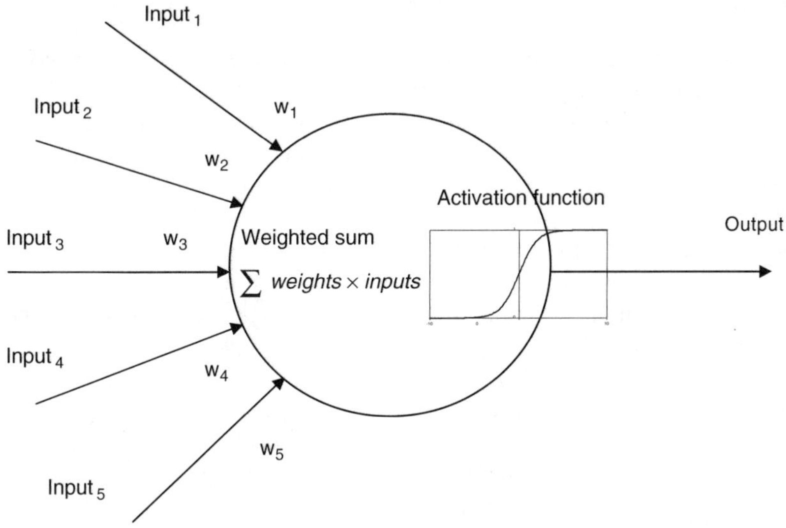

FIGURE 6.4 Execution of a single hypothetical neuron with 5 inputs and logistic activation function.

in turn connect to an output layer that reveals the result of the network's calculations. Each "neuron" takes inputs from the earlier layers, weights them, and sums the weighted inputs. It then passes the weighted sum through an "activation" function (commonly the logistic function) and passes the resulting figure on to each neuron in the next layer.

The crucial point in the creation of a neural network model is the assignment of the large number of connection weights between the neurons. "Training" the network involves the use of a data set for which the outcome values are known and discovering the values of each weight that give a network output as close as possible to the correct one. The trained network can then be presented with new data for which the outcomes are not known, and the network outputs can be used to estimate the unknown outcomes. Training of neural networks is possible because of the discovery that if the derivative of the activation function is known for a neuron, then its partial derivatives can be used to push each of the incoming weights for that neuron in the direction of lower error. By repeating the process many times for all the training patterns, the network will gradually assign optimum values for all the weights. The only requirement of the non-linear output function is that its derivative be easy to calculate — hence the popularity of the logistic function and tanh in many neural networks.

6.4.2 Drawbacks

Artificial neural networks have been criticized as "black boxes." Although this is a somewhat unfair designation, it is true that it is not possible to "read" the internal weights of a trained network. Unlike parametric statistical techniques, there is no direct relationship between the weight given to a particular input and its importance to the model. Although a weight close to zero at the input layer does mean that the network makes little use of that input, it does not necessarily follow that a large weight means a major contribution. It is difficult to use a neural network to quantify the contribution of a given input to the overall model. Remember, though, that neural networks are essentially non-linear — so ambient temperature, for example, may affect the final outcome only when it is extremely hot or cold. A more realistic concern is that the analyst does not really know which aspects of the problem have been captured by the network. If the background environment is changed, it will thus be difficult to predict how the model's usefulness will change. A good deal of empirical testing is required before it is known how useful a given model will be in practice.

6.4.3 Forecasting

A concrete example relevant to waterborne outbreaks might be to train a neural network on a time series data set of a chosen disease measure, such as requests for fecal sample analysis received by a public health laboratory per day. The training outputs would be some future values of the same measure, (say 1, 2, 3, 4, 5, 6, and 7 days ahead). If the network is able to truly generalize the relationships between the past and future values, it could then be used with new data to predict the coming days' numbers.

Training a neural network to generalize for forecasting is not, however, a simple process. In comparison to the creation of auto-regressive models, which use few parameters and fairly direct methods of calculation, neural networks take a long time to train and a lot of computer processing power. There are a number of different network architectures to choose from, and the training process is influenced by a number of different internal network parameters. These include momentum (by which the change in a weight for a given learning step is influenced by the changes during the previous step) and learning rate (which determines how much a weight changes in each training step). So far there are only rules of thumb to guide the network practitioner, and a good deal of empirical experimentation can be required. There is a very real risk that a network will overtrain and be unable to generalize sufficiently to give correct answers on unseen data. This risk can be minimized by validation during training. A randomly selected subset of the training data is reserved before training begins. At regular intervals during training the training is stopped and the accuracy of the network in its current state is tested for the reserved validation set. It is common for a network to continue improving its error against the training set, while the error on the validation set begins to rise again. This is the hallmark of overtraining and indicates that the network should be saved with the weights corresponding to the lowest error on the validation set.

A network trained in this way can often capture the general relationship between the previous behavior of the disease in the region of interest and its neighbors, and the behavior of the disease in the near future. If there are previous outbreaks in the training data set, then the neural network might be able to use that information in the prediction of similar outbreaks in the future. This, plus the fact that the data set need not necessarily be stationary, gives neural networks a potential edge over ARIMA models for prediction.

6.4.4 In Practice

In our own experience, however, neural networks have yet to clearly prove their superiority over other approaches. In many cases the data set turns out to be stationary (or close enough to satisfy an ARIMA model), and then the two types of model tend to give similar results. Even more troublesome — for both kinds of predictive model — is the search for a suitable set of inputs that truly contain the level of information necessary for a useful predictive model. A third practical problem in some cases has been an apparent change in the background environment in which disease events occur. A model that very accurately describes a given time period (and can predict accurately several time points ahead within that time frame) may be no use for predictions in a new time frame.

Neural networks are unlikely to transform the field of disease surveillance in the near future, but they have enough potential advantages over the best alternatives in current use to make them worthy of further investigation.

REFERENCES

1. Stern, L. and Lightfoot, D., Automated outbreak detection: a quantitative retrospective analysis, *Epidemiol. Infect.*, 122, 103, 1999.
2. Centers for Disease Control and Prevention, http://www.cdc.gov/mmwr (home page of the *Morbidity and Mortality Weekly Report*), accessed 27/8/2001.

3. Centers for Disease Control and Prevention, Current trends update: graphic method for presentation of notifiable disease data — United States, 1990, *MMWR,* 40, 124, 1991.
4. Farrington, C. and Beale, A., Computer-aided detection of temporal clusters of organisms reported to the Communicable Disease Surveillance Centre, *Commun. Dis. Rep. CDR Rev.,* 3, R78, 1993.
5. Farrington, C.P. et al., A statistical algorithm for the early detection of outbreaks of infectious disease, *J. R. Statist. Soc.,* 159, 547, 1996.
6. Naus, J.I., The distribution of the size of the maximum cluster of points on a line, *Am. Statist. Assoc. J.,* June, 532, 1965.
7. Wallenstein, S., A test for the detection of clustering over time, *Am. J. Epidemiol.,* 111, 367, 1980.
8. Wallenstein, S., Gould, M.S., and Kleinman, M., Use of the scan statistic to detect time–space clustering, *Am. J. Epidemiol.,* 130, 1057, 1989.
9. Wallenstein, S., Naus, J., and Glaz J., Power of the scan statistic for detection of clustering, *Stat. Med.,* 12, 1829, 1993.
10. Tango, T., The detection of disease clustering in time, *Biometrics,* 40, 15, 1984.
11. Rayens, M. and Kryscio, R., Properties of Tango's index for detecting clustering in time, *Stat. Med.,* 12, 1813, 1993.
12. Page, E., Continuous inspection schemes, *Biometrika,* 41, 100, 1954.
13. Page, E., Cumulative sum charts, *Technometrics*, 3(1), 1, 1961.
14. O'Brien, S. and Christie, P., Do CuSums have a role in routine communicable disease surveillance?, *Public Health,* 111, 255, 1997.
15. Hutwagner, L. et al., Using laboratory-based surveillance data for prevention: an algorithm for detecting *Salmonella* outbreaks, *Emerg. Infect. Dis.,* 3, 395, 1997.
16. Tillett, H.E. and Spencer, I.L., Influenza surveillance in England and Wales using routine statistics. Development of 'cusum' graphs to compare 12 previous winters and to monitor the 1980/81 winter, *J. Hyg.,* 88, 83, 1982.
17. Chatfield, C., *The Analysis of Time Series: An Introduction,* 5th ed., Chapman & Hall, London, 1996.
18. Choi, K. and Thacker, S., An evaluation of influenza mortality surveillance, 1962–1979. I. Time series forecasts of expected pneumonia and influenza deaths, *Am. J. Epidemiol.,* 113, 215, 1981.
19. Choi, K. and Thacker, S., An evaluation of influenza mortality surveillance, 1962–1979. II. Percentage of pneumonia and influenza deaths as an indicator of influenza activity, *Am. J. Epidemiol.,* 113, 227, 1981.
20. Stroup, D., Thacker, S., and Herndon, J., Application of multiple time series analysis to the estimation of pneumonia and influenza mortality by age 1962–1983, *Stat. Med.,* 7, 1045, 1988.
21. Fernandéz-Pérez, C., Tejada, J., and Carrasco, M., Multivariate time series analysis in nosocomial infection surveillance: a case study, *Int. J. Epidemiol.,* 27, 282, 1998.
22. Masters, T., *Practical Neural Network Recipes in C++,* Academic Press, Boston, 1993.
23. Masters, T., *Neural, Novel, and Hybrid Algorithms for Time Series Prediction*, John Wiley & Sons, New York, 1995.
24. Smith, K., Introduction to neural networks and data mining for business applications, *Eruditions*, Emerald, 1999.
25. Rumelhart, D.E., Learning representations by back-propagating errors, *Nature,* 323, 533, 1986.

7 Microbiology and the Investigation of Waterborne Outbreaks: Typing of Norwalk-Like Virus

Carl-Henrik von Bonsdorff and Leena Maunula

CONTENTS

7.1 Introduction....79
7.2 Principles of the Diagnostics of NLVs....80
7.2.1 Methods Available....81
7.2.2 Samples....81
7.2.3 Virus/RNA Concentration....81
7.2.4 Sequencing and Phylogeny....82
7.3 Case Study....82
7.4 Surveillance and Risk Assesment....84
References....84

7.1 INTRODUCTION

This chapter is the first of two that describe the value of microbiological investigations in the examination of waterborne outbreaks. It concentrates on Norwalk-like viruses (NLVs), a cause of diarrhea and vomiting. NLVs are among the most common microbes affecting humans. They are single-stranded RNA viruses, about 30 nm in diameter, and form one of the two human calicivirus genera in the family *Caliciviridae* (Figure 7.1). Like enteric viruses in general, they are characterized by a remarkable physicochemical stability. They are stable in pH ranges from 2 to 9, tolerate heat up to 65°C for 30 min, and apparently free chlorine of 1 mg/l. In cold water, they retain their infectivity for up to a year. All these values are under scrutiny because the NLVs do not grow in any known cell culture, and all the data have been obtained using human volunteers. Adding to their abundance is the fact that the victims produce NLVs in large amounts; their concentration in stool may reach 10^{9-10}/ml and, assuming diarrheal stool volume of 1 liter, the amount of virus excreted by one patient would come close to infecting all of mankind. Furthermore, although the characterization of this newly established virus genus is far from complete, a large number of immunologically distinct NLVs appear to exist. A full grasp of the extent of the genus is hampered by the fact that the "classification" largely rests on genome-based comparisons of rather short stretches of the (polymerase) gene. Rapidly accumulating data on more extensive genome comparisons seem, however, to confirm the tentative clusters as distinct viruses. At present, some 20 different NLVs have been identified.[1,2]

0-8493-1259-0/03/$0.00+$1.50

Nonenveloped, icosahedral, 27-40 nm in diameter
Genome: positive ssRNA, 7.4-7.7 kb

Human caliciviruses:

"Norwalk-like viruses" NLV (Genogroups I and II)

"Sapporo-like viruses" SLV (Genogroup III)

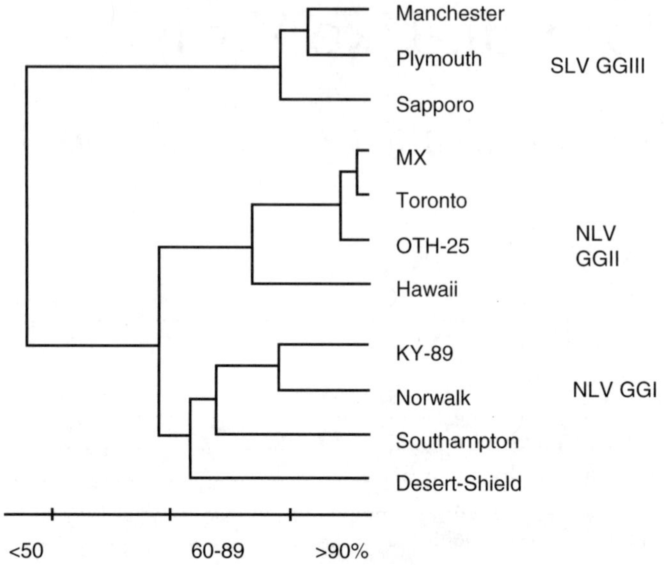

The phylogenetic tree is based on the sequence comparison of the polymerase gene. It shows the high degree of genetic diversity even in this conserved part of the genome.

FIGURE 7.1 General properties of human caliciviruses.

The spread of NLVs is also explained by the observation that immunity to a given NLV is short-lived, lasting for only about 6 months.[3] Thus the epidemiological cohorts at risk are large, and infections and reinfections ensure the vitality of these viruses. In contrast, the well-established diarrheal viruses such as rota-, astro-, and adenoviruses mainly affect small children. Immunity to these viruses is much longer lasting, so symptomatic reinfections are rare.

Based on the genome sequence, the human caliciviruses are divided into two genera: the NLVs and the Sapporo-like viruses (SLVs). For reasons not yet understood, it appears that SLVs mainly affect children, while NLVs affect all age groups. Foodborne outbreaks caused by SLVs, however, have also been noted, and longer observation periods and improved diagnostics may change the present view of the epidemiology.

7.2 PRINCIPLES OF THE DIAGNOSTICS OF NLVS

Since the enteric viruses are produced in large amounts in stool, their demonstration has been straightforward and rather easy. Originally, electron microscopy was found to be a tool that was practical and sensitive enough for their identification. After the characterization of these viruses, immunological tests for antigen demonstration were developed and shown to be the more effective approach.

For caliciviruses in general and NLVs in particular, diagnostic procedures have been quite problematic. Compared to immunological tests, electron microscopy of clinical samples is insensitive even in the most skilled hands. For environmental samples, electron microscopy is totally inadequate. The wide range of immunologically distinct (non-cross-reactive) strains has made antigen detection very difficult. Classification of caliciviruses has been based on genomic characteristics; consequently, diagnostics have evolved around nucleic acid molecular methods; i.e., RT-PCR is still the method of choice. While this method is quite costly for diagnosis in individual patients, it is very useful for environmental studies. The sensitivity of the method is especially important, and additional value is offered by the opportunity for molecular epidemiology by amplicon sequencing.

7.2.1 Methods Available

As pointed out above, diagnostic activity in outbreak investigations should focus on two areas. The easier part of the task is investigation of the patient sample. Handling of the sample is less critical, because the stool contains an excess of viral genome material. There is no need for concentration steps; in fact, dilution is usually beneficial to get rid of possible inhibitors to the PCR reaction. Investigation of the patient sample should always precede the search for viruses in environmental samples (e.g., water). Since NLV identification ultimately is based on sequence recognition, the identity of the virus (sequence) is a prerequisite for optimal sensitivity when testing water.

7.2.2 Samples

For patient samples, stool is the material of choice. Vomit also contains virus in sufficient concentration and can be used as an alternative. In an outbreak situation, five to ten patient samples should be collected. NLV outbreaks are usually very shortlived, and diarrhoeal samples may be difficult to obtain. In an NLV infection, the patient secretes virus for a couple of weeks, and "post-episode" samples can be quite useful. If stool samples have been collected for bacteriological investigations, they can subsequently be used for NLV analysis. This is a good reason why stool samples for bacteriology should be kept for a while and not be discarded immediately after inoculation.

The samples for virological investigation can and should be collected as soon as possible. They can then be stored at –20°C until bacteriological testing has been performed. Some waterborne outbreaks may last for weeks, e.g., if the contamination is prolonged. Under such circumstances, it is advisable to collect patient samples throughout the outbreak to ensure that there is only one causative agent.

The sampling of water will depend on the analytical method employed. Most countries have regulations concerning sample volumes for microbial testing. For viral testing, they have been designed exclusively for (entero)virus culture. Current sampling protocols have not yet taken sufficient account of the introduction of PCR techniques. It is crucial in investigations of waterborne outbreaks to obtain samples early. In outbreak situations, this means when suspicion of contamination first arises. Samples should be collected throughout the distribution network, first from the raw water source, then from the water leaving the waterworks, and finally, depending on the situation, from different parts of the distribution network. It is also advisable to start sampling sewage from the affected area, as this may serve as a measure of the extent of the outbreak. The recommended sample volumes vary between 1 and 50 liters (in some instances, tap water samples of up to 1000 liters are required). If necessary, the samples can be kept refrigerated for weeks (actually for months) prior to testing.

7.2.3 Virus/RNA Concentration

Viruses can be concentrated from water samples in different ways, partly depending on the quality of the water to be analyzed. A considerable reduction in volume can be achieved with different flocculation methods.[4] The use of immunological methods — using antibodies to adsorb viral particles from samples — is very attractive. When magnetic beads are used, the enrichment is technically easy and has been shown to have high efficacy.[5] However, the immunogenic heterogeneity of NLVs seriously restricts the use of this method. Another approach is to bind the virus by its net charge to a (positively) charged surface. The method was used in the past to concentrate poliovirus for subsequent cultivation from tap water and was later adapted to PCR methods.

The method used in our laboratory is essentially the one originally described by Gilgen et al.[7] In this method, a sample of 1 liter is filtered through a positively charged filter and the bound virus is then eluted in 2–3 ml elution buffer. The final sample volume of 100 μl is achieved in a microconcentrator.[8]

Concerning RNA extraction and RT-PCR, there are many examples of suitable RNA extraction protocols as well as primer selections. In all cases, the polymerase gene is the target for amplification. It appears that somewhat higher sensitivity is obtained if both genogroup NLVs are run as separate PCRs. The methods for identifying the PCR product may vary. Band detection in agarose gels may serve as a primary identification. Confirmation can be achieved by hybridization to a probe panel either in a line blot or ELISA-type reaction.[2,9] The hybridization generally increases the sensitivity of detection by 0.5 to 1.0 log as compared to gel electrophoresis. Owing to high variability within the amplicon, hybridization requires many different probes. The benefit is that the probe reaction pattern will already give an idea about the strain's identity. More importantly, if the patient sample reacts weakly to any probe, the amplicon should be sequenced and a fully homologous probe designed for optimal sensitivity. Only then should the water sample be run in PCR.

Ultimately, the methods used must be optimized in each laboratory to give good results. In all presently achieved amplicons, there will be roughly a 65 base common part, the sequence of which serves as a "fingerprint" for each strain. It appears that the variability even over this conserved part of the genome is large enough to offer a quite solid tool for epidemiological purposes. In critical cases, the sequencing can be extended to comprise larger areas of the genome, e.g., the capsid area.

7.2.4 Sequencing and Phylogeny

The sequencing of the PCR product is a rather straightforward task. With the modern capillary sequencers, the sequence can essentially be determined "on-line." When these are not available, the sequencing can be performed manually quite comfortably, since the amplicon is short enough to be revealed in one run. In our early work, we used a biotinylated primer which makes it possible to fix the product to a solid surface for purification and then separate the strands.[9] The obtained sequences have to be trimmed to the same length. There are different programs for sequence comparisons. Figure 7.2 shows a phylogenic tree of Finnish NLV outbreaks in the years 1998–99. Comparable findings have been obtained in many countries and the clusters observed appear likely to be quite universal. Their final number is, however, still unknown.

7.3 CASE STUDY

Even though technical preparedness for adequate analysis of waterborne NLV outbreaks exists, the responsible authorities seem to be insufficiently aware of the analytical possibilities. A major difficulty in this context seems to be the initial detection of an outbreak. The winter vomiting disease, one of the clinical manifestations of NLV infection, is very common in communities because it is highly infectious and is spread from person to person. The usual signals, such as an increase in visits to doctors, are weak and make it difficult to recognize the presence of an epidemic. This was clear in the Finnish outbreak in Heinävesi, where practically all of the 5000 inhabitants of the community were infected during the 3 weeks in which the outbreak peaked.[8] The 30 visits to the health care center due to acute gastrointestinal symptoms were mainly a consequence of the publicity surrounding the outbreak. In this case, water was suspected as the source of the outbreak just in time for adequate sampling. Patient samples were obtained at three points during the outbreak. Water samples were collected from the raw water supply (lake water) and from different parts of

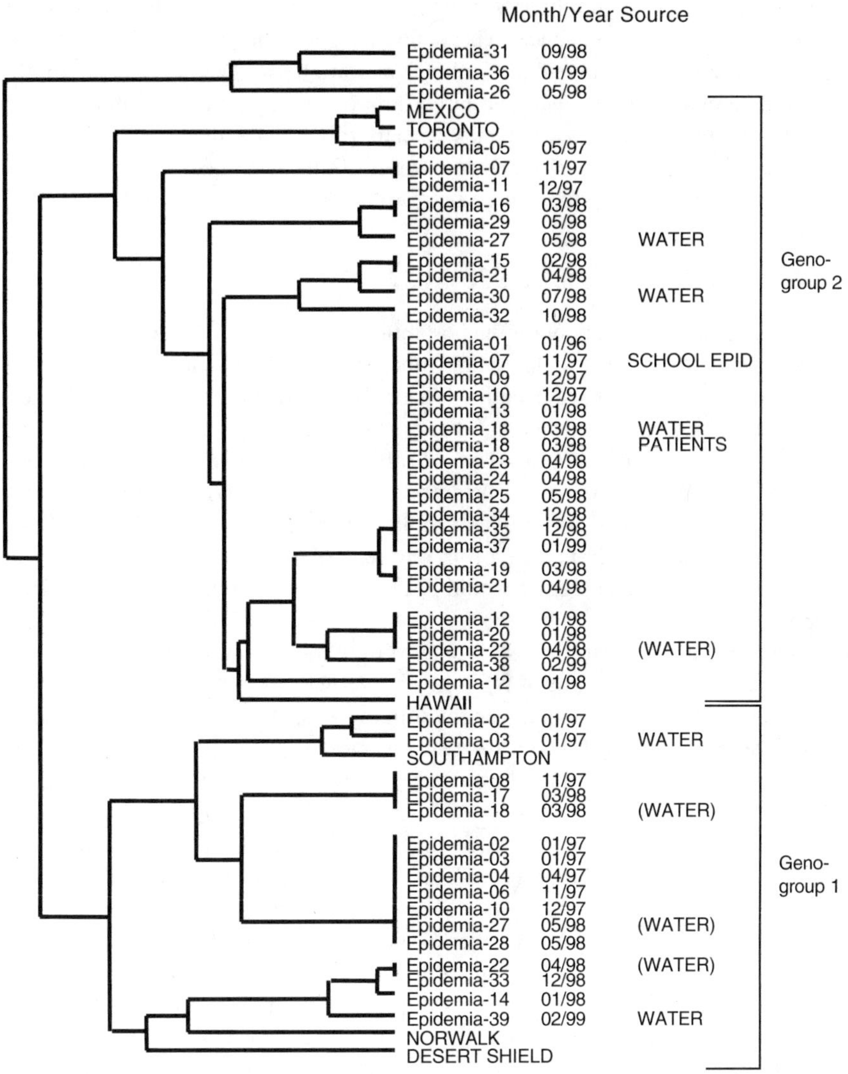

Note the numerous genetic clusters. As a rule, patient samples in a single outbreak show an identical amplicon sequence. Exceptions are seen when sewage contamination from large communities takes place, in which case more than one NLV is often encountered. Only the suspected waterborne outbreaks have been marked. The brackets indicate a second NLV from the same outbreak. Epidemics number 7 and 18 are referred to in the case report.

FIGURE 7.2 Tree diagram based on the amplicon sequence obtained from patient samples of NLV outbreaks that occurred in Finland during 1997–99. (Source: v. Bonsdorff C.H. and Maunula, L., *Duodecim,* 116, 70, 2000. With permission.)

the distribution network. Consumers at distant parts of the network were selected with the hope that the longer retention time would ensure the presence of contaminated water. Sewage samples were also taken for quantitative measurements of the virus. In addition, samples were collected upstream and downstream of the community. Water samples were 1 to 2 liters each, and the sewage samples were just 5 ml. The patient samples contained two NLVs, a dominant genogroup II virus, and a less frequently occurring ggI virus. The latter's reaction to the PCR probes indicated initially that is was Lordsdale-like. The Lordsdale-like ggII virus was found in the raw water in five out of six tap water samples and in the downstream lakewater sample. The ggI virus was not detected in any of the water samples. The amplicon sequencing revealed that all of the ggI and ggII isolates shared an identical amplicon sequence. These findings, together with a thoroughly performed epidemiological survey, clearly defined the outbreak as waterborne. When searching for the possible source of the contamination of the water, a large outbreak was noted in a school in a town some 70 km upstream of Heinävesi. That outbreak was caused by an identical (i.e., Lordsdale-like) ggII NLV (Figure 7.2). Since this virus is quite common in Finland, a more extensive sequence comparison would be needed to trace the source more reliably.

7.4 SURVEILLANCE AND RISK ASSESMENT

The NLV diagnostics serve as a model for the possibilities offered by molecular methods in outbreak investigations and epidemiology. At the same time, such methods can be used for surveillance purposes at the waterworks and have been implemented in some progressive ones. Presently, much of the work is still at the research stage and better standards are needed for the methodology. As a precaution, waterworks at risk could adapt a "rolling sampling" model. Taking weekly 1-liter samples and storing them at +4°C for a time sufficient to detect possible outbreaks (4 to 6 weeks) and then discarding them would not pose a problem in practical terms. This would ensure that samples would be available early in case of an outbreak. At the same time, it would save testing costs. On the other hand, regular testing would not be too cumbersome and costly if it was part of a centralized system.

Another approach is to monitor risks by determining the amount of virus released in sewage. In the case of Heinävesi, the amount of NLV in sewage was 10^5 PCR units/ml after the epidemic peaked, and remained at about 2 logs lower for some weeks. It is clear that such an outbreak is a threat to water users downstream. The testing of sewage, even by quantitative PCR, can be done directly from 100 μl samples and thus does not require concentration steps. Presently, the establishment of automated quantitative PCR for NLVs is hampered by their vast heterogeneity.

Wherever efforts have been made to identify them, NLVs seem to be very common contaminants of water and a frequent cause of outbreaks. This seems to be true for all kinds of water supply systems. Sewage may either contaminate natural raw water supplies, leak directly into drilled wells, or breaks may occur in the distribution network. The methods described here serve as an example of the possibilities both for surveillance and for tracking the source of outbreaks. They also serve as a good model for identifying weaknesses in the water distribution system. Thus, NLVs should be considered as an alternative to the small RNA bacteriophages which are suggested as indicators for viral contamination. The benefit of the latter is that infectious viral particles are monitored rather than just (part of) the viral genome, as is the case with (RT-)PCR.

The medical impact of an NLV outbreak is moderate and therefore often overseen. On the other hand, such an outbreak should serve as a warning for the considerably more serious threat presented by the hepatitis A virus. This virus is not presently endemic in industrialized countries, and population immunity is largely absent. Even limited outbreaks would result in considerable contamination of sewage and most likely in subsequent contamination of receiving water bodies.

REFERENCES

1. Green, K.Y. et al., Taxonomy of caliciviruses, *J. Infect. Dis.*, 181 (Suppl 2), 322, 2000.
2. Vinje, J. and Koopmans, M., Simultaneous detection and genotyping of "Norwalklike viruses" by oligonucleotide array in reverse line blot hybridization format, *J. Clin. Microbiol.*, 38, 2595, 2000.
3. Matsui, S.M. and Greenberg, H.B., Immunity to calicivirus infection, *J. Infect. Dis.*, 181 (Suppl 2), 331, 2000.
4. Grohman, G., Viruses, food and environment, in *Foodborne Microorganisms of Public Health Significance,* Hocking, A.D. et al., Eds., AIFST (NSW Branch), 603.

5. Myrmel, M., Rimstad, E., and Wasteson, Y., Immunogenetic separation of a Norwalk-like virus in artificially contaminated environmental samples, *Int. J. Food Microbiol.,* 62, 17, 2000.
6. Sobsey, M.D. and Jones, B.I., Concentration of poliovirus from tapwater using positively charged microporous filter, *Appl. Environ. Microbiol.*, 37, 588, 1979.
7. Gilgen. M. et al., Three-step isolation method for sensitive detection of enterovirus, rotavirus, hepatitis A virus and small round structured viruses in water samples, *Int. J. Food Microbiol.*, 37, 189, 1997.
8. Kukkula, M. et al., Outbreak of viral gastroenteritis due to drinking water contaminated by Norwalk-like viruses, *J. Infect. Dis.*, 180, 1771, 1999.
9. Maunula L., Piiparinen, H., and v. Bonsdorff, C.-H., Confirmation of Norwalk-like virus amplicons after RT-PCR by microplate hybridization and direct sequencing, *J. Virol. Methods*, 83, 125, 1999.

8 Microbiology and the Investigation of Waterborne Outbreaks: The Use of *Cryptosporidium* Typing in the Investigation of Waterborne Disease

Gordon Nichols and Jim McLauchlin

CONTENTS

8.1 Introduction 87
8.2 Laboratory Methods 88
8.2.1 Method Development 88
8.2.2 Sample Testing 89
8.3 Epidemiological Information from Typing Isolates 89
8.3.1 Outbreaks 90
8.3.2 Geographic Variation and Travel 91
8.3.3 HIV Infection 92
8.4 Taxonomy and Nomenclature 92
8.5 Typing — Prospects for the Future 92
References 94

8.1 INTRODUCTION

Cryptosporidiosis is an important cause of diarrhea or illness throughout the world. The relative resistance of the oocysts to chlorine means that disinfecting water with this chemical is ineffective, and waterborne outbreaks have resulted from inadequate or defective water treatment. Some of these outbreaks have been large, particularly those involving mains drinking water.

The epidemiology of the majority of *Cryptosporidium* cases remains unknown, and so there is a strong imperative to enhance our understanding of this disease. The analysis of microbial typing data provides one approach that is especially useful with *Cryptosporidium* because the host ranges of different types vary. The demonstration that different genotypes have different transmission cycles is important in demonstrating that typing can be used as a tool to examine the epidemiology of cryptosporidiosis.[1,2] It has been possible to gain additional information on possible sources of contamination from genotyping studies. Typing techniques have also been useful in the investigation of waterborne outbreaks, allowing patients' strains to be compared with oocysts detected in animal feces.

0-8493-1259-0/03/$0.00+$1.50

8.2 LABORATORY METHODS

8.2.1 Method Development

When *Cryptosporidium* oocysts first started to be detected in diarrheal patients it was widely thought that they represented a single infecting species, *Cryptosporidium parvum*. They could be differentiated from *C. muris* and *C. baileyi* by microscopically examining the size and shape of the oocysts. In the late 1980s, Western blotting techniques performed on oocyst antigens extracted from human and animal feces were performed using polyclonal antibodies raised in rabbits and mouse monoclonal antibodies (Figure 8.1).[1,3] Isoenzyme thin-layer starch–gel electrophoresis was used to examine electrophoretic differences in malate dehydrogenase, carboxylesterase, lactate dehydrogenase, glucose phosphate isomerase, and phosphoglucomutase.[4,5] The Western blotting techniques demonstrated strain differences in the human and animal isolates studied. The approach was applied to larger numbers of fecal samples, and the results identified significant heterogeneity in the isolates tested. Although a modification of this approach was successfully used in examining cases and in outbreak investigation, the Western blotting approach had a number of problems that made it impractical for routine use.[6,7] Many oocysts were required to get a blotting pattern, the inoculum and gels were difficult to standardize, the resolution was limited, the fecal extraction process may have led to artifacts, and the process was generally unsuitable for screening large numbers of fecal samples. As a result of these difficulties PCR approaches were developed that allowed the rapid extraction of genetic material from *Cryptosporidium* oocysts in feces.[8–10] DNA was extracted using mechanical agitation by a beadbeater and Zirconia beads.[12] Methods were also developed for extracting genetic material from fecal smears on slides.[11] The sensitivity of PCR detection was compared with approximate oocyst counts measured by immunofluorescent microscopy.[12] Using three different genes for detection of *Cryptosporidium* oocysts in 218 patients, TRAP-*C*1 (thrombospondin-related adhesive protein oocyst) was the least sensitive, COWP (*Cryptosporidium* outer wall protein) the next, and 18S rRNA the most sensitive (Figure 8.2). A nested COWP PCR was found to be considerably more sensitive than an unnested reaction, amplifying 18% more positive samples.[13]

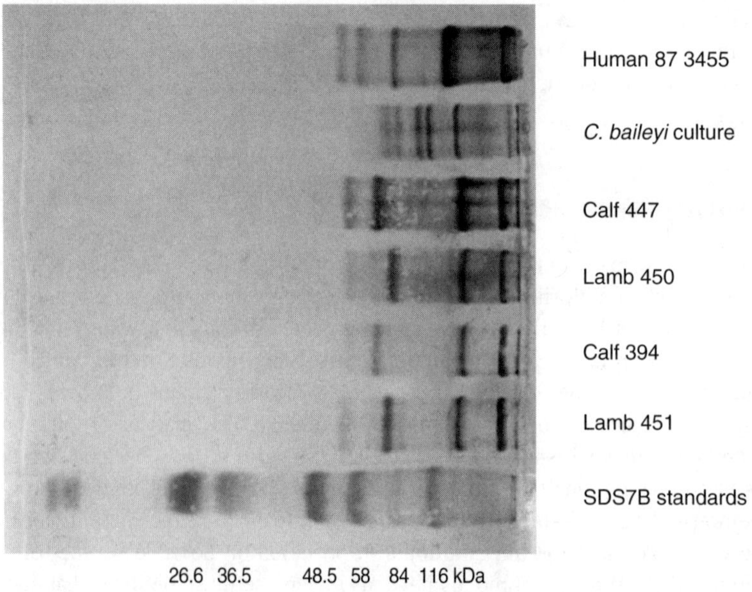

FIGURE 8.1 Western blot of *Cryptosporidium* isolates using FITC-labelled monoclonal antibody MAB C1 and alkaline phosphatase-labelled anti FITC. (Source: Nichols, G.L., McLauchlin, J., and Samuel, D., *J. Protozool.*, 38, 2375, 1991. With permission.)

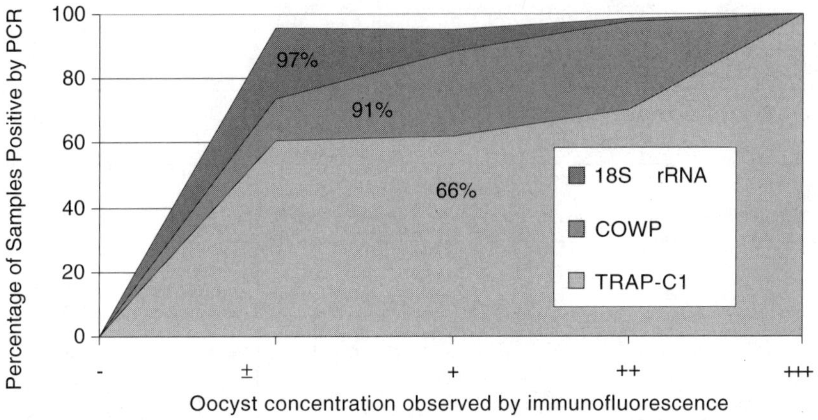

FIGURE 8.2 DNA extraction (method 2) from 218 patients diagnosed as having cryptosporidiosis.

8.2.2 Sample Testing

The development of routine typing for *Cryptosporidium* isolates was based on a number of key features of typing systems. Firstly, the more samples tested, the higher the probability that different types will be detected. Secondly, the greater the number of genes tested, the greater the opportunity to detect differences between strains and the greater confidence in isolate characterization. Thirdly, the more discriminatory the typing method at detecting variations in non-conserved genetic regions, the better the chance of developing subtyping methods that might be epidemiologically useful. In order to meet these criteria we tested large numbers of fecal samples from around the U.K. over an 18-month period between 1998 and 1999 where *Cryptosporidium* had been detected by routine microscopic examination. Samples from family outbreaks and outbreaks linked to drinking water and swimming pools were also tested. In addition, outbreaks were investigated and infections within families were examined. Samples from animals were tested and a few patients were followed up over the course of infection to determine whether isolates were stable over time. Routine surveillance has been continued at the PHLS *Cryptosporidium* Reference Unit.[14] Collecting data in this way meant that seasonal and geographic trends could be established for the surveillance data.

8.3 EPIDEMIOLOGICAL INFORMATION FROM TYPING ISOLATES

From the analyses performed to date it can be concluded that there are a number of species of *Cryptosporidium* in the U.K. that can cause human disease, of which *C. parvum* genotype 2 and *C. parvum* genotype 1 represent over 90% of the isolates.[15] Smaller numbers of *C. meleagridis*, *C. felis*, and *C. canis* strains make up most of the remainder.[16,17] With the seasonal data over 18 months, substantial seasonal variation was observed in the distribution of types (Figure 8.3). *C. parvum* genotype 1 was more common during the late summer period, whereas *C. parvum* genotype 2 was more common in the spring, although several years will need to be studied before consistent seasonal trends can be identified. It has been suggested that cases in the spring are more likely to derive from livestock, and cases in the autumn from people returning from abroad.[15] Over 100 isolates from livestock were tested, but organisms other than *C. parvum* genotype 2 were not detected.[15] Further animal testing will be necessary to identify the full spectrum of species that can infect animals within the U.K. The development of sensitive techniques for detecting and speciating oocysts in environmental waters will allow comparison of isolates from patients in outbreaks with isolates from water.[18]

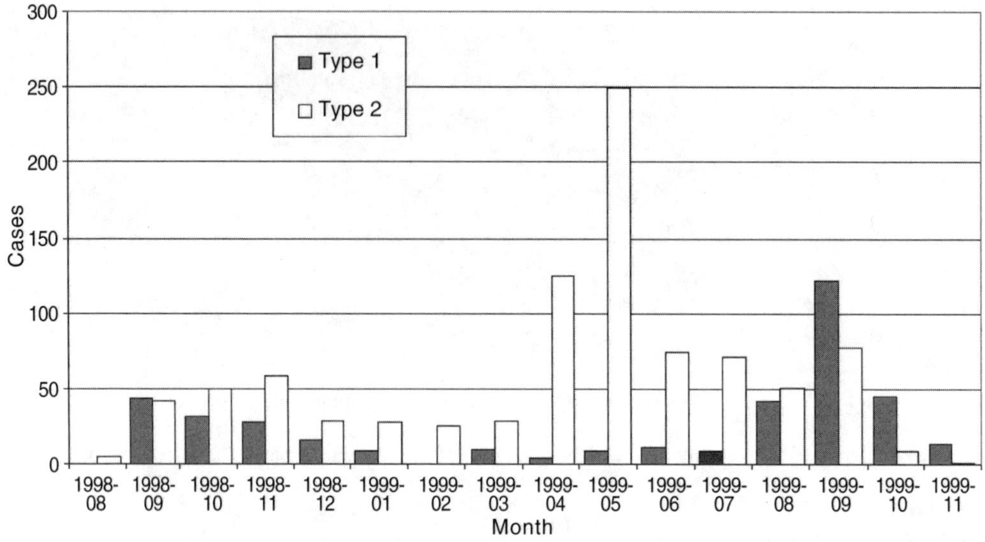

FIGURE 8.3 *Cryptosporidium* types by month including outbreaks.

8.3.1 Outbreaks

Outbreaks caused by *C. parvum* genotype 2 and *C. parvum* genotype 1 have been identified (Table 8.1), and epidemiological evidence suggests that some *C. parvum* genotype 2 outbreaks have resulted from contamination of water supplies with animal feces and some *C. parvum* genotype 1 outbreaks resulted from contamination of drinking water with sewage.[13,15] Swimming pool outbreaks were more frequently associated with dual infections than outbreaks linked to mains drinking water.

Epidemiological typing of bacteria has been useful in the analysis of food poisoning outbreaks because an outbreak strain can be identified that differs from unrelated sporadic cases occurring

TABLE 8.1
Genotyping of Human Isolates of *Cryptosporidium* in Outbreaks of Cryptosporidiosis Linked to Water

Outbreak	Year	Source	Total	*C. parvum* genotype 1	*C. parvum* genotype 2	*C. meleagridis*	*C. parvum* genotype 1 & 2
1	1994	Drinking water	8	8	0	0	0
2	1995	Drinking water	145	140	2	0	3
3	1997	Drinking water	11	11	0	0	0
4	1997	Drinking water	174	158	14	1	1
5	1997	Drinking water	15	15	0	0	0
6	1998	Drinking water	6	0	6	0	0
7	1998	Drinking water	25	0	25	0	0
8	1999	Drinking water	337	4	331	2	0
9	1998	Swimming pool	3	3	0	0	0
10	1999	Swimming pool	6	3	3	0	0
11	1999	Swimming pool	10	0	10	0	0
12	1999	Swimming pool	17	13	1	0	3
13	1999	Swimming pool	20	20	0	0	5
Total			777	375	392	3	12

within the community. In analyzing the data from outbreaks, the nature of *Cryptosporidium* infections may differ substantially from bacterial food poisoning incidents. Unlike outbreaks where a particular *Salmonella* type grows up in a food source and infects many people, *Cryptosporidium* outbreaks are from organisms present in feces, or in water and food contaminated with feces, since this parasite cannot grow outside of the infected host. The result is that without an amplification stage, mixtures of oocysts from different infected people or animals may be swallowed, resulting in mixed infections. This is particularly the case when sewage is the source of contamination, because it is likely to contain organisms from a variety of people infected with different strains. One would assume that people infected from a single infected person (e.g., a food handler or a child in a nursery) might be more likely to be infected by a single type than people infected through water from sewage. There is some evidence for this, and people with dual infections represent a small but significant percentage of cases and their feces infecting a population might cause mixed infections. However, current PCR methodologies are not well suited to detect mixtures. It should also be remembered that a small number of a different isolate in a population might result from a different source, even in an outbreak.

8.3.2 Geographic Variation and Travel

Typing differences are apparent in people returning from abroad. Overall, there was a preponderance of *C. parvum* genotype 1 over *C. parvum* genotype 2, but distribution of cases was different between countries. People returning from Spain had equal percentages of *C. parvum* genotype 2 and *C. parvum* genotype 1, whereas people coming back from Pakistan had predominantly *C. parvum* genotype 1. Travel-associated cryptosporidiosis is seasonal, with a higher incidence in the late summer (Figure 8.4). This coincided with an increase in *C. parvum* genotype 1 in the community at this time of year, possibly resulting from community spread. The demonstration of outbreaks of cryptosporidiosis associated with swimming pools indicates that this is an important route of transmission of cryptosporidiosis within the community, and possibly in travellers (who use pools abroad). The distribution of *Cryptosporidium* types by country varied substantially (Figure 8.5). The seasonality of travel-related cryptosporidiosis varied by country, with Spanish cases more common in late summer and infected people returning from Pakistan in spring and summer as well as the late summer.

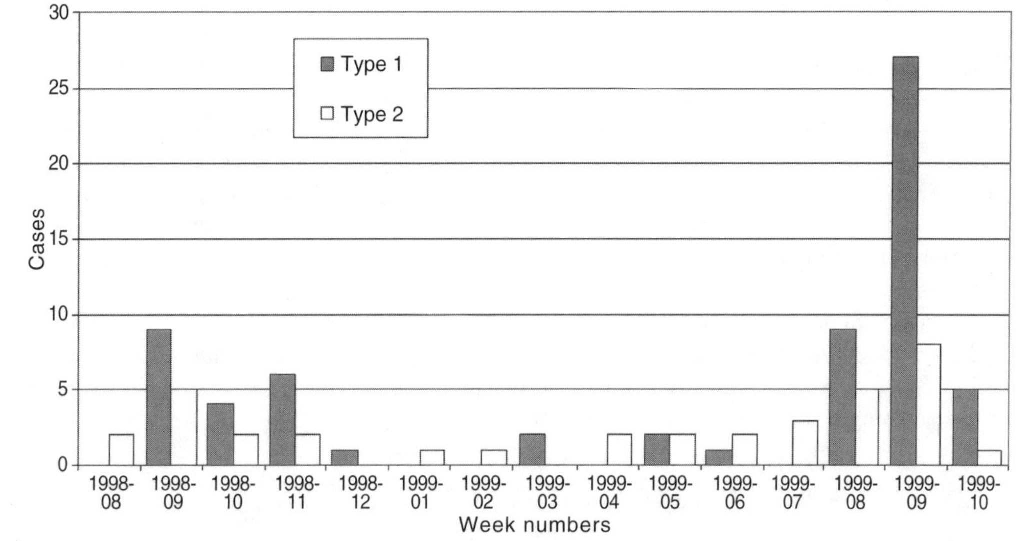

FIGURE 8.4 *Cryptosporidium* types in people returning from outside the U.K.

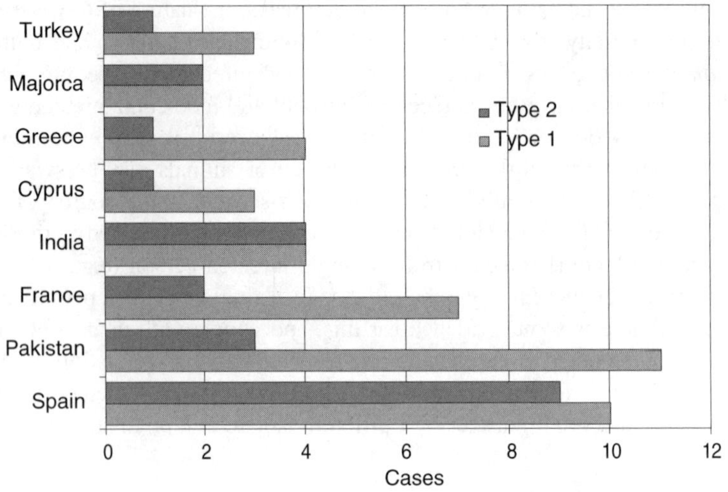

FIGURE 8.5 *Cryptosporidium* types in travellers.

8.8.3 HIV Infection

Typing of *Cryptosporidium* isolates from patients with HIV or AIDS and those from other immunocompromised patients indicate that the types encountered do have the same distribution as those found in immunocompetent people.[16,17,19–21] There is an overrepresentation of non-*C.parvum* isolates, including *C. meleagridis* and *C. felis.*

8.4 TAXONOMY AND NOMENCLATURE

The genotypic differences between *C. parvum* genotype 1 and *C. parvum* genotype 2 are sufficient to constitute their reclassification as separate species. As the first report of *Cryptosporidium* in the small intestine of a mouse (Tyzzer, 1912) was probably *C. parvum* genotype 2[22] and not *C. parvum* genotype 1, the latter should be renamed (*C. hominis* has been suggested). The *C. parvum* genotype 2 should be called *C. parvum,* as much of the literature relates to this organism. There are now a variety of *C. parvum*-like organisms specific to other hosts which show a similar level of diversity and consequently are also likely to justify renaming as separate species. The criteria for naming should include morphological and phenotypic information indicating that the organism belongs to the genus *Cryptosporidium* and genetic information confirming that it belongs to the genus *Cryptosporidium,* but with sufficient genetic differences to mark it as being distinct from other species. Subtyping is revealing substantial variation within both *C. parvum* genotype 1 and *C. parvum* genotype 2. Nomenclature for subtypes will remain somewhat *ad hoc* until a convention for naming these is published. It should be remembered that organisms isolated from an infected animal may be mixed and should be called isolates. Isolates that have been passaged through many animals (e.g., TAMU, Iowa, Moredun) are likely to be more defined and may be called strains, although contamination of animals with other *Cryptosporidium* oocysts remains possible and such strains may well have heterogeneous gene populations (see below). Strains cloned from single sporozoites have not yet been produced.

8.5 TYPING — PROSPECTS FOR THE FUTURE

There are still a number of questions about *Cryptosporidium* that typing may help to answer. Much of the typing work to date has shown differences between organisms that are probably at the species level. More recent studies have indicated variations that are within species.[23–26] It remains unclear whether individual isolates are homogeneous or heterogeneous. Theory would suggest that since each zygote is formed from a separate macrogametocyte and microgametocyte, and the product of this zygote is an oocyst with four sporozoites, then each oocyst should contain two genetically identical sporozoites that are genetically different from the two other genetically identical sporozoites. The zygote is thus a heterozygous diploid stage, but it is likely that each sporozoite is haploid and therefore homozygous (it only has one set of genes). Although there is little experimental evidence to support this, the hypothesis is testable through the development of cloned strains and recombination of such clones with different alleles. A clone produced from a single sporozoite should have a single set of genes unless sporozoites are diploid. Recombination of cloned strains should in addition be able to establish recombination frequencies and confirm genetic linkages generated by other methods. The relatively common occurrence of mixed human infections with *C. parvum* genotype 1 and *C. parvum* genotype 2 suggests that if recombination between these two were possible, these would have been detected. There is no good evidence that this has occurred. However, it highlights the fact that mixed infections, with different subtypes that can recombine, would be possible and indeed likely. If, as we suggest, members of the genus *Cryptosporidium* spp. have a diploid zygote with all other stages being haploid, then the oocysts passed by an infected animal may have a mixed gene pool comprising two or more copies of some alleles.

It is now clear that a variety of *Cryptosporidium* spp. can infect humans both with and without an underlying immunodeficiency. It is also clear that different species have different host specificities, some of which are broad spectrum (*C. parvum* genotype 2), and others narrow (*C. parvum* genotype 1). At present there is no technique for examining the host specificity of isolates other than inoculating a large variety of animals, birds, and other vertebrates. *In vitro* techniques for testing host specificity would be useful. It remains unclear whether the differences relate to the extent to which bile from different hosts will initiate excystation, whether there are specific receptors on the epithelial cells of different host species that the sporozoites/merozoites target, whether there are immune mechanisms that prevent the establishment of infection in some hosts, or whether the nutrition of the parasite is important. At present there is little epidemiological information indicating whether the severity of human disease associated with *C. parvum* genotype 2 differs from that of *C. parvum* genotype 1 or *C. meleagridis*, and whether these differ from mixed infections, although oocyst shedding was found to be longer for *C. parvum* genotype 1 than *C. parvum* genotype 2.[29] It is also unclear whether current methods will reliably detect the majority of mixed infections. There is little evidence to suggest whether the distribution of different *Cryptosporidium* types in humans reflects the extent of exposure to oocysts of different species or differences in human resistance to infection by the different species (as might be represented in an ID50).

More epidemiological evidence is needed to establish what causes much of the sporadic human disease. While drinking water remains a possibility and swimming pools may contribute, evidence may be improved when the several case-control studies of sporadic disease that are under way are published. Epidemiological evidence indicates that different types may be transmitted through different routes. The use of microsatellite loci to subtype isolates may make it possible to establish the sources of infection with greater confidence.[24–26,27,28]

Human volunteer studies conducted in Texas suggest that a proportion of people who have been reinfected with *C. parvum* genotype 2 following a primary infection with the same organism will be symptomatic but may not excrete oocysts.[30,31] This suggests that there could be substantial under-ascertainment of this organism. It is not clear whether the same applies to *C. parvum* genotype 1 or other species that can infect humans.

The approach taken to *Cryptosporidium* typing within the U.K. might well be one that could be applied to other organisms that are not easily cultivable, such as *Giardia*.

REFERENCES

1. Nichols, G.L., McLauchlin, J., and Samuel, D., A technique for typing *Cryptosporidium* isolates, *J. Protozool.*, 38, 2375, 1991.
2. Peng, M.M. et al., Genetic polymorphism among *Cryptosporidium parvum* isolates: evidence of two distinct human transmission cycles, *Emerg. Infect. Dis.*, 3, 567, 1997.
3. McLauchlin, J. et al., Identification of *Cryptosporidium* oocysts by monoclonal antibody, *Lancet*, 1, 51, 1987.
4. Ogunkolade, B.W. et al., Isoenzyme variation within the genus *Cryptosporidium*, *Parasitol. Res.*, 79, 385, 1993.
5. Awad-El-Kariem, F.M. et al., Differentiation between human and animal strains of *Cryptosporidium parvum* using isoenzyme typing, *Parasitology*, 110 (2), 129, 1995.
6. Patel, S., McLauchlin, J., and Casemore, D.P., A simple SDS-PAGE immunoblotting technique using an enhanced chemiluminescence detection system to identify polyclonal antibody responses to complex cryptosporidial antigen preparations following a monoclonal antibody retest and image overlay technique, *J. Immunol. Methods*, 205, 161, 1997.
7. McLauchlin, J. et al., The epidemiology of cryptosporidiosis: application of experimental sub-typing and antibody detection systems to the investigation of water-borne outbreaks, *Folia Parasitol.*, 45, 83, 1998.
8. Patel, S., Pedraza-Díaz, S., and McLauchlin, J., The identification of *Cryptosporidium* species and *Cryptosporidium parvum* directly from whole faeces by analysis of a multiplex PCR of the 18S rRNA gene and by PCR/RFLP of the *Cryptosporidium* outer wall protein (COWP) gene, *Int. J. Parasitol.*, 29, 1241, 1999.
9. Patel, S. et al., Molecular characterisation of *Cryptosporidium parvum* from two large suspected waterborne outbreaks, *Commun. Dis. Public Health*, 1, 231, 1998.
10. Spano, F. et al., PCR-RFLP analysis of the *Cryptosporidium* oocyst wall protein (COWP) gene discriminates between *C. wrairi* and *C. parvum*, and between *C. parvum* isolates of human and animal origin, *FEMS Microbiol. Lett.*, 150, 209, 1997.
11. Amar, C., Pedraza-Díaz, S., and McLauchlin, J., Extraction and genotyping of *Cryptosporidium parvum* DNA from fecal smears on glass slides stained conventionally for direct microscope examination, *J. Clin. Microbiol.*, 39, 401, 2001.
12. McLauchlin, J. et al., Genetic characterization of *Cryptosporidium* strains from 218 patients with diarrhea diagnosed as having sporadic cryptosporidiosis, *J. Clin. Microbiol.*, 37, 3153, 1999.
13. Pedraza-Díaz, S. et al., Nested polymerase chain reaction for amplification of the *Cryptosporidium* oocyst wall protein gene, *Emerg. Infect. Dis.*, 7, 49, 2001.
14. Chalmers, R. and Elwin, K., Implications and importance of genotyping *Cryptosporidium*, *Commun. Dis. Public Health*, 3, 155, 2000.
15. McLauchlin, J. et al., Molecular epidemiological analysis of *Cryptosporidium* spp. in the United Kingdom: results of genotyping *Cryptosporidium* spp. in 1,705 fecal samples from humans and 105 fecal samples from livestock animals, *J. Clin. Microbiol.*, 38, 3984, 2000.
16. Pedraza-Díaz, S. et al., Unusual *Cryptosporidium* species recovered from human faeces: first description of *Cryptosporidium felis* and *Cryptosporidium* "dog type" from patients in England, *J. Med. Microbiol.*, 50, 293, 2001.
17. Pedraza-Díaz, S. et al., *Cryptosporidium meleagridis* from humans: molecular analysis and description of affected patients, *J. Infect,. 42*, 243, 2001.
18. Lowery, C.J. et al., Detection and speciation of *Cryptosporidium* spp. in environmental water samples by immunomagnetic separation, PCR and endonuclease restriction, *J. Med. Microbiol.*, 49, 779, 2000.
19. Guyot, K. et al., Molecular characterization of *Cryptosporidium* isolates obtained from humans in France, *J. Clin. Microbiol.*, 39, 3472, 2001.
20. Morgan, U. et al., Molecular characterization of *Cryptosporidium* isolates obtained from human immunodeficiency virus-infected individuals living in Switzerland, Kenya, and the United States, *J. Clin. Microbiol.*, 38, 1180, 2000.
21. Pieniazek, N.J. et al., New *Cryptosporidium* genotypes in HIV-infected persons, *Emerg. Infect. Dis.*, 5, 444, 1999.

22. Tyzzer, E.E., *Cryptosporidium parvum* (Sp. Nov.), a coccidium found in the small intestine of the common mouse, *Archiv Fur Protistenkunde,* 26, 394, 1912.
23. Caccio, S. et al., A microsatellite marker reveals population heterogeneity within human and animal genotypes of *Cryptosporidium parvum, Parasitology,* 120(3), 237, 2000.
24. Caccio, S., Spano, F., and Pozio, E., Large sequence variation at two microsatellite loci among zoonotic (genotype C) isolates of *Cryptosporidium parvum, Int. J. Parasitol.*, 31, 1082, 2001.
25. Feng, X. et al., Extensive polymorphism in *Cryptosporidium parvum* identified by multilocus microsatellite analysis, *Appl. Environ. Microbiol.*, 66, 3344, 2000.
26. Liu, C. et al., A random survey of the *Cryptosporidium parvum* genome, *Infect. Immun.,* 67, 3960, 1999.
27. Aiello, A.E. et al., Microsatellite analysis of the human and bovine genotypes of *Cryptosporidium parvum, J. Eukaryot. Microbiol.,* 46, 46S, 1999.
28. Carraway, M., Tzipori, S., and Widmer, G., A new restriction fragment length polymorphism from *Cryptosporidium parvum* identifies genetically heterogeneous parasite populations and genotypic changes following transmission from bovine to human hosts, *Infect. Immun.*, 65, 3958, 1997.
29. Xiao, L. et al., Identification of 5 types of *Cryptosporidium* parasites in children in Lima, Peru, *J. Infect. Dis.,* 183, 492, 2001.
30. Chappell, C.L. et al., Infectivity of *Cryptosporidium parvum* in healthy adults with pre-existing anti-*C. parvum* serum immunoglobulin G, *Am. J. Trop. Med. Hyg.,* 60, 157, 1999.
31. Okhuysen, P.C. et al., Susceptibility and serologic response of healthy adults to reinfection with *Cryptosporidium parvum, Infect. Immun.*, 66, 441, 1998.

9 Engineering Considerations in the Investigation of Waterborne Outbreaks

Kim R. Fox

CONTENTS

9.1 INTRODUCTION

"The main point is that disease-germs shall not be present in our drinking water" is a quotation from a 1913 handbook on drinking water filtration.[1] That same statement holds true today and is a main concern of water treatment utilities around the world. The importance of maintaining a microbially safe drinking water is emphasized by the problems when breakdowns have occurred. The largest recorded waterborne disease outbreak in the United States was the cryptosporidiosis outbreak in Milwaukee in 1993.[2] The etiologic agent for this outbreak was *Cryptosporidium parvum*. At that time, *Cryptosporidium* was not regulated in drinking water, as the importance of this pathogen in the cause of waterborne disease was only starting to be understood. A considerable amount of research has been done on *Cryptosporidium* (analytical techniques, removal capabilities, inactivation procedures, and infectious dose) since that outbreak, and more will be done. Although *Cryptosporidium* was the organism of concern in Milwaukee, other emerging pathogens will probably become the focus of the future.

In every water system where microbial quality is a concern, source water quality, water treatment, and microbial monitoring are essential aspects in maintaining safe drinking water. Today, most drinking water systems practice the multiple barrier concepts as part of their overall plans for providing safe water.

In locations where waterborne disease outbreaks have occurred, engineering investigations can be used to determine what barriers may have failed. By making this determination, guidance can be given to the water industry to prevent future outbreaks from occurring.

In most cases, the engineering investigation takes place some time after the outbreak has occurred. An outbreak is normally identified when local physicians or health officials begin to see an increase in specific diseases or symptoms. The increase in disease (or symptoms) may prompt

0-8493-1259-0/03/$0.00+$1.50

health officials to determine whether the numbers coming in are abnormal for a particular situation. If the disease is then thought to be possibly water related, an engineering investigation should be done. This investigation may complement any epidemiological study that is being done, and engineers and epidemiologists should work together to determine what may have been the problem.

This chapter will use three case studies to show what happened in three different outbreaks as examples of engineering investigations.

9.2 THE MULTIPLE BARRIER CONCEPT

The premise behind the multiple barrier concept is that one should utilize multiple barriers in a drinking water system to prevent pathogens (or other contaminants) from reaching the consumer. If one barrier were to collapse, then the other barriers would be there to minimize pathogen presence in the treated water. Although the exact combination of barriers may differ between locations, the barriers can be classified as follows: (1) source water protection, (2) water treatment facilities, (3) disinfection and distribution, and (4) education.

Source water protection refers to providing the best source water possible prior to treatment. This may involve such steps as controlled usage of the watershed, sewage outfall minimization, wellhead protection, reservoir storage prior to treatment, and any other technique to reduce contamination of the source water. Source water protection may also include use of alternative sources if better source waters can be made available.

The water treatment facilities barrier encompasses all water treatment techniques including (but not limited to) simple slow sand filters, advanced enhanced coagulation processes, and membrane systems. The treatment plant must be designed and operated correctly to provide the contaminant barrier.

Disinfection and distribution processes are normally the final physical/chemical barriers where inactivation of microorganisms can occur. The disinfection barrier is more that just the disinfection provided at the water treatment plant. This barrier may also include maintaining a disinfectant residual out in the distribution system to limit regrowth of microorganisms and to provide a limited barrier against subsequent contamination (i.e., cross-connection contamination). Distribution system maintenance is essential in maintaining the integrity of the drinking water. Contamination can occur at any location throughout a distribution system, and proper operation and maintenance must be done to minimize problems.

The final barrier is not a physical barrier to contamination but is a controlling factor in maintaining and providing safe drinking water. Education is an important factor for all water systems. The education barrier crosses all the other barriers. Without proper operation and maintenance, the first three barriers will not operate correctly. Education of water utility personnel and management, public officials, and water consumers is an important aspect of maintaining safe water.

9.3 THE ENGINEERING INVESTIGATION OF WATERBORNE OUTBREAKS

In order to demonstrate the use of engineering studies in the investigation of waterborne outbreaks, we will describe three outbreaks that have occurred within the United States.

9.3.1 GIDEON, MISSOURI

A waterborne disease outbreak was identified in Gideon, Missouri (U.S.) beginning in late 1993.[3] The etiological agent for this outbreak was *Salmonella typhimurium,* and it was estimated that over 600 people were affected with diarrhea. The initial epidemiological data indicated that drinking water had been a factor. At that time, the Water Supply and Water Resources Division

(WSWRD) of the United States Environmental Protection Agency (USEPA) was asked to make an engineering investigation of the drinking water system. Gideon is a small town with a population of approximately 1100. The drinking water system at the time of the outbreak was well water that was pumped into the distribution system. There were several elevated storage tanks located in the distribution system. No disinfection was used in the drinking water at the time of the outbreak, and the safety of the supply was dependent on the single barrier of source water protection. Prior to the involvement of the team from USEPA but after detection of the outbreak, the town began adding chlorine to the water.

The team from USEPA conducted a small sanitary survey of the system and found areas of possible concern. This survey included sampling for microorganisms throughout the system along with checking for chlorine residuals. These samples showed inconsistencies with chlorine residuals and high levels of heterotrophic bacteria in various portions of the distribution system. *Salmonella typhimurium* was identified in a few of the water samples. Birds roosting in elevated storage tanks were thought to have caused the drinking water contamination. There was evidence (bird feathers, bird nests, and bird fecal material) in the tanks that birds had in fact been inside the storage facilities. Just prior to the initial outbreak, the town's maintenance crew had done a complete flushing of the system in order to alleviate taste and odor complaints. It was speculated that the flushing of the system drained the storage facilities down to their lowest levels. This allowed stagnant water in the bottom of the storage tanks to be mixed into the system and caused the contamination.

In order to show that this is what may have happened, the team from USEPA modelled the town's distribution system. In this model the system's layout, demand, pump information, storage tanks, and flushing information were entered into a program known as EPANET. This information was used to generate graphs such as those in Figure 9.1.

Figure 9.1 shows the water distribution from each storage tank after the flushing program. Overlays of locations of incidence of disease were placed onto this map. The incidence of disease and the propagation of water from one of the storage tanks showed that one contaminated tank may have caused the outbreak. As the tank was drained during the flushing program, the stagnant water at the bottom of the storage tank was mixed into the incoming water. This newly contaminated water was then dispersed out into the distribution system.

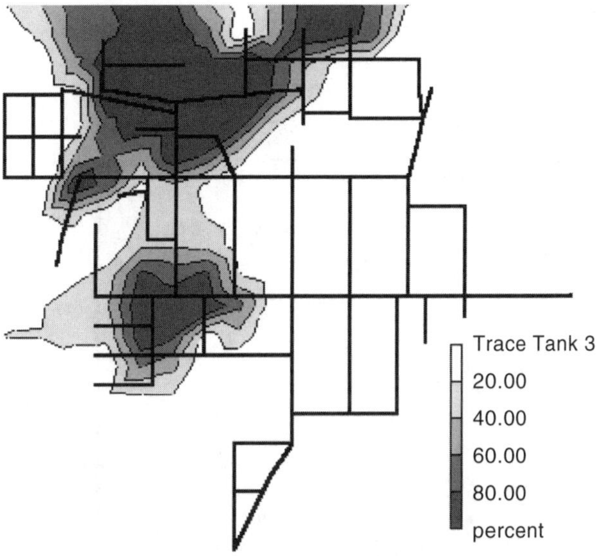

FIGURE 9.1 Gideon, Missouri propagation map.

9.3.2 Karl Meyer Hall

Karl Meyer Hall is a residency dormitory for the Cook County Hospital in Chicago, Illinois. In July, 1994 a number of physicians and employees living in the residency dormitory became ill and could not report for work. The symptoms for the reported illnesses were watery stools, fatigue, and anorexia. The epidemiological data suggested either the salad bar in the dormitory cafeteria or the drinking water. After a few months of discussion, the WSWRD was asked to make an engineering assessment of the drinking water situation in Karl Meyer Hall.

The dormitory was a twelve-story building connected to the municipal drinking water supply. There had been no evidence of increased disease in surrounding buildings or in the area, nor had there been any concerns about the municipal drinking water in other locations. This investigation centered on that building. Prior to Chicago's putting in complete water treatment, it was not uncommon for individual buildings to have their own treatment trains. This dormitory originally took water from the municipal distribution system and sent that water through pressure sand filters. After the sand filters, the water was pumped to two storage tanks located in the penthouse area of the building. The storage tanks provided the volume of water and the pressure needed for the dormitory residents.

Once Chicago staring fully treating its water, many buildings removed their treatment devices. In this case, the filters remained on-line and had not been maintained for at least 10 years. No backwashing or maintenance of any kind had been done. Many of the people involved did not believe that the filters were still connected. The engineering investigation showed that the filters were indeed still connected, and all the building's water was still going through them. Although these filters had not been maintained for 10 years, water samples after passing through the filters showed residual chlorine levels similar to those before the filters.

A further investigation of the storage tank facilities in the penthouse area provided more information. The epidemiological data showed that residents had indicated that on the day prior to the onset of disease there were reports of low water pressure and cloudy water. Maintenance records showed that the raw water pump in the basement had stopped working that day and had to be repaired. A diagram of one of the two storage tanks is shown in Figure 9.2.

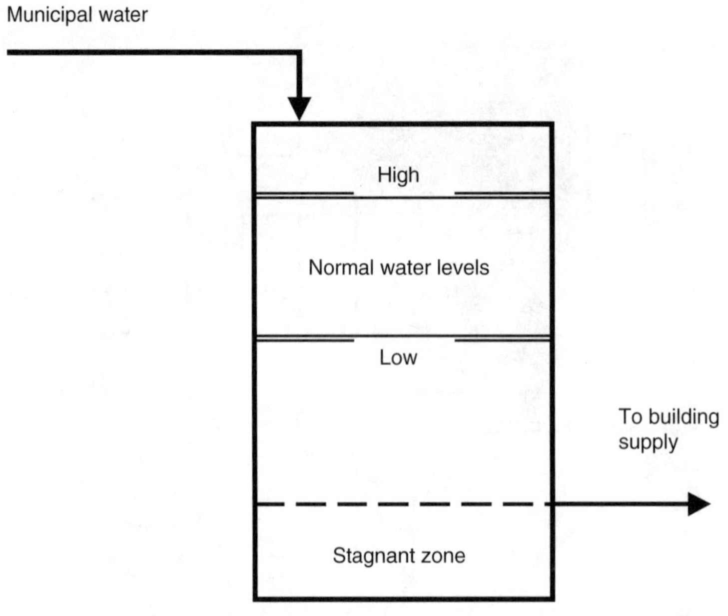

FIGURE 9.2 Karl Meyer Hall storage tank.

Investigation of the storage tanks showed evidence of bird fecal contamination. The tanks, although inside the building, were uncovered. Windows in the penthouse were broken and bird feathers and fecal material were on pipes and structures above the tanks. When the pump in the basement stopped, normal water usage drained the tank to the building feed line. At this point, no more water was available to the residents. When the pump was repaired and water was again flowing into the storage tank, the stagnant zone at the bottom of the storage tank was mixed into the system. The mixing caused the cloudy water reports and allowed for contaminated water to be distributed throughout the facility.

The etiological agent was not fully identified in this outbreak, and the initial studies showed it to be blue-green algae. Follow-up studies have suggested that *Microsporidia* may have been the agent.

Since that outbreak, the filters and storage tanks were removed. Local health officials also began a process to check all buildings for similar situations in order to prevent repeat performances.

9.3.3 Milwaukee, Wisconsin

In early 1993, Milwaukee, Wisconsin reported a sharp increase in the number of people attending health care services with diarrhea. It was also reported that there were shortages of over-the-counter drugs for diarrhea control at local pharmacies. On April 6, a doctor ordered a parasitic analysis on a patient's fecal specimen. *Cryptosporidium* was detected in the fecal smear, and local and state officials were notified of the *Cryptosporidium* detection. A concurrent survey of diarrhea cases in local nursing homes indicated that residents in nursing homes in the southern part of the city were 14 times more likely to have had diarrhea than those in the northern part of the city.

In addition to the nursing home survey, turbidity problems at the southern water treatment plant also implicated drinking water and this plant as being suspect in the cryptosporidiosis outbreak. At that point, the southern (Howard) plant was shut down. All of the drinking water for Milwaukee was supplied by the northern (Linwood) plant under a boil water order at that time.

The closure of the Howard Water Treatment Plant (HWTP), the boil water order, the magnitude of the number of reported diarrhea cases, and the media attention all helped to focus water utility personnel, engineers, scientists, government officials, and rule-making bodies on this waterborne outbreak. Follow-up surveys have indicated that as many as 403,000 people may have been ill during the Milwaukee incident.[2]

During the initial stages of the outbreak, the City of Milwaukee requested the assistance of the WSWRD to provide technical support. A USEPA team familiar with filtration processes and with the removal of *Cryptosporidium* oocysts by filtration went to Milwaukee. The team concentrated its efforts on evaluating the operational and monitoring data available from the southern HWTP. The goal was to assess how (from an engineering standpoint) *Cryptosporidium* may have passed into the water treatment facility.

The source water for Milwaukee, Wisconsin, is Lake Michigan (City of Milwaukee, 1992). The city's water is treated at two water treatment facilities: the northern-situated Linwood treatment plant and the southern HWTP. Both treatment facilities treat Lake Michigan water by conventional water treatment processes (coagulation, sedimentation, filtration, and disinfection). The Linwood facility has a water treatment capacity of 275 million gallons per day (MGD) and the Howard treatment facility has a filtration capacity of 100 MGD. During typical operation, the Linwood plant supplies the northern two-thirds of the water district. The HWTP supplies the remaining one-third. A large mixing zone exists in the distribution system between the two treatment facilities, but the general flow of water is northern or southern. The initial investigation linked the cryptosporidiosis outbreak to drinking water treated at the Howard treatment facility, resulting in temporary shutdown of the facility. The EPA team focused its efforts on understanding the operation of the Howard treatment plant.

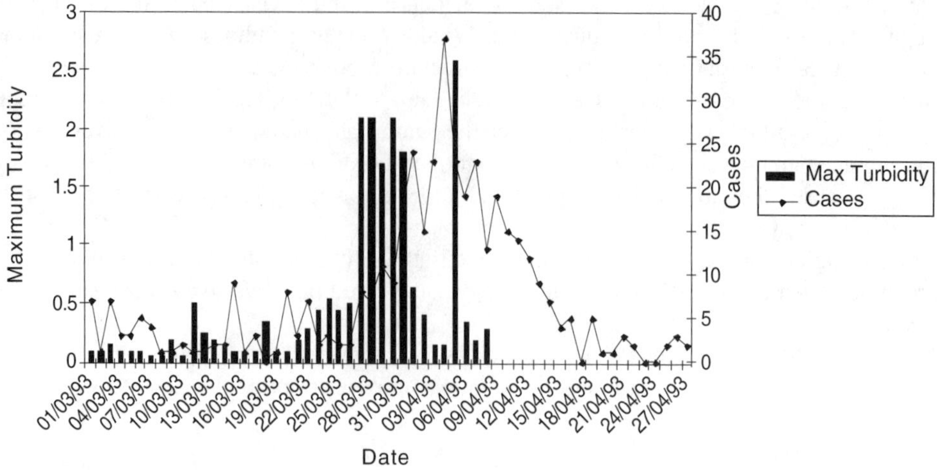

FIGURE 9.3 Maximum daily turbidity and number of cases during Milwaukee outbreak.

The HWTP is a conventional coagulation/sedimentation/filtration facility. A complete description can be found in Fox and Lytle.[4] Alum (aluminum sulfate) was the coagulant used until August, 1992. At that time, the facility switched to polyaluminum chloride (PACL). The switch to PACL was done with the belief that a benefit of higher finished water pH for corrosion control would be met as well as reduced sludge volume and improved coagulation effectiveness in cold raw water conditions. Before switching to PACL, the city consulted with the chemical manufacturer, Wisconsin DNR, and other communities receiving Lake Michigan water and using PACL.

In the time frame immediately preceding March 1993, the HWTP was consistently producing a low turbidity final water (daily averages of 0.1 NTU or less). During the period of March 18 through April 8 (the plant was shut down on April 8), the effluent turbidity from the HWTP was highly variable, ranging from 0.1 to 1.7 NTU (Figure 9.3). The team was asked to look at what caused the higher turbidity levels to occur. At all times during this period, effluent water samples were negative for coliforms and met the Wisconsin DNR regulations for turbidity.

The HWTP receives a highly variable quality of influent water (from Lake Michigan) to be processed through the plant. During the time period of March 18 through April 8, the raw water turbidity levels ranged from 1.5 to 44 NTU. Total coliforms ranged from <1 CFU/100 mL to around 3200 CFU/100 mL in the raw waters. All effluent water samples were negative for coliforms. Average raw water turbidity levels for previous months were around 3 or 4 NTU and influent coliform levels were < 20 CFU/100 mL.

During the time period investigated, plant facility personnel responded to turbidity changes throughout the treatment processes by adjusting coagulant dosages. Coagulation dosage adjustments were also made to compensate for coagulation demands resulting from taste- and odor-controlling treatment. Throughout the period, coagulant dose adjustments were continuously being made to meet the demands of raw water quality.

Although the coagulant dosages were being adjusted, filter effluent turbidities on several occasions exceeded turbidity values that were achieved in previous months. As the coagulant doses approached what might be optimum dosages for the particular raw water conditions, improvements in settled water turbidities and filter effluent turbidities were achieved. This pattern was seen twice. The first time was when PACL was the primary coagulant at the HWTP. The second time was when the primary coagulant was switched back to alum on April 2, 1993. The improvements in filter effluent turbidity demonstrated that the plant was fully capable of producing low turbidity water under optimal chemical coagulation conditions (i.e., dosages applied) even when challenged with high turbidity raw water.

There are several factors that may have increased the time to reach the optimum coagulant dosages for low filter effluent turbidities during this time. One of these factors may include a lack of historical use records for PACL. The previous coagulant had been used for almost 30 years. The new coagulant had only been used for a short time and the historical records were not fully developed. The optimum chemical dosages were sought through laboratory testing and consultation with DNR and the chemical supplier to achieve the lowest turbidity possible. The coagulant adjustments were made based on all available data.

Another important factor is the time required to see a result in the treated water quality after chemical adjustment. With a short residence time for the water in the plant and a rapidly changing influent water quality, dosage optimization was difficult.

During the higher effluent turbidity episodes, greater numbers of particulates passed through the HWTP as evidenced by the higher turbidity values exiting the plant clearwell. Although a greater number of particulates passed through the plant, this does not necessarily mean that *Cryptosporidium* oocysts passed through the plant. This does, however, suggest that if a large number of oocysts were present in the source water at this time, the likelihood of passage would increase. There is no way to know for sure that this scenario resulted in *Cryptosporidium* oocysts' passage. Monitoring for this organism is not a common practice in the drinking water supply industry and is not required in Wisconsin by the Wisconsin Administration Code.

9.4 DISCUSSION

Each of the case studies presented here has shown different areas that were responsible for the waterborne disease outbreaks. Each outbreak is different, and the engineering investigation needs to be based on what is present at that location. Drinking water plant personnel and authorities need to work under the assumption that pathogens are always present in their source water. By using that assumption, aggressive water treatment is suggested and operation and maintenance practices should be maintained.

Proper engineering investigations should be done as soon as possible during a suspected waterborne disease outbreak. In many cases, an outbreak may not be identified until it is over, and thus the investigation is not concurrent with the outbreak. Getting the investigation started as soon as possible will allow for a better opportunity to find contaminated samples. Although it is best to begin the engineering investigation during an outbreak, most investigators need to realize that much of their work will be done after the outbreak has ended. The team must understand that the conditions may have changed, and what is there now may not have been there when the problem occurred.

The engineering investigations can show where and how the pathogens got through the barriers. Information gathered in those investigations, if disseminated, can be used by water authorities to prevent similar outbreaks from occurring. Follow-up investigations are essential to maintaining safe drinking water.

REFERENCES

1. Hazen, A., *The Filtration of Public Water-Supplies*. 1st ed., John Wiley & Sons, New York, 1913.
2. MacKenzie, W.R. et al., A massive outbreak in Milwaukee of *Cryptosporidium* infection transmitted through the public water supply, *New Engl. J. Med.*, 331, 161, 1994.
3. Clark, R.M. et al., Tracking a *Salmonella serovar typhimurium* outbreak in Gideon, Missouri: role of contamination propagation modelling, *J. Water SRT — Aqua*, 45, 171, 1996.
4. Fox, K.R. and Lytle, D.A., The cryptosporidiosis outbreak in Milwaukee: investigation and recommendations, *JAWWA*, 88, 1996.

10 Causes of Waterborne Outbreaks Reported in the United States, 1991–1998

Gunther F. Craun, Rebecca L. Calderon, and Nena Nwachuku

CONTENTS

10.1 Introduction....105
10.2 Drinking Water Outbreaks....106
10.2.1 Public Water Systems....106
10.2.1.1 Type of System and Water Source....106
10.2.1.2 Outbreak Etiologies, System Type, and Water Source....107
10.2.1.3 Water System Deficiencies, System Type, and Water Source....108
10.2.1.4 Water Quality during Outbreaks in Public Water Systems....110
10.2.2 Individual Water Systems....111
10.3 Recreational Water Outbreaks....111
10.4 Discussion....114
10.4.1 Waterborne Outbreaks and Deficiencies in Public Water Systems....114
10.4.1.1 Groundwater Systems....114
10.4.1.2 Distribution System Contamination....114
10.4.1.3 Protozoan Outbreaks....115
10.4.1.4 Outbreaks and Coliforms....115
10.4.2 Recreational Water....116
10.5 Conclusions....116
References....117

10.1 INTRODUCTION

In this article we review information from 230 waterborne outbreaks reported in the United States during the period 1991 to 1998. More than 443,000 cases of illness occurred during outbreaks in 41 states and three U.S. territories. An estimated 764 hospitalizations and 60 deaths occurred. Most (55%) of the outbreaks were associated with contaminated drinking water. Of the 126 drinking-water outbreaks, 109 were reported in public water systems, and 17 were reported in individual water systems. An additional 104 (45%) outbreaks were associated with recreational water activities, which were primarily swimming. The U.S. disease surveillance system is discussed in Chapter 3 and also in various reports.[1–6]

Most reported outbreaks are associated with water used or intended for drinking or domestic purposes, but outbreaks are also associated with the ingestion of water not intended for consumption (e.g., the use of contaminated springs and creeks by backpackers and campers, and ingestion of

0-8493-1259-0/03/$0.00+$1.50

water while swimming). Recreational waters encompass swimming pools, water parks, and naturally occurring fresh and marine surface waters. Although the surveillance system includes whirlpool- and hot tub-associated outbreaks of dermatitis, these outbreaks are not evaluated in our analysis. The surveillance system does not include waterborne outbreaks that occur on cruise ships operating from U.S. ports and outbreaks caused by contamination of water or ice at its point of use (e.g., a contaminated water faucet or serving container). We did, however, include in our analysis outbreaks caused by contaminated ice and water in containers; these outbreaks are classified under miscellaneous deficiencies.

10.2 DRINKING WATER OUTBREAKS

10.2.1 Public Water Systems

In the United States, public water systems are classified as either community or non-community water systems and are regulated by the Environmental Protection Agengy (EPA).[7–16] A community water system serves year-round residents of a community, subdivision, or mobile-home park that has 15 or more service connections or an average of 25 or more residents. A non-community water system is used by the general public for greater than 60 or more days per year and has at least 15 service connections or serves an average of 25 or more persons. Of the approximately 170,000 public water systems in the United States, 55,000 (32%) are community systems and 115,000 (68%) are non-community systems. Community water systems serve some 243 million persons. Millions of persons use non-community systems while traveling or working in the United States. Non-community water systems are also classified as non-transient (20,000 systems) and transient (95,000 systems). Non-transient systems (e.g., in factories and schools with their own water systems) serve 25 or more persons for at least 6 months of the year. Transient non-community water systems do not serve at least 25 of the same persons over 6 months per year (e.g., restaurants, rest stops, and parks).

Each public water system associated with a waterborne outbreak was classified as having one of the following deficiencies: untreated surfacewater; untreated groundwater; treatment deficiency (e.g., temporary interruption of disinfection, inadequate disinfection, and inadequate or no filtration); distribution system deficiency (e.g., cross-connection, contamination of water mains during construction or repair, and contamination of a storage facility); and unknown or miscellaneous deficiency (e.g., contaminated ice, containers, or bottled water). Water sources are identified as either surfacewater or groundwater. Systems that use both surfacewater and groundwater sources were classified according to either the affected water source or the primary water source.

10.2.1.1 Type of System and Water Source

Forty-seven waterborne outbreaks and 422,298 illnesses were reported in community water systems; 62 waterborne outbreaks and 6562 illnesses were reported in non-community systems. A single outbreak of cryptosporidiosis in Milwaukee was responsible for 403,000 cases of illness and an estimated 50 deaths in 1993. This outbreak is the largest reported in the United States since the collection of statistics began in 1920.

Over 156,000 (92%) public water systems primarily rely on groundwater sources; 74 (68%) of the outbreaks in public systems were associated with groundwater sources (Table 10.1). Slightly more than 13,000 (8%) systems use surfacewater sources, and 24 (22%) outbreaks occurred in water systems that used surfacewater sources. A water source was not identified for 8 outbreaks in non-community systems and 3 waterborne outbreaks in community systems. These 11 outbreaks were unrelated to source water quality and were caused by either contamination of the distribution system, contaminated ice, or a contaminated water storage container.

Twenty-two (47%) outbreaks in community systems occurred in systems using groundwater. Twenty of these systems used well water, one obtained water from a spring, and one used water

TABLE 10.1
Waterborne Outbreaks Reported in U.S. Drinking Water Systems by Type of System and Water Source, 1991–1998

	Number of Waterborne Outbreaks			
Water Source	Community Systems	Non-Community Systems	Individual Systems	All Water Systems
Groundwater[a]	22	52	11	85
Surfacewater[b]	22	2	1	25
Unknown	3	8	5	16
Totals	47	62	17	126

[a] Surfacewater = lakes, reservoirs, rivers, streams
[b] Groundwater = wells and springs

from both well and spring sources. Twenty-two (47%) outbreaks also occurred in community systems using surfacewater. Fifty-two (84%) of the outbreaks reported in non-community systems occurred in systems using groundwater; 47 systems used well water, and 5 used spring water. Only 2 (4%) outbreaks occurred in non-community systems that used surfacewater, probably reflecting the few non-community systems that use surfacewater sources.

10.2.1.2 Outbreak Etiologies, System Type, and Water Source

Seventeen (16%) outbreaks were classified as acute chemical poisoning, while a bacterial, viral, or protozoan etiology was identified in 43 (39%) outbreaks (Table 10.2). In 49 (45%) outbreaks, an infectious agent was suspected but not identified. Of 31 outbreaks in community systems with a known or suspected infectious etiology, 13 (42%) were associated with groundwater sources, 15 (48%) with surfacewater sources, and 3 (10%) with unknown water sources (Table 10.2). Chemical contaminants caused 41% of the outbreaks in community groundwater systems while *Giardia* and

TABLE 10.2
Etiology of Waterborne Outbreaks, 1991–1998; Number of Outbreaks by Type of Water System and Water Source

	Community Water Systems			Non-Community Water Systems		
Etiological Agent	Surface-water	Ground-water	Unknown Source	Surface-water	Ground-water	Unknown Source
Undetermined	5	1	1	1	36	5
Chemical	7	9				1
Giardia	6	4			3	
Cryptosporidium	3	3	1	1	1	
Norwalk-like virus	1	1				
Campylobacter		1			2	1
Salmonella, non-typhoid		1				
Escherichia coli O157:H7		1			3	1
Shigella		1			5	
Vibrio cholerae			1			
Hepatitis A virus					1	
Plesiomonas shigelloides					1	
Total	22	22	3	2	52	8

TABLE 10.3
Etiology of Waterborne Outbreaks; Cases of Illness by Type of Water System and Water Source, 1991–1998

	Community Water Systems			Non-Community Water Systems		
Etiological Agent	**Surface-water**	**Ground-water**	**Unknown Source**	**Surface-water**	**Ground-water**	**Unknown Source**
Undetermined	10,210	18	67	250	4789	101
Chemical	104	409				2
Giardia	1,937	49			128	
Cryptosporidium	403,343	4294	77	27	551	
Norwalk-like virus	148	594				
Campylobacter		172			51	7
Salmonella, non-typhoid		625				
E. coli O157:H7		157			39	27
Shigella		83			484	
Vibrio cholerae			11			
Hepatitis A virus					46	
Plesiomonas shigelloides					60	
Total	415,742	6401	155	277	6148	137

Cryptosporidium caused 32% of the outbreaks. In community surface water systems, *Giardia* and *Cryptosporidium* caused more outbreaks (41%) than chemical contaminants (32%).

Of 61 infectious disease outbreaks in non-community systems, 52 (85%) were associated with groundwater sources; 2 (3%) occurred in systems with surface-water sources, and 7 (11%) occurred in systems with unknown water sources. In non-community systems using groundwater, most (69%) outbreaks were of undetermined etiology. *Giardia* and *Cryptosporidium* caused 4 (8%) outbreaks in non-community groundwater system; the remaining outbreaks were caused by bacterial (21%) or viral (2%) agents.

Sixteen (34%) outbreaks in community systems and one (2%) outbreak in non-community systems were caused by chemical contaminants. Of the 16 outbreaks of acute chemical poisoning in community systems, 7 occurred in groundwater systems and 9 occurred in surfacewater systems. Most (69%) chemical outbreaks in community systems were due to contamination of the distribution system. High copper levels due to corrosive water were identified in 7 outbreaks. Cross-connections and back-siphonage (nitrate, soap concentrate, and fluoride) caused 4 outbreaks. Five (29%) outbreaks were related to inadequate control of chemical addition (fluoride, sodium hydroxide, chlorine). One outbreak of copper poisoning occurred in a non-community system. Almost 99% of the illnesses in community system outbreaks were associated with surfacewater systems; most occurred during the *Cryptosporidium* outbreak in Milwaukee (Table 10.3). Outbreaks in non-community systems caused 6562 illnesses, 94% of which occurred in systems using groundwater; 75% of the illnesses reported in non-community groundwater systems were of undetermined etiology. Non-community system outbreaks were, on average, much smaller than community system outbreaks. Outbreaks in non-community systems caused 106 illnesses per outbreak compared to 420 illnesses per outbreak in community systems (8985 per outbreak if the Milwaukee outbreak is included).

10.2.1.3 Water System Deficiencies, System Type, and Water Source

Distribution system deficiencies including corrosive water were the most frequent (36%) cause of outbreaks in community systems. Contaminants entered the distribution systems through cross-connections, back-siphonage, poorly protected distribution storage facilities, and during construction and repairs to pipes. The remaining outbreaks in community systems were associated with

TABLE 10.4
Waterborne Outbreaks and Deficiencies in Public Water Systems Surfacewater Sources, 1991–1998

	Community Systems Surfacewater Source		Non-Community Systems Surfacewater Source	
Type of Contamination	**Outbreaks**	**Percent**	**Outbreaks**	**Percent**
Untreated surface water	0	0	0	0
Inadequate or interrupted disinfection; disinfection only treatment	4	18	1	50
Inadequate or interrupted filtration	4	18	0	0
Distribution system contamination	9	41	0	0
Inadequate control of chemical feed	2	9	0	0
Miscellaneous/unknown	3	14	1	50
Total	22	100	2	100

inadequately treated groundwater (22%) or surfacewater (17%), inadequate control of chemical feed (11%), and miscellaneous/undetermined causes (14%). In non-community water systems, 63% of 62 reported outbreaks occurred in groundwater systems that were inadequately treated. Non-community outbreaks were also associated with distribution system deficiencies (13%), unfiltered surfacewater (2%), and miscellaneous or undetermined causes (22%).

Of the 24 outbreaks reported in public systems using surfacewater, 22 (92%) occurred in community water systems (Table 10.4). Distribution system contamination was also the most (41%) frequently identified deficiency in community surfacewater system outbreaks. Inadequate disinfection of unfiltered water and inadequate filtration caused 36% of the outbreaks in community surfacewater systems.

Of the 74 outbreaks reported in public systems using groundwater, 52 (70%) occurred in non-community water systems (Table 10.5). In community groundwater systems, 5 (23%) outbreaks were associated with untreated water, whereas 18 (35%) outbreaks in non-community groundwater systems were associated with untreated water. In non-community systems that used untreated well water, 10 (56%) outbreaks were caused by the overflow or seepage of sewage through soil or rock, and 2 (11%) were caused by contaminated surface runoff and improper construction. In 6 (33%)

TABLE 10.5
Waterborne Outbreaks and Deficiencies in Public Water Systems Groundwater Sources, 1991–1998

	Community Systems Groundwater Source		Non-Community Systems Groundwater Source	
Type of Contamination	**Outbreaks**	**Percent**	**Outbreaks**	**Percent**
Untreated groundwater	5	23	18	35
Inadequate or interrupted disinfection; disinfection only treatment	3	14	21	40
Inadequate or interrupted filtration	1	4	0	
Distribution system contamination	8	36	8	15
Inadequate control of chemical feed	3	14	0	
Miscellaneous/unknown	2	9	5	10
Total	22	100	52	100

outbreaks, the source of contamination was not determined. When all deficiencies are combined, 41% of outbreaks in community groundwater systems were attributed to inadequate or no treatment. In non-community groundwater systems, these same deficiencies caused 75% of outbreaks.

10.2.1.4 Water Quality during Outbreaks in Public Water Systems

The EPA's total coliform rule (TCR) requires public water systems to routinely monitor their tap water for total coliforms.[7,8] Water quality information was available from routine surveillance records for 45 outbreaks. In the 12-month period before these 45 outbreaks, only 5 (22%) community and 2 (9%) non-community systems had violated the EPA's coliform limit.

Water quality information collected during the outbreak investigation was reviewed for 78 known or suspected infectious disease outbreaks to determine how frequently coliforms were detected in water systems during an outbreak investigation and whether the detection of coliforms was associated with certain types of water systems or etiological agents. Excluded from this analysis were the 14 outbreaks associated with contaminated faucets, bottled water, contaminated ice, and water contaminated in storage containers. In many of the investigations, more coliform samples were collected than would be required by the TCR for routine monitoring purposes, and the samples were collected during a relatively short period of time. Often water samples were collected during a 1- to 2-week period. Water samples were usually collected during the early stages of an outbreak. In several investigations, samples were not collected until 2 to 4 weeks after the beginning of the outbreak. In one outbreak, water samples were collected 2 months after the beginning of the outbreak. In several investigations, water samples were collected from water sources rather than the distribution system. For example, in non-community systems, coliform information from well water samples was available for seven outbreaks where the well was not disinfected. In these seven outbreaks, information from source water samples was used as a substitute for tap water samples. Because the well water was not treated, it was presumed that tap water samples, if they had been collected, would likely be of similar quality.

Information about the presence of coliform bacteria in the water system during the investigation was available for 72 (92%) outbreaks in public water systems (Table 10.6). Total coliforms were detected during 50 outbreaks. In 15 outbreaks where only 1 water sample was collected, the sample was found to be coliform positive. In 6 outbreaks, 1 positive sample was found among the 2 to 20 samples collected. In outbreaks where coliforms were not detected, as few as 2 and as many as 44 samples were collected. Total coliforms were detected during the investigation of 83% of non-community system outbreaks but only 46% of community system outbreaks. Total coliforms were detected during the investigation of 44 (88%) outbreaks caused by bacteria, viruses, and unidentified

TABLE 10.6
Total Coliform Data Collected during Waterborne Outbreak Investigations, Public Water Systems, 1991–1998[a]

	Number of Outbreaks			
Water System	Outbreaks of Known or Suspected Infectious Etiology	Outbreaks with Total Coliform Data	Outbreaks where Total Coliforms were Detected	Outbreaks where Total Coliforms were Not Detected
Community	27	26	12	14
Non-community	51	46	38	8
Totals	78	72	50	22

[a] Excluded from analysis are chemical outbreaks and outbreaks associated with contaminated bottled water, ice, faucets, containers, and water recreation.

agents but during only 5 (26%) outbreaks caused by *Giardia* or *Cryptosporidium*. Water samples were tested for fecal coliforms in 44 outbreaks, of which 36 (82%) were positive.

10.2.2 Individual Water Systems

In the United States, some 24 million persons (9%) rely on individual water systems which are not owned or operated by a water utility and serve less than 15 connections or less than 25 persons. Individual water systems are not regulated by the EPA. Each state or county develops regulations for these systems. Outbreaks associated with individual water systems are less likely to be recognized than outbreaks in public water systems, and only 17 outbreaks and 161 illnesses were reported for these water systems. Most outbreaks (65%) and illnesses (88%) occurred in individual systems using well water (Table 10.7). Etiological agents that caused outbreaks in individual systems were similar to those that caused outbreaks in public water systems. Six (35%) outbreaks were caused by high nitrate and lead. In 3 outbreaks, single cases of methemoglobinemia were reported, and high levels of nitrate were found in the wells. In one outbreak, a reverse-osmosis membrane filter reduced nitrate levels in the water source but levels were still high enough to cause illness.[4] Another 3 single-case outbreaks involved infants with high blood lead levels.[5] These cases were detected through a lead screening program. Water stored at the homes of the infants was found to be corrosive; lead was leaching from fittings and lead-soldered seams in the storage tanks. Total coliforms were found in water samples collected during the investigation of 9 (82%) of 11 outbreaks of known or suspected infectious etiology. Water samples were tested for fecal coliforms in 6 outbreaks and were detected in 5 of these. Six (55%) outbreaks of known or suspected infectious etiology were associated with untreated, contaminated well water. In one outbreak, inadequate disinfection was provided for well water. A shigellosis outbreak was associated with water that was contaminated during storage, and a giardiasis outbreak with the use of untreated surface water. In the remaining two outbreaks, no water source was identified.

10.3 RECREATIONAL WATER OUTBREAKS

State and local governments have jurisdiction over recreational water. The operation, disinfection, and filtration of public swimming and wading pools are regulated by state and local health departments. For fresh waters (e.g., lakes, ponds) used for swimming, the EPA has established a guideline for microbial water quality.[21] However, states and localities can have either more or less stringent guidelines or regulations. Authorities usually post warning signs to alert potential bathers about

TABLE 10.7
Etiology of Waterborne Outbreaks in Individual Water Systems Outbreaks and Cases of Illness by Water Source, 1991–1998

	Outbreaks			Cases of Illness		
Etiological Agent	Surface-water	Ground-water	Unknown Source	Surface-water	Ground-water	Unknown Source
Undetermined	0	2	1	0	43	8
Chemical	0	3	3	0	3	5
Giardia	1	1	0	2	10	0
Cryptosporidium	0	2	0	0	39	0
E. coli	0	1	0	0	3	0
Shigella	0	1	1	0	33	5
Hepatitis A virus	0	1	0	0	10	0
Total	1	11	5	2	141	18

TABLE 10.8
Etiology of Recreational Waterborne Outbreaks, Outbreaks, and Cases of Illness by Type of Water Source, 1991–1998

	Outbreaks				Cases of Illness			
Etiological Agent	Lake	Swim Pool[a]	River	Other[b]	Lake	Swim Pool	River	Other[b]
Cryptosporidium	3	19		1	429	9477		369
Naegleria	9		4	4	9		4	4
E. coli O157:H7	9	2			293	44		
Shigella	11			1	1216			9
Undetermined	8	1	1	1	1016	100	15	61
Giardia	3	5	1		59	187	6	
Schistosoma	6			1	173			30
Pseudomonas		5				162		
Leptospira	2				381			
Norwalk-like virus	2			1	48			55
Chemical		2				29		
Salmonella, non-typhoid		1				3		
Adenovirus	1				595			
Total	54	35	6	9	4219	10002	25	528

[a] Includes wading pools and pools and other activities at water parks.
[b] Water slide park, dunking booth, hot spring, canal, fountain, ocean, unknown.

poor water quality. Signs are posted until water quality improves. Outbreaks of gastroenteritis, dermatitis, meningoencephalitis, conjunctivitis, and leptospirosis associated with water recreation were reported in 29 states and one U.S. territory. An estimated 14,774 persons became ill in the 104 reported outbreaks. Most (51%) outbreaks were associated with swimming and bathing activities in lakes, ponds, and reservoirs, but a significant number of outbreaks (33%) were associated with swimming or wading pools at various locations including community centers, parks, water theme parks, motels, country clubs, daycare centers, schools, and hospitals (Table 10.8).

Eleven (11%) of the 104 water recreation outbreaks were acute gastroenteritis of undetermined etiology. In each of the other outbreaks, an etiological agent was identified. Most outbreaks (69%) associated with swimming and wading pools were caused by *Cryptosporidium* and *Giardia*. *Cryptosporidium* was responsible for 9477 (64%) cases of illness and 23 (22%) outbreaks (Table 10.8). Nineteen (83%) of the 23 outbreaks caused by *Cryptosporidium* were associated with chlorinated, filtered pool water, and only 3 outbreaks were associated with swimming in lake water. Three cryptosporidiosis outbreaks and 8475 cases of illness occurred in water-theme parks. One cryptosporidiosis outbreak occurred at a zoo, where 369 persons became ill after playing in a sprinkler fountain.[1] The fountain was originally designed as a decorative fountain and had become a popular interactive play area for children. Water was sprayed through the air, drained through grates, collected, passed through a sand filter, and chlorinated and recirculated.

Two bacterial pathogens, *Shigella* and *Escherichia coli* O157:H7, were the most frequently identified etiological agents for outbreaks associated with swimming at lakes and ponds (Table 10.8). *E. coli* O157:H7 caused 11 (11%) outbreaks; 9 (82%) of these occurred while swimming in lakes. One of the remaining two *E. coli* gastroenteritis outbreaks was associated with swimming in a poorly maintained and poorly chlorinated indoor pool. The other *E. coli* outbreak occurred at a watertheme park where 7 of 23 ill persons developed hemolytic uremic syndrome, and one died. A fecal accident in a children's pool at the water park was suspected to be the source of the outbreak. Low chlorine levels were documented and could have been inadequate to inactivate the bacteria. *Shigella* caused 12 outbreaks (12%), 11 of which were associated with swimming in lake water. One *S. sonnei* outbreak where 9 persons became ill was associated with a wading pool that included a sprinkler fountain. The system recirculated chlorine-treated water, and many diaper-aged children were observed sitting in the wading pool.

Three outbreaks of gastroenteritis caused by Norwalk-like virus were reported; two were associated with swimming in lakes and one with bathing in hot springs. In all three outbreaks, the water was found to contain fecal coliforms, but the source of the virus was not identified. An outbreak of salmonellosis was reported among persons using a scuba dive pool that had been filled with fish.

Three outbreaks of *Schistosoma* dermatitis (swimmer's itch) were associated with swimming in Oregon lakes; in two outbreaks, geese were the suspected source of these parasites. Other outbreaks of schistosomal dermatitis occurred after swimming in lakes in New Jersey, Utah, and Wyoming. One dermatitis outbreak was associated with swimming in ocean water in Delaware, where local snails were found to contain cercariae of *Austrobilharzia variglandis*, an avian schistosome implicated as a cause of cercarial dermatitis.[4] Two outbreaks of chemical dermatitis were associated with incorrect dosing of chemicals to adjust the pH of swimming pool water and the addition of chemicals to remove excess chloramines.

In 1991, an outbreak of leptospirosis was associated with swimming in a rural pond in Illinois. *Leptospira interrogans* was found in urine specimens and in pond water. A second outbreak of leptospirosis occurred among competitors in a triathlon in Illinois during 1998.[1] Three hundred and seventy-five persons became ill after swimming in a lake, and 28 persons were hospitalized. This is the largest outbreak of leptospirosis ever reported in the United States.

Six (6%) outbreaks of conjunctivitis were reported. Adenovirus serotype 3 was implicated from clinical and water samples collected in an outbreak of conjunctivitis, pharyngitis, and fever. Five swimming-pool-associated outbreaks of conjunctivitis, otitis, and rash were caused by *Pseudomonas*.

Seventeen persons diagnosed with primary amebic meningoencephalitis died. Nine of these single-case outbreaks were associated with swimming in lakes or ponds. The remaining cases were associated with swimming in rivers and canals, facial immersion in a water puddle during a fight,[4] and bathing in a hot spring that had been associated with two previous cases. *N. fowleri* infections are generally acquired during the summer months, when the temperature of fresh water is favorable for the multiplication of the organism. The ameba can enter a person's body through the nasal passages when water is forced up the nose, especially during underwater swimming and diving.[1]

Information was available about the source of contamination and other factors that may have contributed to the outbreak for 40 recreational outbreaks, including 15 outbreaks associated with swimming pools and 21 associated with lakes or ponds (Table 10.9). Poor maintenance and oper-

TABLE 10.9
Causes of Waterborne Disease Outbreaks Associated with Recreational Water

Source of Contamination or Deficiency	Number of Outbreaks
Fecal accident or ill bather	13
Children in diapers	8
Poor maintenance, inadequate treatment or operation of swimming or wading pool	9
Bather overload or crowding	3
Floods	1
Livestock	1
Geese	2
Seepage or overflow of sewage	3
Total	40

ation (e.g., inadequate chlorination or filtration, excessive application of pool chemicals) were identified in 9 (60%) of 16 outbreaks associated with swimming or wading pools. Fecal accidents and use of pools by diaper-age children were suspected or identified in 6 (40%) outbreaks. Outbreaks associated with lakes, ponds, rivers, canals, and other waters used for recreational purposes were caused by a variety of problems. Fecal accidents and sick bathers were responsible for 9 (43%) of 21 lakewater-associated outbreaks. Other suspected causes included contamination from diapers (19%), animal waste contamination (14%), sewage contamination of the bathing area (14%), and overcrowding of bathers (10%). Flood waters contaminated a canal that was used by children for swimming in one outbreak. In the remaining two outbreaks with information about contamination, diaper-age children playing in spray fountain pools were suspected to be sources of contamination. In the 12 outbreaks where fecal accidents were identified or suspected, 5 outbreaks were caused by *E. coli* O 157:H7 and 3 were caused by *Shigella*; the remaining outbreaks were caused by *Cryptosporidium* (2), Norwalk-like virus (1), and an undetermined agent (1). In the 8 outbreaks where diaper-age children were suspected sources of contamination, outbreaks were caused by *Cryptosporidium* (3), *Shigella* (3), and undetermined agents (2).

10.4 DISCUSSION

10.4.1 Waterborne Outbreaks and Deficiencies in Public Water Systems

Almost half of the outbreaks reported in public water systems were attributed to inadequate or no treatment of groundwater. Distribution system deficiencies caused almost one-fourth of the outbreaks in public systems. Inadequate or no filtration of surfacewater caused less than 10% of outbreaks reported in public systems. Although coliforms were found during the investigation of 46% of community and 83% of non-community system outbreaks, surveillance records showed that only 22% of community and 9% of non-community systems that experienced outbreaks had violated the EPA's coliform limit in the 12-month period before the outbreak. Thus, meeting the EPA's coliform limits may not provide a good indication of the potential for an outbreak.

10.4.1.1 Groundwater Systems

Most outbreaks in groundwater systems were associated with contaminated, untreated groundwater (32%) and inadequate or interrupted disinfection (32%). These two deficiencies were also responsible for most (74%) of the illnesses reported in groundwater outbreaks. In community groundwater systems, inadequate or no water treatment was responsible for 41% of the outbreaks and 70% of the illnesses reported. In non-community groundwater systems, 40% of the outbreaks were caused by inadequate water disinfection; these outbreaks were responsible for 78% of the illnesses reported. Adequate, continuous disinfection of groundwater is required to reduce the occurrence of outbreaks, particularly for small systems where intermittent contamination of wells and springs is difficult to detect or prevent. Wells and springs should also be protected from sources of contamination such as surface runoff, septic tank effluents, and sewage discharges. Periodic sanitary surveys, along with appropriate corrective measures and a hydrogeologic assessment, can help identify systems with the highest possibility of fecal contamination. The EPA has proposed requirements for sanitary surveys,[16] disinfection of groundwater, and source water monitoring for *E. coli,* coliphage, or enterococci.

10.4.1.2 Distribution System Contamination

Twenty-five waterborne outbreaks in public water systems were attributed to contaminants that entered the distribution system; 17 of these occurred in community systems. Eight (47%) of 17 distribution system outbreaks in community systems and 5 (63%) of eight outbreaks in non-community systems were associated with cross-connections or problems with backflow prevention devices (i.e., they had not been installed, had been inappropriately installed, or had been inadequately maintained). Other outbreaks were caused by contaminants entering through mains and storage facilities or leaching of metals from plumbing and pipes because of corrosive water. Increased attention should be paid to maintaining the integrity of the distribution system, reducing corrosion byproducts, and preventing contamination from cross-connections and backsiphonage, inadequately protected storage reservoirs and tanks, and the repair and construction of water mains. The maintenance of a chlorine residual throughout the system can help protect against some sources of distribution system contamination and warn of potential contamination. When decreased residual levels are detected in a routine monitoring program, water system operators should initiate investigations to identify sources of contamination.

10.4.1.3 Protozoan Outbreaks

In recent years, there have been decreased reports of cryptosporidiosis outbreaks caused by contaminated surfacewater and increased reports of outbreaks in groundwater systems. Outbreaks of giardiasis continue to be associated with both surface- and groundwater systems. During 1991 to 1994, four of seven outbreaks of cryptosporidiosis and five of nine outbreaks of giardiasis were associated with groundwater contamination. Two giardiasis outbreaks were reported in 1995; one occurred in a filtered, disinfected surfacewater system and the other in an unfiltered surfacewater system. In 1997 and 1998, three outbreaks were caused by *Giardia*; one occurred in a chlorinated, unfiltered surfacewater system and two in wellwater systems. No waterborne outbreaks during 1995 to 1997 were attributed to *Cryptosporidium*; two outbreaks in 1998 were caused by sewage contamination of well water.

Giardia and *Cryptosporidium* continue to pose waterborne risks in the United States, and the occurrence of outbreaks in groundwater systems emphasizes the importance of assessing the potential for contamination of groundwater by sewage and surfacewater. Groundwater sources contaminated by protozoa are considered to be under the direct influence of surfacewater and are subject to the filtration requirements of the Surface Water Treatment Rule (SWTR).[13] The continued occurrence of giardiasis outbreaks in surface water systems emphasizes the importance of requiring water systems to meet turbidity standards and other provisions of the SWTR.[13] More stringent EPA regulations for acceptable turbidity values for surfacewater systems have become effective since the Milwaukee outbreak in 1993,[14,19] and many water utilities have joined the Partnership For Safe Water,[20] which helps treatment plants consistently achieve good removal of microbes and turbidity.

10.4.1.4 Outbreaks and Coliforms

Water contamination was documented in the majority of systems during the outbreak investigation. During outbreak investigations in 1991 to 1998, total coliforms were detected in 69% of the outbreaks reported and in 52 and 87% of outbreaks in community and non-community systems, respectively. These findings are similar to those reported in previous studies.[17,18] During 1983 to 1992, coliforms were detected in the investigation of 73% of outbreaks reported. In both 1991–1998 and 1983–1992, coliforms were detected during most of the outbreaks caused by bacteria and unidentified agents, but during relatively few outbreaks caused by protozoa.

Water samples collected during or just after a contamination event that results in an outbreak may not be applicable to the utility of routine monitoring required by the TCR to identify water systems that may be vulnerable to waterborne outbreaks because water sampling was frequently more intensive. Also, water samples were usually collected within 2 to 4 weeks after the contamination event. In some investigations, contamination was sufficiently large that a single sample was positive for coliforms. In other investigations, no coliforms were detected even though a large number of samples were collected, emphasizing that water contamination sufficient to cause an outbreak can be short-lived. Thus, the timing of sample collection, as well as the number of samples collected, should be considered when developing routine monitoring protocols.

As noted earlier, few public water systems that reported an outbreak had exceeded total coliform limits in the 12 months before the outbreak. The EPA's TCR requires the collection of a minimal number of water samples for small community and non-community systems. For example, for community systems that serve 1000 or fewer persons only a single coliform sample must be collected each month. For systems serving 1001 to 4900 persons, only 2 to 5 samples per month are required. A large or continuous source of contamination would be necessary to detect coliforms during routine monitoring when so few samples are collected. One, or even five coliform samples collected during the month will not likely detect short-lived, intermittent contamination events.

10.4.2 Recreational Water

The unintentional ingestion of a single mouthful of contaminated water while swimming can cause illness, even in non-outbreak settings.[22,23] Most recreational outbreaks occurred while swimming in lakes and swimming pools and were caused primarily by either bather overload, fecal accidents, or children in diapers. Swimming pool outbreaks were associated with inadequate treatment and poor maintenance and operation. Outbreaks attributed to bacteria were associated primarily with fresh water (i.e., lakes). In contrast, most of the outbreaks caused by *Cryptosporidium* and *Giardia* were associated with chlorinated, filtered pool water.

The EPA has published criteria for evaluating the quality of both marine and fresh water used for recreation.[21,24] Fresh and marine waters are subject to contamination from sewage discharges, watershed runoff from agricultural and residential areas, and floods. Microbial monitoring has been recommended for recreational areas potentially contaminated by sewage. Overt fecal accidents and soiled bodies can also cause fecal contamination of the water; however, the utility of routinely monitoring water for fecal contamination caused by bathers has not been established. Efforts have focused on providing adequate toilet and diaper-changing facilities at recreational areas, requiring showers before bathing, and limiting the number of bathers. Although difficult to enforce, an important measure is to prevent persons, especially young children, from entering recreational waters if they are experiencing or convalescing from a diarrheal illness. Limiting the amount of water forced into the nasal passages during jumping or diving (e.g., holding the nose or wearing nose plugs) could reduce the risk for primary amebic meningoencephalitis.

Cryptosporidium and *Giardia* are resistant to disinfection at levels generally used in swimming pools, and some pool filtration systems might not be effective in removing oocysts. Even pools with filters and disinfection practices capable of removing or killing these parasites may require several hours to completely recirculate the pool water once it becomes contaminated. Swimmers remain at risk until all of the water is recirculated through an effective water treatment process.

10.5 CONCLUSIONS

Although the reporting of outbreaks is incomplete, waterborne outbreak surveillance data can identify the types of water systems, their deficiencies, and the respective etiological agents associated with the outbreaks, and thus the surveillance is useful for evaluating the adequacy of current source water protection strategies, water treatment technologies, drinking and recreational water regulations, and for influencing research priorities. Because the surveillance system is voluntary and does not include data for sporadic cases of disease that may be waterborne, the statistics do not reflect the true incidence of waterborne outbreaks or disease, and observed trends in the occurrence of waterborne outbreaks may be a reflection of surveillance activities of local and state health agencies.

REFERENCES

1. Barwick, R.S. et al., Surveillance for waterborne-disease outbreaks — United States, 1997–1998, *MMWR*, 49 (No. SS-4), 1, 2000.
2. Levy, D.A. et al., Surveillance for waterborne-disease outbreaks — United States, 1995–1996, *MMWR*, 47 (No. SS-5), 1, 1998.
3. Kramer, M.H. et al., Surveillance for waterborne-disease outbreaks — United States, 1993–1994, *MMWR,* 45 (No. SS-1), 1, 1996.
4. Moore, A.C. et al., Surveillance for waterborne disease outbreaks — United States, 1991–1992, *MMWR,* 42 (No. SS-5), 1, 1993.
5. Herwaldt et al., Waterborne-disease outbreaks, 1989–1990, *MMWR,* 40 (No. SS-3), 1, 1991.
6. Craun, G.F., Ed., *Methods for the Investigation and Prevention of Waterborne Disease Outbreaks*, U.S. Environmental Protection Agency, EPA publication no. 600/1–90/005a, Cincinnati, OH, 1990.
7. 40 CFR Parts 141 and 142, Drinking water: national primary drinking water regulations; total coliforms (including fecal coliforms and *E. coli*); final rule, *Fed. Reg.*, 54, 27544, 1989.
8. 40 CFR Parts 141 and 142, Drinking water: national primary drinking water regulations; total coliforms; corrections and technical amendments; final rule, *Fed. Reg.*, 55, 25064, 1990.
9. 40 CFR Part 141, Water programs: national interim primary drinking water regulations, *Fed. Reg.*, 40, 59566, 1975.
10. Pontius, F.W. and Roberson, J.A., The current regulatory agenda: an update, *J. Am. Water Works Assoc.,* 86, 54, 1994.
11. Pontius, F.W., Implementing the 1996 SDWA amendments, *J. Am. Water Works Assoc.,* 89, 18, 1997.
12. 40 CFR Parts 141 and 142, Drinking water: national primary drinking water regulations; filtration, disinfection; turbidity, *Giardia lamblia*, viruses, Legionella, and heterotrophic bacteria; final rule. *Fed. Reg.*, 54, 27486, 1989.
13. U.S. Environmental Protection Agency, Guidance Manual for Compliance with the Filtration and Disinfection Requirements for Public Water Systems Using Surface Water Sources, Contract No. 68–01–6989, Washington, D.C., 1991.
14. 40 CFR Parts 141 and 142, National primary drinking water regulations: enhanced surface water treatment requirements; proposed rule, *Fed. Reg.*, 59, 38832, 1994.
15. 40 CFR Part 141, National primary drinking water regulations: monitoring requirements for public drinking water supplies: *Cryptosporidium, Giardia*, viruses, disinfection byproducts, water treatment plant data and other information requirements; proposed rule, *Fed. Reg.*, 59, 6332, 1994.
16. U.S. Environmental Protection Agency, Ground Water Rule Deliberative Document, Washington, D.C., November 23, 1999.
17. Craun, G.F., Berger, P.S., and Calderon, R.L., Coliform bacteria and waterborne disease outbreaks, *J. Am. Water Works Assoc.,* 89(3), 96, 1997.
18. Batik, O., Craun, G.F., and Pipes, W.O., Routine coliform monitoring and waterborne disease outbreaks, *J. Environ. Health*, 45, 227, 1983.
19. MacKenzie, W.R. et al., A massive outbreak in Milwaukee of *Cryptosporidium* infection transmitted through the public water supply, *N. Engl. J. Med.*, 331, 161, 1994.
20. Renner, R.C. and Hegg, B.A., Self-assessment guide for surface water treatment plant optimization, American Water Works Association Research Foundation, catalog no. 90736, Denver, CO, 1997.
21. Dufour, A.P., *Health Effects Criteria for Fresh Recreational Waters*, U.S. Environmental Protection Agency, EPA publication no. 600/1–84–004, Research Triangle Park, NC, 1984.
22. Calderon, R.L., Mood, E.W., and Dufour, A.P., Health effects of swimmers and nonpoint sources of contaminated water, *Int. J. Environ. Health Res.*, 1, 21, 1991.
23. Seyfried, P.L. et al., A prospective study of swimming-related illness. I. Swimming-associated health risk, *Am. J. Public Health*, 75, 1068, 1985.
24. Cabelli, V.J., *Health Effects Criteria for Marine Recreational Waters*, U.S. Environmental Protection Agency, EPA publication 600/1–80–031, Research Triangle Park, NC, 1983.

11 *Cryptosporidium* in England and Wales

Mike Waite and Peter Jiggins

CONTENTS

11.1 Introduction....119
11.2 Early Regulatory Framework....120
11.2.1 Applicability of the Early Regulations to Outbreaks of Cryptosporidiosis....122
11.3 New Regulations on *Cryptosporidium* in Water....122
11.3.1 1995 Torbay Cryptosporidiosis Outbreak....122
11.3.2 Legislative Response to the Torbay Outbreak....123
11.3.3 Experience with New Regulatory Approach....124
11.4 Conclusions....125
References....125

11.1 INTRODUCTION

As was discussed in Chapter 5, outbreak investigations can have far-reaching effects on society. This chapter is effectively about the impact of an outbreak on water quality legislation within the United Kingdom (U.K.). It also illustrates the potential use of outbreak reports.

The first outbreak of cryptosporidiosis in the U.K. in which public drinking water supplies were recognized as being implicated occurred in 1988 in Scotland. Shortly after that outbreak there was a large outbreak in England, peaking in early 1989, affecting parts of Oxfordshire and Wiltshire. In that outbreak there were over 500 laboratory-confirmed cases and possibly as many as 5000 cases in total. Up to June 2000 there have been around 30 cryptosporidiosis outbreaks where the public water supply possibly has been implicated. At the time of the first outbreaks, water supply was mostly in the public sector, although there were a number of long-established private companies supplying the public with drinking water. England and Wales were served by 10 regional water Authorities, which were largely based on river catchments. Their primary responsibility was for the unified management of the water cycle — that is to say, the supply of drinking water; the collection and treatment of sewage; the quality of rivers and the drainage of land into those rivers; and abstractions of water from rivers, lakes, and underground. The legislative framework did not provide specifically for punitive sanctions in the event of outbreaks of waterborne disease as it might reasonably have been presumed that the public sector acted in the best interests of the public at all times. This legislative weakness was highlighted when a large amount of aluminum sulphate was accidentally added to the public water supply in Camelford southwest of England in 1989. It became apparent that it was possible under water-related legislation at that time to prosecute successfully the responsible water authority for the impact of the discharged water on fish in a watercourse, but not for its effect on those who consumed it.

0-8493-1259-0/03/$0.00+$1.50

11.2 EARLY REGULATORY FRAMEWORK

With the passing of the 1989 Water Act, most of the responsibilities of the Regional Water Authorities in England and Wales were transferred to new private companies.[1] In addition to the transfer of responsibilities, the act made a number of other changes to the law that were intended to protect the interests of the public:

1. Created a new offense of suppling water that is unfit for human consumption, which was intended to remedy the weakness demonstrated by the events at Camelford.
2. Three regulatory bodies were established for England and Wales with broad responsibilities:
   a. Office of Water Services (OFWAT): financial regulation of the water industry.
   b. National Rivers Authority (NRA) (later to become part of the Environment Agency): quality of surface- and groundwaters and control of abstraction from and discharge to waters.
   c. Drinking Water Inspectorate (DWI): quality of drinking water supplies.

The act bestowed powers and imposed duties on the secretary of state, as well as empowering him to appoint technical assessors to act on his behalf in respect to matters relating to drinking water quality. The DWI was established to carry out that role. (Subsequent references to the DWI in this chapter should be read as referring to the powers or duties of the secretary of state as administered by DWI on his behalf.)

Under the power to make regulations given to the secretary of state under Section 65 of the act, the Water Supply (Water Quality) Regulations 1989 were made.[2] These regulations, which have since been the subject of a number of amendments,[3–7] gave effect to the requirements of the relevant EC Directive on the quality of water intended for human consumption, as well as imposing a number of national standards.[8] Contravention of the regulations is not an offense, but DWI has a duty to initiate enforcement action unless any contravention is considered trivial or is unlikely to occur again. Enforcement action by the DWI need not proceed if the water company gives a legal undertaking to take steps to remedy the contravention in the shortest practicable time.

The Water Act 1989 was replaced in 1991 by a number of separate acts, the regulation of the water companies being contained in the Water Industry Act 1991 (WIA), which presently remains in force.[9]

In addition, the secretary of state issued the Water Undertakers (Information) Direction 1990 (the Information Direction), which requires water companies to provide a range of information necessary for the DWI to determine whether the companies were complying with their duties under the regulations.[10] This direction, which is a legally enforceable instrument, was reissued and updated in 1992 and again in 1998.[11,12] As well as requiring the provision of information regarding sampling and analysis, it requires notification of events related to drinking water quality, as detailed in Table 11.1, to the DWI.

The nature of the information required is shown in Table 11.2.

The direction also requires a full report within 1 month of the event, which must contain at least the information specified in Table 11.3.

With this information the DWI carries out a full investigation to determine whether the company has contravened Section 70 of the WIA, and, if so, whether it is likely to be able to demonstrate the statutory defense of having taken "all reasonable steps and exercised all due diligence for securing that the water was fit for human consumption." The DWI then institutes proceedings where appropriate. It also determines whether the company has contravened any of its enforceable duties under the regulations or the information direction, and initiates enforcement action where necessary.

To facilitate these investigations, the DWI may obtain reports from local authorities, health authorities, the Environment Agency, the incident management team, and, when one is convened, the outbreak control team (see below).

TABLE 11.1
Notification Requirements of the Water Undertakers (Information) Direction 1992

- Any event which, by reason of its effect or likely effect on the quality ... of drinking water supplied by it, gives rise, or is likely to give rise, to a significant risk to the health of persons to whom the water is supplied.
- Any other matter relating to the supply of water which:
  1. Is of national significance
  2. Or has attracted ... significant national or local publicity
  3. Or ... has caused, or is likely to cause, significant concern to persons to whom the water is supplied
- Notification must be by telephone, fax, or e-mail as soon as possible, and in writing within 72 hours of first notification.

TABLE 11.2
Water Undertakers (Information) Direction 1992 Requires a Report within 72 Hours Which Must Include:

- Particulars of the event
- Assessment of likely effect on water quality
- Any information available as to cause
- Particulars of actions taken or proposed
- List of person notified (other than customers)
- Copies of any press notices issued

TABLE 11.3
Water Undertakers (Information) Direction 1992 Requires a Full Report Within 1 Month, Which Must Include:

- Update on information required in the 72-hour report
- Details of any sampling carried out
- Copies of any reports provided to the water company by its medical, scientific, or technical advisors, any local authority and district health authority
- Assessment of the effectiveness of actions taken and of liaison with the local authority, district health authority, emergency services, and the public
- Statement of proposals, if any, for further actions identified as necessary or desirable in light of the event
- Any other relevant information

At the conclusion of the DWI's investigations, it notifies the company, local authorities, and other interested parties of its findings and where it considers there are lessons to be learned, which may be of general importance, it conveys these to all water companies. It may also publish a full public report on major incidents.

11.2.1 Applicability of the Early Regulations to Outbreaks of Cryptosporidiosis

Following the 1989 cryptosporidiosis outbreak, a committee of experts was set up to advise on steps to be taken to minimize the risk of waterborne outbreaks of cryptosporidiosis and the management of outbreaks when they occur. The reports were aimed not only at water companies, but also at local authorities and health professionals. This committee under the chairmanship of Sir John Badenoch produced its first report in July 1990 (Badenoch 1) and a second report in 1995 (Badenoch 2).[13,14] Following the death of Badenoch, the committee produced a third report in 1998 under the chairmanship of Professor Ian Bouchier.[15] These reports have no legal standing, but water companies were encouraged and expected to follow their recommendations, and the DWI carried out inspections to confirm that companies were doing so.

However, there were no standards relating specifically to *Cryptosporidium* other than the so-called "catch-all" regulation 3(3)(a), which specified that for water to be wholesome it must not "contain any element, organism, or substance (other than a parameter) at a concentration or value which would be detrimental to public health." Not being a parameter, there was no requirement to monitor water supplies for *Cryptosporidium*, although some monitoring by spot samples did take place. In the event of the detection of *Cryptosporidium* oocysts in a public water supply, it would have been a matter of expert opinion as to whether the numbers detected in the water would be detrimental to public health.

Among the many recommendations of the committee of experts in its first report was the establishment of an outbreak control team (OCT) in each health authority area. The OCT should be chaired by the relevant director of public health or his nominee, normally the consultant in communicable disease control (CCDC), with representatives of the water company, directors of environmental health, a consultant microbiologist, and the area control of infection nurse. Other experts should be co-opted as necessary. Whenever there is evidence of increased levels of cryptosporidiosis in the community, the OCT should be convened and initiate investigations. These investigations should include an epidemiological investigation into the possible source of the infections.

It was anticipated by the DWI and others that in the event of an outbreak of cryptosporidiosis which was shown by the epidemiological investigations of the OCT to be strongly associated with water supply, the expert report would form the basis of evidence in support of any subsequent prosecution.

11.3 NEW REGULATIONS ON *CRYPTOSPORIDIUM* IN WATER

11.3.1 1995 Torbay Cryptosporidiosis Outbreak

An outbreak of cryptosporidiosis occurred in August and September, 1995. The outbreak was recognized by an increase in the number of confirmed cases of the disease being reported by microbiology laboratories in parts of South and West Devon. The CCDC convened the OCT as soon as the outbreak was recognized and an epidemiological study was planned and executed. Because the outbreak was in a popular holiday area around the town of Torquay, many of the cases occurred in persons who were not local residents and had returned home in the incubation period of the disease, becoming ill after their return (see Chapter 12). Therefore, it was necessary to collect data from laboratories throughout the country.

It was decided at the outset that a case–control study was neither practical nor necessary and a descriptive study was carried out. It was apparent from the beginning that cases showed an association with water supplies from Littlehempston Water Treatment Works. By the end of the outbreak there had been 575 cases identified, of which 500 completed questionnaires, usually by telephone interview, but in some instances during home visits. Of these, 479 met the case definition and were analyzed. Because some areas were served by Littlehempston water alone, others received a blended mixture, and yet others received no Littlehempston water at all, it was possible to calculate a relative risk and trend, and both the relative risk of 9.8 and the trend were shown to be significant at $p < .0000001$.

Oocysts were also detected in the treated water from Littlehempston Treatment Works. The DWI concluded that there were aspects of the operation of the treatment process that could be criticized and the company was unlikely to be able to demonstrate that it had exercised all due diligence, as there had been particularly an earlier outbreak in 1992 in the same area in which an association with Littlehempston water was suggested by an epidemiological study, which was not robust.

The DWI carried out its own assessment of the incident and initiated a prosecution, taking the OCT report as evidence that water unfit for human consumption had been supplied and the case went to the Crown Court in September 1997.[16] The OCT report and, in particular, the epidemiological study were not produced for the purpose of prosecution, but solely as part of managing and understanding the outbreak. Nevertheless, it was believed that the report could be presented in evidence, as it was scientifically sound and reached very clear conclusions.

The presiding judge considered arguments regarding the admissibility of the report and ruled that in order for it to be accepted, the defense would have to have the opportunity to controvert every single piece of information used. To be able to do that, every single piece of information used in the compilation of the OCT report would have to be available in evidence and to be supported by signed statements, so that the persons responsible were open to questioning by the defense. This would have meant that for every diagnosed case a complete chain of signed statements from the general practitioner who saw the patient, through the laboratory analysis to the reporting of the result, and, hence, through to the completion of the questionnaire by the patient and its subsequent handling and processing would have to be presented. This had not been done and to do it would have been almost impossible — every patient would have had to waive medical confidentiality and agree to give evidence in court if required. The judge, therefore, using the discretion allowed to him, ruled the report inadmissible. No further evidence was given and the company was acquitted of all charges.

A further problem, which was not tested, is that for a successful conviction it is necessary to prove beyond reasonable doubt that an offense was committed. In this case, the alleged offense was of supplying water that was unfit for human consumption through pipes to premises. Had the report been accepted, it could have proved that some of the water supplied had for some of the time been unfit as evidenced by the cases. However, it was necessary to prove that an individual premises had been supplied with unfit water and that an individual had suffered in consequence. As there were 479 cases meeting the case definition for whom questionnaires had been completed, there were potentially 479 individual offenses. A number of sample cases had been brought, and each one would have to be considered by the court in isolation.

The normal incidence of cryptosporidiosis in the area at that time of the year was 15 cases, and in the outbreak there were approximately 500 cases. It follows that any individual case had a 15 in 500, or 3%, chance of being part of the normal seasonal incidence. It is unlikely that the court would accept a 3% possibility of no association with drinking water as establishing beyond reasonable doubt that any individual case was directly caused by drinking water. Therefore, it is likely that even if 479 charges had been brought, in no individual case could it have been shown beyond reasonable doubt that the water was responsible for the infection.

It appeared that the regulatory framework was not adequate to enable successful prosecution for the supply of water unfit for human consumption by virtue of causing cases of a disease which was endemic in the population.

11.3.2 Legislative Response to the Torbay Outbreak

It was clearly unacceptable to have a situation in which it was relatively straightforward to secure conviction of a water company for supplying water rejected by consumers on the grounds of discoloration, but not when water supplied gave rise to cryptosporidiosis. It was considered that it would not be realistic for an epidemiological study in the event of a future large outbreak, such as Torbay, to meet the standards of evidence as indicated by the judge. An alternative approach was required to restore public confidence in the regulation of water companies.

It is obvious that for cryptosporidiosis to be contracted from drinking water, oocysts must be present in the water. It was decided then that it should be made an offense not to achieve a suitably low level of oocysts in a water supply, regardless of whether any disease could be shown to ensue. It is recognized that conventional treatment cannot be guaranteed to remove all oocysts and that a zero standard would therefore be unrealistic. Also, there is insufficient data available at this time to set an acceptable concentration of oocysts based on likely health effects. For those reasons it was decided to set a treatment standard which should be capable of being met by any conventional treatment plant operating correctly. In addition, such evidence as was available suggested that events leading to the passage of significant numbers of oocysts through treatment were frequently of short duration and, thus, likely to be missed by spot sampling. New regulations regarding *Cryptosporidium* (Regulations 23A and 23B) were added to the regulations by means of the Water Supply (Water Quality) (Amendment) Regulations 1999.[7]

These new regulations required water companies to carry out a risk assessment for all water sources to determine if there was a risk of *Cryptosporidium* oocysts being present in water entering the supply, and submit that assessment to the DWI. The DWI has accepted that any works in which all the water passes through sufficient treatment plant capable of removing or retaining all particles greater than 1 micron, and where this process is subject to continuous monitoring and shutdown on failure, will not require continuous monitoring for oocysts. Where that assessment established a risk, the water company had to submit a program of works to ensure compliance with the new treatment standard and to institute a program of monitoring and reporting to demonstrate compliance with it. The new treatment standard is that a continuous sample at a flow rate of not less than 40 liters/h shall be taken each day and, when analyzed in accordance with the specified regulatory procedures, shall not be shown to contain more than an average of 1 oocyst/10 liters.

These new additional regulations came into force on June 30, 1999 with risk assessments to be completed by October 1, 1999, programs submitted by January 31, 2000, and monitoring to start on April 1, 2000. Because of the way the regulations were drafted, water companies were not legally obliged to institute continuous monitoring until any treatment enhancements deemed necessary had been implemented. Nevertheless, many companies instituted monitoring before they were required to and provided details of their operational sampling to the DWI. (The 1985 EC Drinking Water Directive was replaced in 1998 and new Water Supply [Water Quality] Regulations were made in December 2000 to give effect to the new directive.[17,18] These regulations retained the requirements in respect to the treatment standard, risk assessment, and continuous monitoring for *Cryptosporidium*.)

11.3.3 Experience with New Regulatory Approach

Of the 1388 water treatment works in use in 2000, 332 were identified as being at risk. Of these, 95 were either abandoned or "mothballed," while of the remainder, compliance monitoring was in place at 155 waterworks by June 2001 and operational sampling was being carried out at the other 82.

The regulations lay down stringent requirements covering sampling and analysis to ensure that results of analysis are acceptable as evidence in a court of law.

Between April 1, 2000 and June 30, 2001, 63,798 samples were analyzed and oocysts were detected in 4320 (6.8%) of these, the positive samples being taken from 108 different sites. Of the positive samples, 93.6% were found to have no more than 0.1 oocysts in 10 liters, and only 7 samples, from only 2 sites, breached the standard of 1 oocyst in 10 liters. The highest concentration found was 4.91 oocysts in 10 liters. A small but significant number of samples initially reported as contravening the treatment standard were subsequently shown not to have contained *Cryptosporidium*. In none of the instances in which the treatment standard was exceeded was there any evidence of lack of diligence. Since the new regulatory regime was instituted, in no instance, where there has been continuous monitoring of a treatment works, has there been any evidence of cases of cryptosporidiosis in which the treatment works has been implicated.

This new monitoring requirement will ensure that in the event of any future outbreak of cryptosporidiosis associated with a water treatment works there will be real-time data available regarding oocysts in the supply at the time infection probably occurred. It will also provide valuable data regarding the extent of exposure to *Cryptosporidium* via public drinking water supplies.

11.4 CONCLUSIONS

There is a reasonable public expectation that there should be effective punitive sanctions available against private companies that fail in their duty of care, causing the public to suffer in consequence. This expectation extends to water supply companies. It was considered that the 1989 Water Act made adequate provisions by creating the offense of supplying water unfit for human consumption, but when this was tested in the courts it proved wanting because of the difficulties in meeting the legal standard of proof. Information which is perfectly adequate for an epidemiological study need not be adequate for presentation in court, and to obtain information suitable for legal presentation may well prejudice the epidemiological study. Patient cooperation may well be reduced if there is the possibility of being required to give evidence in court. To remedy this, new regulations were made which required compliance with a treatment standard of less than an average of 1 oocyst in 10 liters of water leaving a treatment works in any 24 hours. They also required continuous sampling at all treatment works where there was a perceived risk of oocysts being present in the treated water.

These new regulations have required water companies to take a close look at their sources and in many cases they have abandoned small sources which were seen as being at significant risk of containing oocysts. They have also obtained and developed expertise in the ecology, isolation, and enumeration of *Cryptosporidium* oocysts. The monitoring programs are also capable of providing information about the occurrence of *Giardia* in water supplies. The outcome of this enforced change in legislative approach has been that water companies' attention is very much focused on *Cryptosporidium,* and a valuable database of the frequency and extent of occurrence of *Cryptosporidium* oocysts in water supplies is accumulating. It is also perhaps not coincidental that since the advent of the new regulation there have been no outbreaks of cryptosporidiosis in which public water supplies have been implicated. In the event of future such outbreaks, information should be available concerning numbers of oocysts entering a supply at the time infections were contracted rather than only from the time the outbreak was detected.

REFERENCES

1. Water Act 1989, HMSO, London, 1989.
2. Water Supply (Water Quality) Regulations 1989 — SI 1147, HMSO, London, 1989.
3. Water Supply (Water Quality) (Amendment) Regulations 1989 — SI 1384, HMSO, London, 1989.
4. Water Supply (Water Quality) (Amendment) Regulations 1991 — SI 1837, HMSO, London, 1991.
5. Water Supply (Water Quality) (Amendment) Regulations 1991 — SI 2790, HMSO, London, 1991.
6. Water Supply (Water Quality) (Amendment) Regulations 1996 — SI 3001, HMSO, London, 1996.
7. Water Supply (Water Quality) (Amendment) Regulations 1999 — SI 1524, Stationery Office, London, 1999.
8. Council Directive 80/778/EEC of 15 July 1980 relating to the quality of water intended for human consumption, *Official J. Eur. Comm.*, L229, 11, 1980.
9. Water Industry Act 1991, HMSO, London, 1991.
10. Water Undertakers Information Direction 1990, HMSO, London, 1990.

11. Water Undertakers Information Direction 1992, HMSO, London, 1992.
12. Water Undertakers Information Direction 1998, Stationery Office, London, 1998.
13. Badenoch, J., *Cryptosporidium* in Water Supplies, Report of the group of experts, HMSO, London, 1990.
14. Badenoch, J., *Cryptosporidium* in Water Supplies, Second report of the group of experts, HMSO, London, 1995.
15. Bouchier, I., *Cryptosporidium* in Water Supplies, Third report of the group of experts, HMSO, London, 1998.
16. Waite, W.M., Assessment of Water Supply and Associated Matters in Relation to the Incidence of Cryptosporidiosis in Torbay in August and September 1995, Report of the Drinking Water Inspectorate, London, 1997.
17. Council Directive 98/83/EEC of 13 November 1998 on the quality of water intended for human consumption, *Off. J. Eur. Comm.*, L330, 32, 1998.
18. Water Supply (Water Quality) Regulations 2000 — SI 3184, Stationery Office, London, 2000.

Section 3

Investigation of Sporadic Waterborne Disease

Jamie Bartram

INTRODUCTION

The final section of the book focuses on waterborne disease transmission outside of detected or detectable "outbreaks." As has already been noted in the general introduction to this book, waterborne disease is among the top rank of disease burden globally and this burden of disease is concentrated on children and the poor. A common theme that emerged from several of the chapters in this section is that a large proportion, and probably the vast majority, of waterborne disease burden arises outside of detected outbreaks. This statement contrasts with the view, predominant until only a few years ago and still periodically heard, that the failure to detect outbreaks of waterborne disease illustrates that this route of disease transmission is largely conquered in industrialized countries.

Some authors in this section also explore the use to which resulting information might be put. These include: demonstrating association of a disease or pathogen transmission with a route of exposure; assessing population dose-response; direct testing of interventions; standard setting; identifying areas requiring management attention; and contributing to understanding the local, national, or global burden of disease (and thereby contributing to policy development). Understanding of both disease burden and the cost-effectiveness of interventions is increasingly called for to guide policymaking in industrialized countries and has much to offer in making the best use of limited resources in developing countries.

Quality of data and information is a recurrent theme in this section. The failure to consider intended use during study design is seen as a significant problem and was emphasized quite strongly at the Basingstoke meeting. Each of the methods discussed in this section has its strengths and weaknesses. No one method is best in all situations, and each approach has a particular value and purpose for waterborne disease epidemiology. The idea of "suitability for purpose" as the key criteria for quality demands on data and information repeatedly arises. A common concern emerging in several chapters and discussions relates to the design of studies to provide usable information. A general sense emerges that much supportive evidence of limited direct use was and continues to be produced. The general conclusion supports the need to concentrate resources on studies of suitable quality, designed to produce data for specific uses and targeted upon key "information poor" areas.

The point is made very clearly in Chapter 12 that outbreak-related cases probably represent a relatively small proportion of waterborne disease burden. This chapter addresses the contribution that improved analysis of data from existing surveillance systems can make to understanding waterborne disease. The chapter emphasizes the importance of waterborne transmission of one particular pathogen, *Cryptosporidium*. It also highlights the potentially large proportion of all cases of this organism that are associated with clusters (36%). Only very few of these clusters were identified as outbreaks and investigated at the times they occurred. Many of these clusters of cases may represent undetected waterborne outbreaks. This chapter, as well as several of the other chapters in this section, suggest that the term "sporadic" for such disease is a misnomer and that outbreak detection is unlikely to pick up other than large events.

Most of the remaining chapters in this section concern themselves with specific epidemiological approaches to the investigation of non-outbreak-related cases of infection that may be waterborne.

In Chapter 13, the authors describe the use of geographical information systems (GIS). The application of GIS allows the team to overlay the geographical distribution of cases and the characteristics of the water and the distribution system, and analyze the data to determine if any relationships exist between the variables. In order to make the best use of GIS, current and complete information on cases (e.g., postcodes), water quality (e.g., concentrations of *Escherichia coli*), and characteristics of the distribution system (e.g., water flows, pressures, etc.) must be available.

Chapter 14 describes the design of time series analyses, where changes in time of water quality data are compared with variation in measures of human illness. The most well-known example of this approach has been the association of cases of gastroenteritis in the community as measured by attendance at medical centers or sales of antidiarrheal drugs, with water turbidity.

Chapter 15 describes the contribution that sero-epidemiological studies are making to our understanding of waterborne disease. As they are being used in waterborne disease epidemiology, sero-epidemiological studies draw their conclusions by comparing the prevalence of antibodies to specific pathogens in different populations or in the same population at different times. As such, they are variations of the geographical and time series analyses discussed in the previous two chapters using antibody positivity as an indicator of past infection rather than other measures of current illness.

The three approaches discussed in Chapters 13 to 15 are effectively ecological studies that measure population rather than individual exposure to the risk factor and compare it in time or geographically with average incidence (or sero-prevalence) within the population. Because such studies do not generate information on exposure of individuals, such studies are potentially subject to bias because of the "ecological paradox." The focus of the following three chapters is on studies that investigate individuals.

Chapter 16 is the first chapter that uses more traditional analytical epidemiological studies and concentrates on case–control studies. Case–control studies have already been addressed in the context of outbreak investigations in Chapter 5. In the context of sporadic disease, case–control studies have a number of advantages in that they can provide information on the contribution of a wide range of risk factors to disease. On the other hand, it is usually only feasible to design case-control studies around single pathogens. Also, case–control studies depend on the efficiency of case ascertainment, and as such they are not really suitable for determining the total burden of disease due to drinking water, even for the particular pathogen under investigation.

The type of prospective study discussed in Chapter 17 can begin to address the issue of disease burden by recording illness in individuals. The individuals are usually chosen to allow comparisons of illness with individuals with different quality water supplies. Such studies can also allow the impact of changes in water quality on health to be addressed. However, it can be difficult in such studies to fully control for potential confounding variables.

Chapter 18 discusses the impact of intervention studies, where the impact of public health interventions on health is studied. Three types of intervention study are discussed. In the first type, the impact of prior interventions is studied, as in the impact of drinking bottled water during an outbreak of waterborne disease. This is, in effect, a variation on the case–control study design. The second type looks at the impact of implementing population-wide interventions, such as building a new treatment works, on health. As currently used, this is a form of ecological study and has many of the same potential problems as discussed in Chapters 13 and 14. The third type is the randomized controlled trial (RCT), where people are randomly chosen to receive a particular intervention such as a point of use filter, and then keep a diary recording their health. RCTs are generally believed to be the best measure of disease burden from drinking water. However, they are expensive to perform and can only detect common illnesses. Studies aimed at detecting the impact of interventions on specific waterborne pathogens would probably require far too many participants to be justifiable.

The final chapter (Chapter 19) broadens the focus once again away from waterborne disease in developed nations to waterborne disease in the developing world. This chapter initially considers the development of our understanding of the global burden of waterborne disease and its impact on children in developing nations. The chapter then discusses many of the additional problems facing the epidemiologist in designing epidemiological studies in developing nations. These difficulties include the multiplicity of water sources and the general background of poor sanitation in many areas. This chapter also points out the wider range of potential diseases, such as dracunculiasis and schistosomiasis, associated with water in developing nations.

12 Using Existing Surveillance-Based Data

Gordon Nichols

CONTENTS

12.1 Introduction.......131
12.2 *Cryptosporidium* Surveillance within England and Wales.......132
 12.2.1 Screening.......132
 12.2.2 Surveillance Data.......133
 12.2.3 Typing.......134
 12.2.4 Age Distribution.......134
 12.2.5 Clusters.......135
 12.2.6 Outbreak Surveillance.......136
 12.2.7 Seasonality.......137
 12.2.8 Regional Variations.......137
12.3 The Value of Surveillance.......138
References.......140

12.1 INTRODUCTION

Numerous approaches have been used to link water with disease. Routine surveillance, as with other techniques that can be used for linking water consumption with infection, has its advantages and disadvantages. Surveillance is a useful starting point to categorize the salient features of infectious diseases so that control and prevention strategies can be developed and implemented.

Infectious disease surveillance relies on two main elements: the microbiology and the epidemiology of the implicated organisms (Figure 12.1). The prerequisites of surveillance include the need to be aware that an organism exists, development of methods for demonstrating the presence of the organism, and adoption of these methods widely throughout the laboratory system. Once adopted, an adequate quality assurance scheme is necessary to ensure the consistency of laboratory testing. It is necessary to develop screening criteria to determine which specimens should be tested for the particular organism. The person who decides on the screening criteria for individual samples varies from country to country. In countries where private laboratories predominate, decisions about what tests should be conducted on a sample are often strongly clinician-driven. In countries with a predominantly publicly funded laboratory system, the laboratory may play a stronger role in deciding what tests should be performed. The policy and practice of general practitioners, in relation to sending fecal samples to laboratories, can vary substantially. Differences in the follow-up of infected patients and the family contacts by environmental health officers and others can also affect surveillance. It is important to have expertise and understanding of the organism being studied, and to develop suitable systems of confirmation and typing.

On the epidemiological side of surveillance, routine reporting criteria need to be established. There must be case reporting to local public health professionals and to a national surveillance

0-8493-1259-0/03/$0.00+$1.50

Microbiology

- Organism awareness
- Method development
- Method adoption
- Quality assurance
- Screening criteria
- Who decides on screening
- GP policy and practice
- EHO follow-up
- Expertise and understanding
- Confirmation and typing service

Epidemiology

- Routine reporting criteria
- Local reporting and surveillance
- National case reporting
- Outbreak detection, investigation, and reporting
- Enhanced surveillance
- Sentinel sites
- Analysis of outbreaks
- Expert groups/reports
- International activity

FIGURE 12.1 The elements of surveillance.

center. There also needs to be local and national assistance for detecting, investigating, and reporting outbreaks. A system for conducting enhanced surveillance where it is deemed to be useful is also necessary. In this respect, sentinel laboratories (laboratories that have a particular remit for the collection of surveillance data) can be invaluable. There needs to be a system for the analysis and reporting of outbreaks, and expert groups and reports can be useful. Finally, international surveillance and collaboration has proved valuable in building a wider understanding of the epidemiology of diarrheal diseases and further cooperative work on water-related disease will be useful in the future.

12.2 *CRYPTOSPORIDIUM* SURVEILLANCE WITHIN ENGLAND AND WALES

12.2.1 Screening

Although *Cryptosporidium* was first recognized as a human pathogen in 1976, it was not until the early 1980s that suitable staining techniques were developed which could be used to demonstrate *Cryptosporidium* oocysts in human fecal samples. In particular, the development of the modified Ziehl-Neelsen auramine and safranin methods led to an ability to screen large numbers of fecal samples rapidly.[1–3] Subsequent development of an FITC-labeled monoclonal antibody did not greatly improve human cryptosporidiosis surveillance because the method is more cumbersome and time-consuming than other staining methods for fecal screening.[4] It did, however, allow small numbers of oocysts to be detected in water samples, and surveillance of water supplies at significant risk of containing oocysts is now part of U.K. law (see Chapter 11). As with many newly described fecal pathogens, many people initially looked for the organism only in children.

However, it was soon clear that adults could also be infected and many laboratories started screening all fecal samples for this pathogen. A study of cryptosporidiosis in six laboratories was undertaken in 1987[5] and the results of this study were used to suggest screening criteria for all laboratories.[6] These have been developed and incorporated into the PHLS Standard Operating Procedure (B.SOP 30) that recommends "routine screening of all diagnostic stools for *Campylobacter, Salmonella, Shigella,* and *Cryptosporidium* species, and for *Escherichia coli* O157 of all diarrheal (semiformed or liquid) stools." The recommended methods are auramine phenol and modified Ziehl-Neelsen (B.SOP 31).[1,2]

12.2.2 Surveillance Data

Data on the surveillance of cryptosporidiosis in England and Wales shows a steady increase in reporting between 1983 and 1989 (Figure 12.2). This increase reflects the number of laboratories looking for and reporting *Cryptosporidium* cases to National Surveillance. Large waterborne outbreaks in 1989 were responsible for the high number of cases in that year and annual reporting rates have remained fairly stable since. Comparison of *Cryptosporidium* reporting with the reporting of other enteric pathogens shows a substantial increase in *Salmonella* and *Campylobacter* over this time period with little change in *Cryptosporidium* cases. Representation of the annual data hides a lot of detail on the seasonal occurrence of cryptosporidiosis (Figure 12.3). Broadly speaking, weekly data over this time period show a strongly seasonal trend with peaks of cases in the spring and autumn.

A number of elements to enteric pathogen surveillance exist within England and Wales (see Chapters 2 and 3). Routine surveillance data is generated through laboratory reports to the Communicable Disease Surveillance Centre (CDSC) in London. This contains both microbiological and epidemiological data. Outbreaks are investigated locally or in collaboration with national experts. Outbreak surveillance is conducted by sending out forms to public health physicians and environmental health officers, and collecting information on risk factors and other epidemiological data. With some enteric pathogens, clinical surveillance has been useful. This is true of hemolytic uremic syndrome associated with *E. coli* O157, where pediatric surveillance has been useful. Special studies are conducted at intervals on particular pathogens to try and gain information on risk factors and demographic data. Cases are now recorded in international databases for certain specific enteric pathogens (*Salmonella* and *E. coli* O157), allowing the detection of international outbreaks.[7–10] In addition to these exercises, a large study of infectious intestinal disease within the community was published recently.[11–13] This study included a general practice component involving 459,975 person

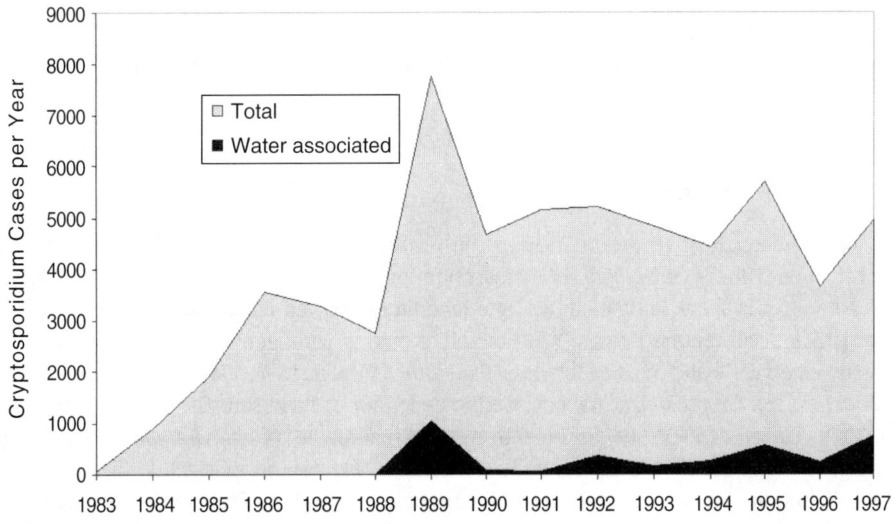

FIGURE 12.2 Cryptosporidiosis in England and Wales, 1983–1997.

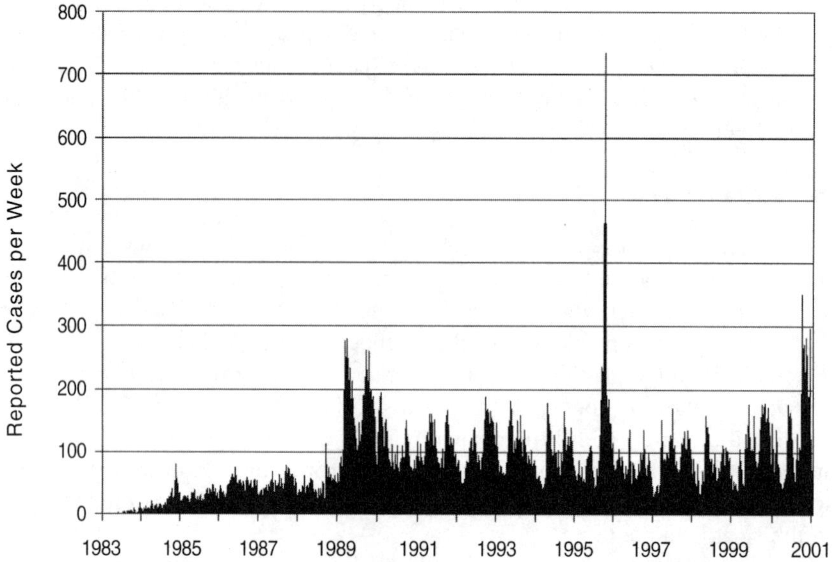

FIGURE 12.3 Cryptosporidium reports in England and Wales by reporting date, 1983–2000.

years of data (8770 people), and a community study involving 4026 person years (781 people) and data. This study calculated the number of cases within the community that were missed by surveillance. With *Salmonella*, there were 3.2 cases in the community for every case reported to the CDSC; with *Campylobacter*, there were 7.6 community cases for everyone reported to surveillance; and for Norwalk-like virus (NLV), there were 1500 cases per case reported.

12.2.3 Typing

Typing has proved very useful in the surveillance of many bacterial enteric pathogens. The routine typing of *Salmonella* isolates over the past 40 years has demonstrated the rise and fall in occurrence of different specific serotypes and phage types. In particular, the rise and fall of *Salmonella enteritidis* PT4 associated with infected chickens has been well documented. Approaches to *Cryptosporidium* typing have been investigated for the past 10 years.[14–16] However, the epidemiological value of *Cryptosporidium* typing has only been realized within the past 5 years with the development of rapid and reproducible genetic methods[17,18] and their application to large numbers of samples.[19–27] Details of these are dealt with in Chapter 8.

12.2.4 Age Distribution

Routine surveillance can give useful information on the age distribution of patients with diarrheal diseases. Infection with *Cryptosporidium* is most commonly detected in children (Figure 12.4). Analysis of results from 45,678 fecal samples in a single laboratory showed *Cryptosporidium* in one-year olds represented 15% of all reported cases. With the other enteric pathogens, the maximum percentage of cases in any one-year band was much less than this (*Shigella* 8%, *Giardia* 7%, *Salmonella* 5%, *Campylobacter* 5%). *Cryptosporidium* occurred in under 5% of fecal samples in all age groups, which was similar to *Giardia* (5%), but different from other pathogens (*Campylobacter* 15%, *Salmonella* 10%, *Shigella* 10%). As this study examined feces from all age groups in a standardized way it clearly shows that infection is much more commonly detected in children than adults. It remains unclear whether the big difference between the incidence in children and adults is due to immunological or developmental facters, differences in exposure to oocysts, or possibly that infected adults do not produce detectable numbers of oocysts in their feces if they have been exposed to *Cryptosporidium* previously.

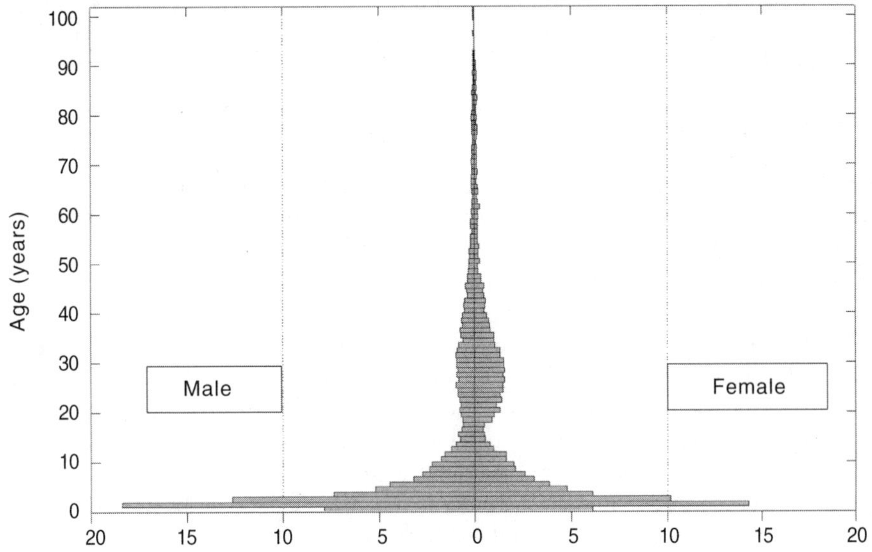

FIGURE 12.4 Age distribution of patients with cryptosporidiosis.

12.2.5 Clusters

Cryptosporidium cases were plotted per day and during the period of 1989 to 1997 (Figure 12.5). In trying to determine the role of waterborne disease, a simple technique was developed for determining local clusters of cases. A cluster was defined as 10 or more cases occurring within a 4-week period, and was determined by day in a rolling fashion. There were 540 local clusters

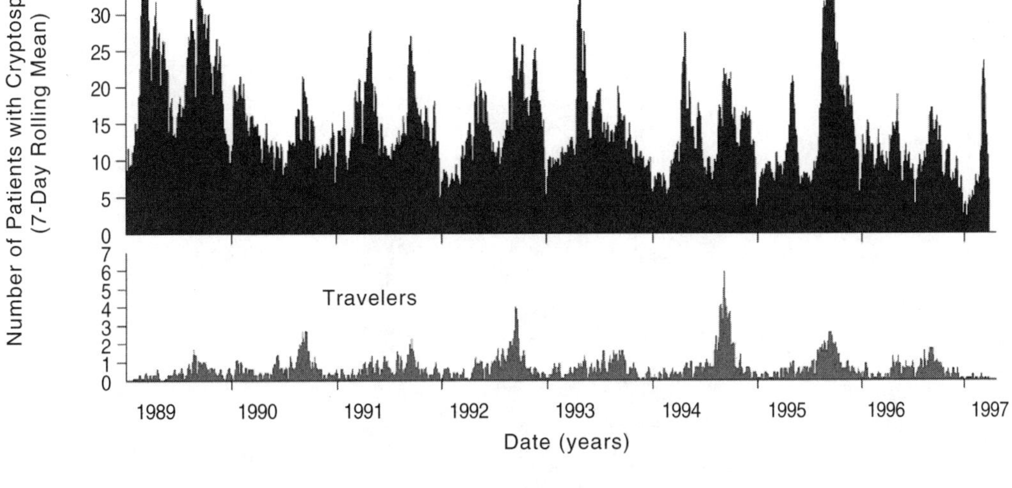

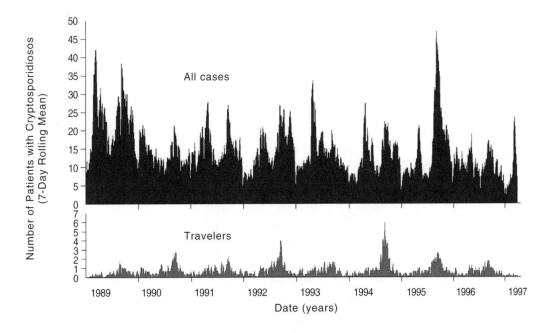

FIGURE 12.5 Cryptosporidiosis cases per day in England and Wales, 1989–1997. Total travel-related cases.

identified, and the cases within these clusters represented 36% of all cases. Direct comparison of databases for outbreaks and clusters was not possible, but it is likely that most outbreaks were within the cluster group.

12.2.6 Outbreak Surveillance

There has been a system of outbreak surveillance for cryptosporidiosis since the first cases in 1983, but routine outbreak surveillance was improved in 1992 with forms being sent to the people investigating all outbreaks of gastrointestinal infection. A general outbreak is defined as two or more cases derived from a common source and excludes family outbreaks. Between 1983 and 1997 there were 80 general outbreaks of cryptosporidiosis in England and Wales, including a number of published ones (Table 12.1). Of the 80 outbreaks, 43 were linked with water, including 25 with a strong, probable or possible association with mains supplies; 3 were linked with private water supplies, and 7 with swimming pools. The remainder were poorly substantiated because there was also contact with farm animals. *Campylobacter* remains the commonest cause of outbreaks associated with private supplies (Said et al., submitted), and routine monitoring indicates that these supplies contravene the microbiological standards much more frequently (over 20% for *E. coli*) than public mains supplies (0.1%). In addition there were 9 outbreaks associated with farms, and 1 milk-borne outbreak. The percentage of cases occurring in outbreaks between 1989 and 1997 ranged from 2 to 20% of cases per year (mean 8%) of all cases. Those linked to mains drinking water outbreaks ranged from 1 to 17% (mean 6%) of cases per year.

One of the consistent problems of outbreak investigation is that small outbreaks are much more difficult to detect than large ones, and the evidence that the outbreak is derived from a common source is more difficult to provide than for a large outbreak. With the evidence from the cluster detection (above), it is likely that there are a much larger number of small outbreaks, most of which go undetected.

TABLE 12.1
Outbreaks and Cases of Cryptosporidiosis in England and Wales 1983 to 1997

Year	Number of Outbreaks	Drinking Water Outbreaks[a]	Total Outbreak Cases	Total Drinking Water Cases[a]	Total Cases in England and Wales	Outbreak Cases as a Percentage of the Total	Drinking Water Outbreak Cases as a Percentage of the Total[a]
1983	1	0	16	0	61	26	0
1984	1	0	19	0	876	2	0
1985	3	0	60	0	1875	3	0
1986	4	0	98	0	3560	3	0
1987	1	0	69	0	3277	2	0
1988	2	0	102	0	2750	4	0
1989	6	3	1090	1042	7768	14	13
1990	4	2	92	49	4682	2	1
1991	9	2	93	46	5165	2	1
1992	12	4	549	343	5211	11	7
1993	9	3	358	164	4832	7	3
1994	7	2	373	257	4432	8	6
1995	5	1	612	575	5691	11	10
1996	4	3	244	236	3660	7	6
1997	12	5	874	743	4321	20	17
Total	80	25	4649	3455	58161	8	6

[a]Cases include those with a strong probable or possible association with public drinking water.

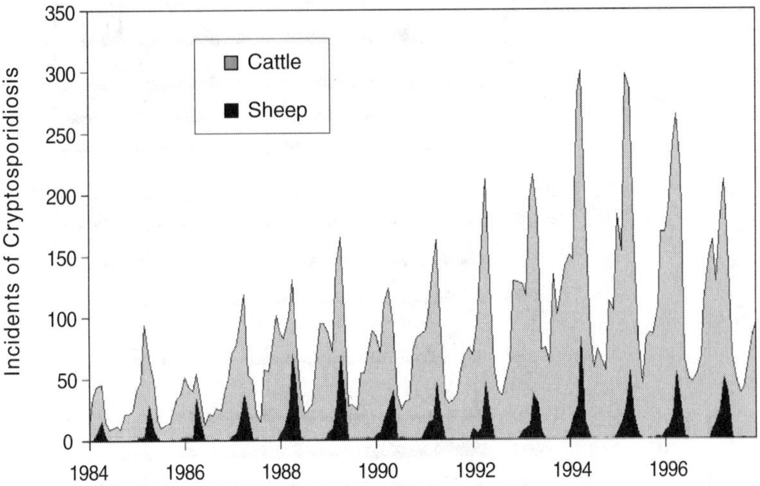

FIGURE 12.6 Incidents of cryptosporidiosis in cattle and sheep in the U.K.

12.2.7 Seasonality

When examining surveillance records for temporal trends, the date of reporting is often used. However, there can be a substantial delay between the start of the patient's illness and when the laboratory detection of *Cryptosporidium* is reported. For most patients, the date of onset is not recorded and the most reliable surrogate is the specimen collection date. When data are plotted using the specimen collection date (Figure 12.5), a clear seasonal trend is apparent with peaks of infection in the spring and late summer/autumn and troughs in mid-summer and winter. The causes for these spring and autumn peaks of cases remains unproven, but suggestions have been made. The spring increase may result from direct or indirect exposure to oocysts derived from newborn lambs and calves that are frequently infected with *Cryptosporidium*.[20,28,29] The incidents of cryptosporidiosis reported by the Veterinary Service show similar seasonal trends, particularly with sheep (Figure 12.6). Similarly, the autumn increase may result from increased community spread from infected people returning from abroad.[20] The seasonal distribution of cryptosporidiosis in people returning to England and Wales from abroad shows a late summer/autumn peak that reflects when most people go on holiday (Figure 12.5). The reason for spread within the community is unclear, but could be facilitated by small outbreaks linked to swimming pools (Rooney et al., awaiting submission).

12.2.8 Regional Variations

The analysis of data by laboratory and region showed dramatic local fluctuations in cases that may or may not be identifiable in national figures as an outbreak. Clearly the large outbreaks usually have a significant impact on national cases, but smaller outbreaks may not cause an increase above background in the national figures. For this reason local surveillance is paramount in the detection of outbreaks, particularly the smaller ones. The seasonal trends can still be observed in some of the regions (Figure 12.7), but are not clearly discernable at the laboratory level. National variations in incidence by the Health Authority are strongly influenced by local outbreaks (Figure 12.8). The national data are therefore a compilation of trends that differ between geographic areas. Despite this, there have been occasions where an outbreak has extended beyond local bounds. This occurred in an outbreak in Oxford and Swindon in 1989 to 1990 when there was an increase in cases in the regions adjacent to the outbreak regions,[30] and more spectacularly in 1995 when there was a national increase in cases at the same time as a waterborne outbreak in a popular tourism area in Devon.[15]

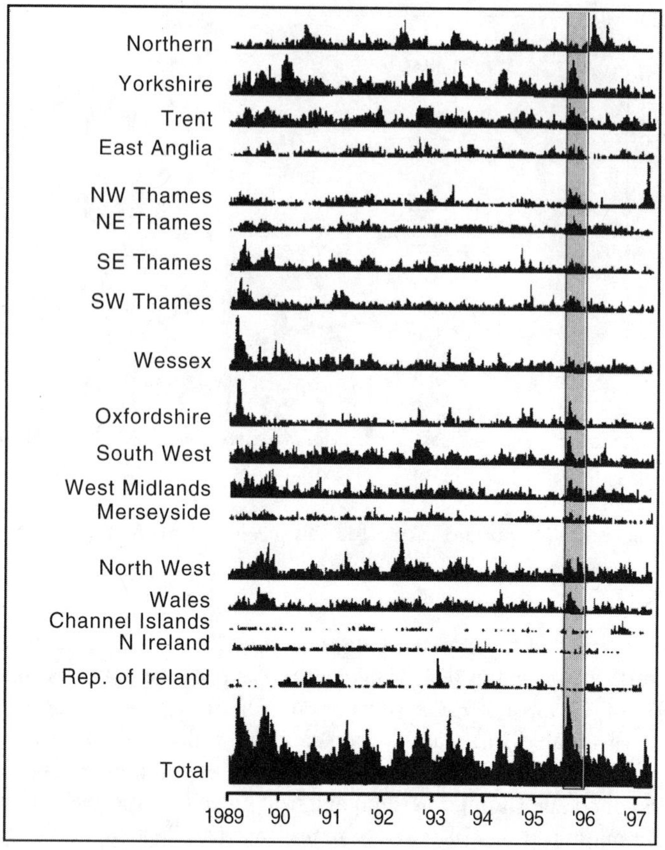

FIGURE 12.7 Cryptosporidiosis in England and Wales by region, 1989–1997. Note: bar represents the large outbreak in South West of England.

12.3 THE VALUE OF SURVEILLANCE

Surveillance has a number of advantages over other approaches for examining the epidemiology of enteric infections such as cryptosporidiosis. Firstly, the development of standardization in the diagnosis and reporting of infections allows both large and small outbreaks as well as sporadic infections to be monitored in real time so that interventions can be undertaken. The detailed microbiology and typing of isolates can allow detailed epidemiology to be conducted. Ascertainment (the extent to which surveillance covers the whole population) is inevitably incomplete, although it has improved over the years. Despite this, surveillance across the country could still be further improved. The approach that has been used in England and Wales has enhanced surveillance in stages. The data from outbreaks and routine surveillance have allowed the generation of hypotheses that can be tested and fed back into disease prevention, particularly in relation to waterborne disease. The routine surveillance data can examine regional variations in prevalence and detect otherwise unrecognized outbreaks.

A large study of infectious intestinal disease in England and Wales showed that some pathogens suffer from worse under-ascertainment than cryptosporidiosis, particularly NLV.[12] This is probably because there is poor laboratory detection for some pathogens. The ongoing series of human volunteer studies on cryptosporidiosis indicate that prior infection with *Cryptosporidium* offers a degree of protection against infection with a small infecting dose of oocysts but will not protect against a larger infecting dose.[31–38] Furthermore, in those volunteers who were symptomatic, there were few oocysts shed in feces.[33,37] The assumption from this is that there could be a substantial

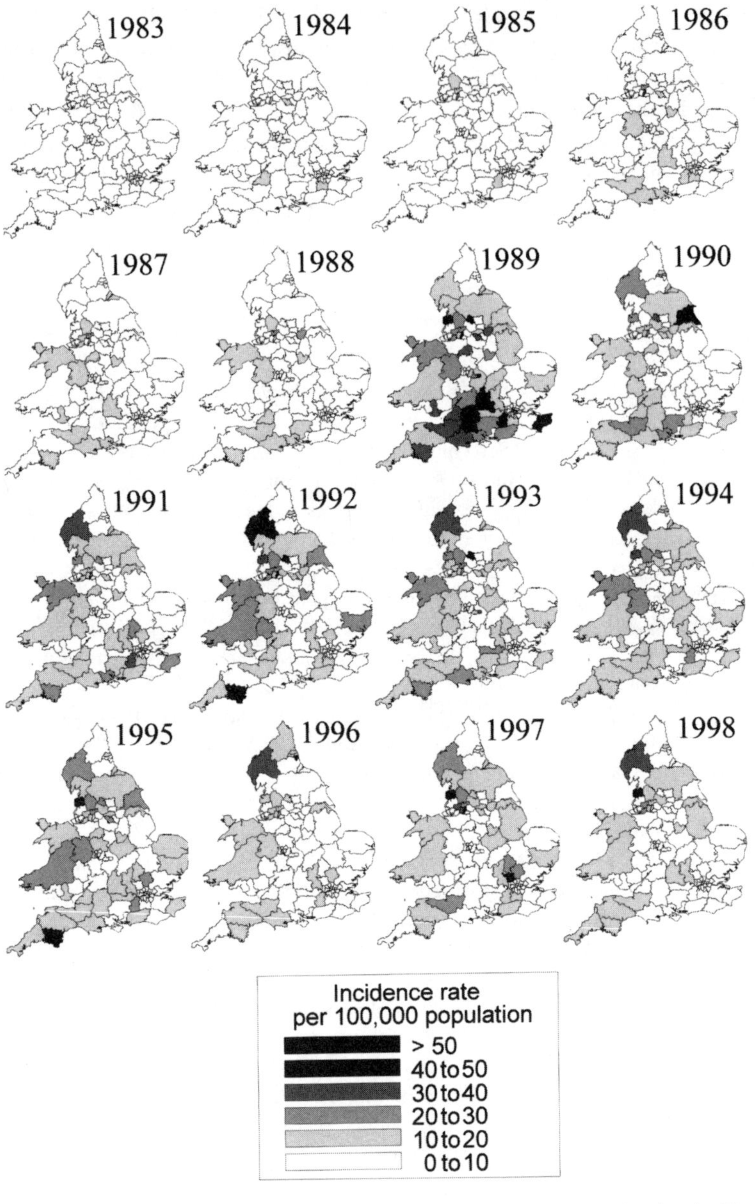

FIGURE 12.8 Geographical incidence of cryptosporidiosis by health authority in England and Wales, 1983–1998.

number of people who are infected and symptomatic but who will not excrete oocysts in detectable numbers. Alternative strategies may be required to determine whether current surveillance is underdiagnosing a substantial number of cases (see Chapter 17).

It can be difficult to estimate the overall burden of infection associated with drinking water consumption from the routine surveillance data. From the reported outbreaks, around 6% of the total cases were linked to drinking water outbreaks, with around 90% of cases having no identified source. While waterborne outbreaks are clearly important and can cause widespread illness as well as severe logistical problems for the water providers, the sources of infection in the 90% of cases that are not occurring in detected outbreaks remain unclear. The recognition that 36% of cases occur in clusters (which includes the outbreaks) hints that many small outbreaks are undetected as such. In a retrospective study of an area in Northwestern England with a history of outbreaks of waterborne cryptosporidiosis, it was suggested that many more outbreaks had been missed than had been detected at the time.[39] Further improvements in local surveillance may be necessary to investigate this problem. The remaining 64% of cases are largely sporadic. The reason for these cases cannot easily be explained by the surveillance conducted to date. While low-level contamination of drinking water has been suggested as a source of these cases, this hypothesis remains untested. Infections from swimming pools, person-to-person transmission, or contaminated food are equally plausible.

REFERENCES

1. Henriksen, S.A. and Pohlenz, J. F., Staining of *Cryptosporidia* by a modified Ziehl-Neelsen technique, *Acta Vet. Scand.*, 1981.
2. Nichols, G.L. and Thom, B. T, Screening for *Cryptosporidium* in stools, *Lancet,* 1, 734, 1984.
3. Baxby, D., Blundell, N., and Hart, C.A., The development and performance of a simple, sensitive method for the detection of *Cryptosporidium* oocysts in faeces, *J. Hyg. (Lond.),* 93, 317, 1984.
4. McLauchlin, J. et al., Identification of *Cryptosporidium* oocysts by monoclonal antibody, *Lancet,* 1, 51, 1987.
5. Public Health Laboratory Service Study Group, Cryptosporidiosis in England and Wales: prevalence and clinical and epidemiological features, *B.M.J.,* 300, 774, 1990.
6. Casemore, D.P. and Roberts, C., Guidelines for screening for *Cryptosporidium* in stools: report of a joint working group, *J. Clin. Pathol.*, 46, 2, 1993.
7. Hastings, L. et al., Salm-Net facilitates collaborative investigation of an outbreak of *Salmonella tosamanga* infection in Europe, *Commun. Dis. Rep. CDR Rev.,* 6, R100, 1996.
8. Killalea, D. et al., International epidemiological and microbiological study of outbreak of *Salmonella agona* infection from a ready to eat savoury snack — I: England and Wales and the United States, *B.M.J.,* 313, 1105, 1996.
9. Lyytikainen, O. et al., Molecular epidemiology of an outbreak caused by *Salmonella* enterica serovar *newport* in Finland and the United Kingdom, *Epidemiol. Infect.,* 124, 185, 2000.
10. Threlfall, E.J. et al., Molecular fingerprinting defines a strain of *Salmonella* enterica serotype *anatum* responsible for an international outbreak associated with formula-dried milk, *Epidemiol. Infect.*, 121, 289, 1998.
11. Sethi, D. et al., A study of infectious intestinal disease in England: plan and methods of data collection, *Commun. Dis. Pub. Health,* 2, 101, 1999.
12. Tompkins, D.S. et al., A study of infectious intestinal disease in England: microbiological findings in cases and controls, *Commun. Dis. Public Health,* 2, 108, 1999.
13. Wheeler, J.G. et al., Study of infectious intestinal disease in England: rates in the community, presenting to general practice, and reported to national surveillance, *B.M.J.*, 318, 1046, 1999.
14. Awad-El-Kariem, F.M. et al., Differentiation between human and animal strains of *Cryptosporidium parvum* using isoenzyme typing, *Parasitology,* 110, 129, 1995.
15. McLauchlin, J. et al., The epidemiology of cryptosporidiosis: application of experimental sub-typing and antibody detection systems to the investigation of water-borne outbreaks, *Folia Parasitol.*, 45, 83, 1998.
16. Nichols, G.L., McLauchlin, J., and Samuel, D., A technique for typing *Cryptosporidium* isolates, *J. Protozool.*, 38, 237S, 1991.
17. Caccio, S. et al., A microsatellite marker reveals population heterogeneity within human and animal genotypes of *Cryptosporidium parvum, Parasitology,* 120, 237, 2000.
18. Peng, M.M. et al., Genetic polymorphism among *Cryptosporidium parvum* isolates: evidence of two distinct human transmission cycles, *Emerg. Infect. Dis.,* 3, 567, 1997.
19. McLauchlin, J. et al., Genetic characterization of *Cryptosporidium* strains from 218 patients with diarrhea diagnosed as having sporadic cryptosporidiosis, *J. Clin. Microbiol.,* 37, 3153, 1999.

20. McLauchlin, J. et al., Molecular epidemiological analysis of *Cryptosporidium* spp. in the United Kingdom: results of genotyping *Cryptosporidium* spp. in 1,705 fecal samples from humans and 105 fecal samples from livestock animals, *J. Clin. Microbiol.,* 38, 3984, 2000.
21. Patel, S. et al., Molecular characterisation of *Cryptosporidium parvum* from two large suspected waterborne outbreaks, *Commun. Dis. Public Health,* 1, 231, 1998.
22. Pedraza-Diaz, S., Amar, C., and McLauchlin, J., The identification and characterisation of an unusual genotype of *Cryptosporidium* from human faeces as *Cryptosporidium meleagridis, FEMS Microbiol. Lett.*, 189, 189, 2000.
23. Bonnin, A. et al., Genotyping human and bovine isolates of *Cryptosporidium parvum* by polymerase chain reaction-restriction fragment length polymorphism analysis of a repetitive DNA sequence, *FEMS Microbiol. Lett.*, 137, 207, 1996.
24. Khramtsov, N.V. et al., Presence of double-stranded RNAs in human and calf isolates of *Cryptosporidium parvum, J. Parasitol.*, 86, 275, 2000.
25. Spano, F. et al., PCR-RFLP analysis of the *Cryptosporidium* oocyst wall protein (COWP) gene discriminates between *C. wrairi* and *C. parvum*, and between *C. parvum* isolates of human and animal origin, *FEMS Microbiol. Lett.,* 150, 209, 1997.
26. Sulaiman, I.M., Xiao, L., and Lal, A.A., Evaluation of *Cryptosporidium parvum* genotyping techniques, *Appl. Environ. Microbiol.*, 65, 4431, 1999.
27. Xiao, L. et al., Species and strain-specific typing of *Cryptosporidium* parasites in clinical and environmental samples, *Mem. Inst. Oswaldo Cruz*, 93, 687, 1998.
28. Sayers, G.M. et al., Cryptosporidiosis in children who visited an open farm, *Commun. Dis. Rep. CDR Rev*, 6, R140, 1996.
29. Evans, M.R. and Gardner, D., Cryptosporidiosis outbreak associated with an educational farm holiday, *Commun. Dis. Rep. CDR Rev.*, 6, R50, 1996.
30. Richardson, A.J. et al., An outbreak of waterborne cryptosporidiosis in Swindon and Oxfordshire, *Epidemiol. Infect.*, 107, 485, 1991.
31. Moss, D.M. et al., The antibody response to 27-, 17-, and 15-kDa *Cryptosporidium* antigens following experimental infection in humans, *J. Infect. Dis.,* 178, 827, 1998.
32. Chappell, C.L. et al., *Cryptosporidium parvum*: intensity of infection and oocyst excretion patterns in healthy volunteers, *J. Infect. Dis.,* 173, 232, 1996.
33. Chappell, C.L. et al., Infectivity of *Cryptosporidium parvum* in healthy adults with pre-existing anti-*C. parvum* serum immunoglobulin G, *Am. J. Trop. Med. Hyg.,* 60, 157, 1999.
34. DuPont, H.L. et al., The infectivity of *Cryptosporidium parvum* in healthy volunteers, *N. Engl. J. Med.*, 332, 855, 1995.
35. Okhuysen, P.C. et al., Prophylactic effect of bovine anti-*Cryptosporidium* hyperimmune colostrum immunoglobulin in healthy volunteers challenged with *Cryptosporidium parvum, Clin. Infect. Dis.*, 26, 1324, 1998.
36. Okhuysen, P.C. et al., Virulence of three distinct *Cryptosporidium parvum* isolates for healthy adults, *J. Infect. Dis.*, 180, 1275, 1999.
37. Okhuysen, P.C. et al., Susceptibility and serologic response of healthy adults to reinfection with *Cryptosporidium parvum, Infect. Immun.*, 66, 441, 1998.
38. White, A.C. et al., Interferon-gamma expression in jejunal biopsies in experimental human cryptosporidiosis correlates with prior sensitization and control of oocyst excretion, *J. Infect. Dis.,* 181, 701, 2000.
39. Hunter, P.R., Syed, Q., and Naumova, E.N., Possible undetected outbreaks of cryptosporidiosis in areas of the North West of England supplied by an unfiltered surface water source, *Commun. Dis. Public Health,* 4, 136, 2001.

13 Geographical Information Systems

Friederike Dangendorf, Susanne Herbst, Martin Exner, and Thomas Kistemann

CONTENTS

13.1 INTRODUCTION

As recent research papers have shown, geographic information systems (GIS) are often used to study the epidemiology of infectious diseases.[1–5] They have rarely been applied, however, to the epidemiology of waterborne disease. Nevertheless, GISs have proved to be extremely useful in assessing health risks in population-based studies of the epidemiology of drinking water-related disease. Aral and Maslia[6] demonstrated the utility of applying GIS to the analysis of human exposure to contaminated drinking water. They showed that contamination due to volatile organic compounds (VOCs) in groundwater reservoirs was distributed via the supply network and used GIS tools to estimate the extent of contamination and the location of exposed populations.

Nuckols et al.[7] also illustrated the advantage of using a GIS application for drinking water epidemiology. They compared two supply areas with different disinfection practices and examined the impact of varying levels of trihalomethanes (THM) on birth weight and other reproductive outcomes. Demographic and epidemiological data were entered into the GIS and linked with water quality modelling to provide new insights into the spatial distribution of disease.

Studies of water quality using GIS most often deal with chemical contaminants.[8] It is obvious that GIS techniques are also useful for analyzing waterborne infectious diseases caused by a variety of pathogens.

A GIS is essentially a complex computer system designed to enter, store, manage, analyze, model, and map spatial information. It enables new forms of communication, not only among researchers but also throughout entire communities.[9,10] With regard to the monitoring of waterborne diseases, the data sets comprise not only epidemiological data but also information about water supply, water treatment, and distribution. Linking large quantities of epidemiological and water supply data to geographical objects is the basic objective of an efficient, task-specific GIS.

0-8493-1259-0/03/$0.00+$1.50

This chapter presents a GIS approach that has been used to analyze the distribution of gastrointestinal infections through the water supply in the region of Rhein-Berg (Northrhine-Westphalia, Germany).

It is astonishing that information on waterborne diseases and outbreaks is rarely available in Germany. In countries with similarly high standards of water supply, waterborne outbreaks and infections occur. In the period 1986 to 1996, a total of 778 outbreaks were reported in 19 European countries.[11] Sweden reported 53 outbreaks and England and Wales 20, but none were reported in Germany. The last waterborne epidemics reported were a shigella outbreak in 1979 in Munich-Ismaning, a typhoid outbreak in 1980 from Jena, and a rotavirus outbreak in 1981 in Halle.[12]

There may be several explanations. Drinking water in Germany may be of a higher quality than most other European countries, so that waterborne diseases and outbreaks do not occur. Cases of waterborne infections and outbreaks may not be identified as waterborne, and therefore not reported. The surveillance system for waterborne infectious diseases in Germany may be inadequate. German consumption habits may be different from those in other countries.

This chapter looks specifically at how the authors have used GIS to relate gastrointestinal infections to information on water quality and distribution. The question is whether waterborne gastrointestinal infections do occur and under what circumstances. The main objective is to examine the hypothesis that spatial variations in the incidence of gastrointestinal diseases in the study area are linked with different drinking water sources. The first results of a retrospective study carried out in 1997 and 1998 in the Rhein-Berg district (state of Northrhine-Westphalia, Germany) are presented. The project was supported by the local public health department and the Association of Drinking Water Reservoirs (ATT Arbeitsgemeinschaft Trinkwassertalsperren e.V.).

GISs are used to estimate exposure to and location of diseases. Some examples of visualized epidemiological data are presented. In addition, the first steps in developing a surveillance system for waterborne diseases are discussed: collecting the relevant databases and integrating them into the system.

13.2 METHODS

13.2.1 Study Area and Water Supply Data

The Rhein-Berg district, situated near Cologne on the Rhine River, extends over 440 km^2. It has a population of 272,000 and is divided into two regions with different sources of drinking water supply. The Rhein-Berg district has 42 subdistricts. In the north and south subdistricts, the drinking water comes from surface reservoirs. In the west, the main water supply is provided from groundwater sources (Figure 13.1).

The concept of "hazard analysis critical control point" (HACCP), which was developed to ensure food safety and later applied to drinking water, was used to determine the structure of the water supply in Rhein-Berg.[13] To assess the safety of the drinking water, data about sources of the drinking water supply, water companies, water service areas, treatment, and distribution were collected. Existing district- and state-level databases on the monitoring of water quality in the state of Northrhine-Westphalia were used. Data covered by TEIS (drinking water data recording and information system at the local level) and TWDB (drinking water database at the state level) include data on water companies, private wells, feeding points, sampling sites, water delivery, microbiological and chemical parameters tested, and test results. Additional data were collected by contacting the water companies to obtain information on the distribution network (length per inhabitant, connected households).

13.2.2 Public Health Data

Gastrointestinal infections are used as a non-specific disease indicator for the epidemiological data set.[14] Various types of pathogens can cause diarrhea, and in Germany gastrointestinal infections are notifiable. For the epidemiological database, all pathogens that may cause diarrhea, except

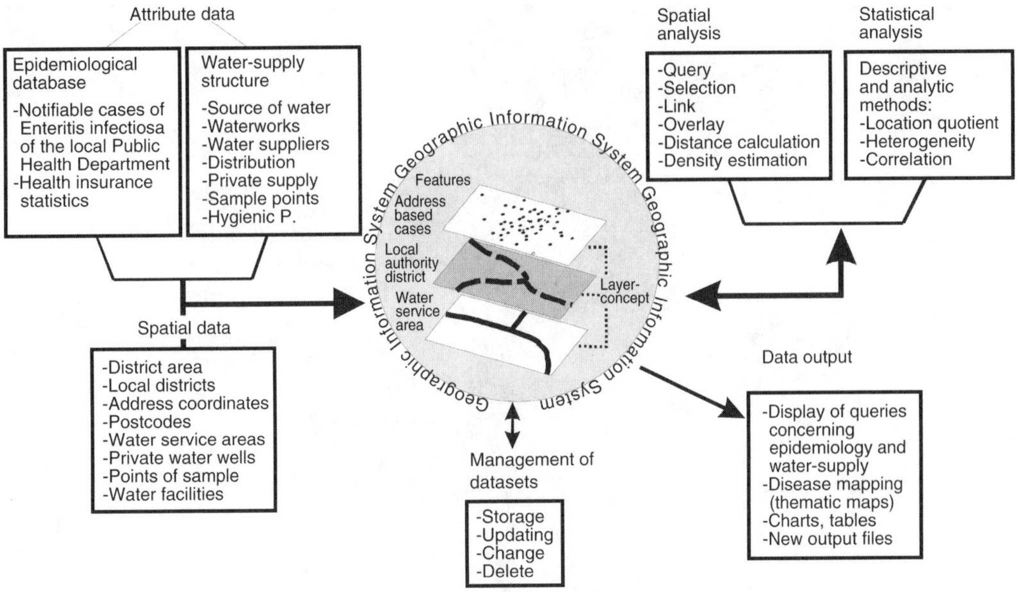

FIGURE 13.1 Concept of GIS processing concerning epidemiological surveillance of waterborne infectious diseases.

Salmonella and *Shigella*, which are most often foodborne or associated with traveling, were taken into account.

The pathogens most frequently notified in the register of the public health department (national or local health departments) are *Campylobacter* spp., adenovirus and rotavirus, *Yersinia* spp., and EHEC. The data are available for the period 1988 to 1998. Since they had not been computerized, this had to be done.

In addition to the public health department data, health insurance data were available. The health insurance company statistics include subscribers reported sick due to diarrhea. The data for the period 1993 to 1998 was exported from an existing database.

13.2.3 Analytical Methods

The collected databases were integrated into a GIS in order to analyze the spatial dimensions of the data. The basic GIS software chosen was ArcView® from Environmental Systems Research Institute (ESRI), Inc., Redlands, CA. Figure 13.2 shows how the GIS can present relatively complex spatial data in an easily understandable graphical manner.

The first step in a GIS project is to collect the relevant databases. The spatial data are the most important component of a GIS and determine its effectiveness. Data were obtained at different levels: district and service areas, address coordinates, and postcode areas. GIS techniques provide instant links between attribute and spatial data (SQL connections, import files).

Spatial data is related to point, polygon, and line objects. The layer concept of the GIS makes it possible to overlay different feature levels and use GIS tools such as query, selection, distance calculation, and buffer functions. Additional descriptive, analytical, and statistical methods were integrated into the system. To analyze the epidemiological data set for spatial variation, the location quotient and the Poisson probability distribution, which are commonly used in disease mapping, were applied.[15,16] Regions with low or high values of disease rates were visualized to give a view of the distribution of disease.

Spatial autocorrelation models are important tools for detecting clusters of cases and showing disease rates across the study area and interactions between neighboring districts.[17] The area-based

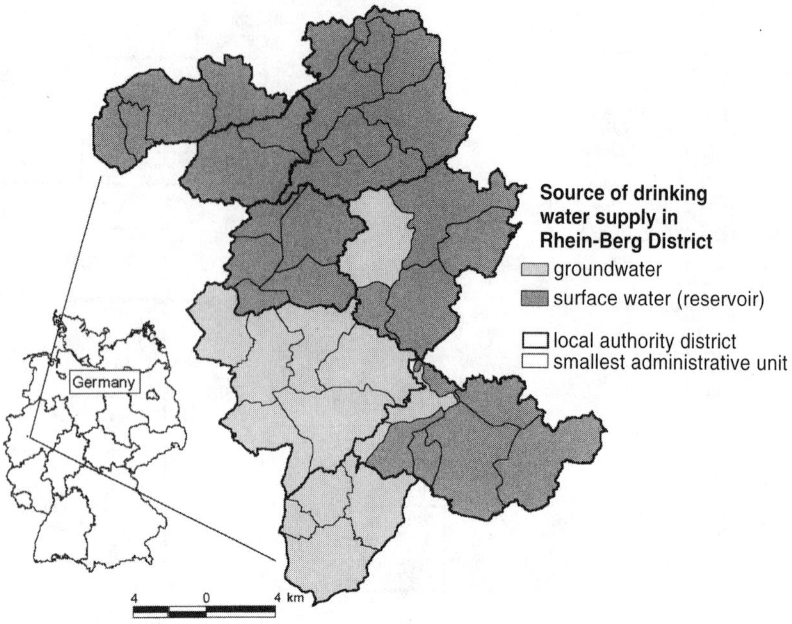

FIGURE 13.2 Origin of drinking water in the study area of Rhein-Berg district, Germany.

Moran's I autocorrelation method was used to determine subdistrict incidence rates. It includes the weight of neighborhood units with the weight $W_{ij} = 1$ if $i \neq j$ and where i and j are adjacent and 0 if not.[18] This geostatistical analysis was carried out with the statistics software S-plus® which provides a linkage to ArcView®.

The hypothesis that the distribution of incidences of enteritis may be linked to the water supply is verified by correlation methods. The Pearson's product-moment correlation statistic and the partial correlation are used to measure the association between the variables.[19,20]

Besides the variable "enteritis incidence rate," parameters characterizing the water supply are evaluated. To determine the population potentially exposed, the number of people provided with surface- or groundwater supply and the amount of private supply are calculated.

Maps, graphs, charts, tables, and export files can be produced as output of the enteritis information system (EIS). Graphically presented data, especially maps, provide new insights on the distribution of disease. Because the results of interactive query are displayed directly on screen, it is easier to interpret the spatial relation of the different data sets.

13.3 RESULTS

With 99.6% of the population connected to the public grid, the supply of drinking water in Rhein-Berg district is overwhelmingly dominated by the public supply. The location of private wells integrated by their coordinates into the GIS shows that they vary among the 42 subdistricts. Merging the two layers revealed that private supply ranges between 0.6 and 6.0% in rural districts.

The public supply is produced by five waterworks and is distributed by 27 water-supply companies (Figure 13.3). Of these, 23 deliver more than 5000 m^3 of drinking water a year. The size of the service areas in the study area ranges between 87.75 km^2 and 0.14 km^2. Especially in the north, many small water providers indicate the persistence of earlier water supply structures. In the south, each supply almost fully equates to a local authority area. Of the five waterworks, three use groundwater, and two use surface water.

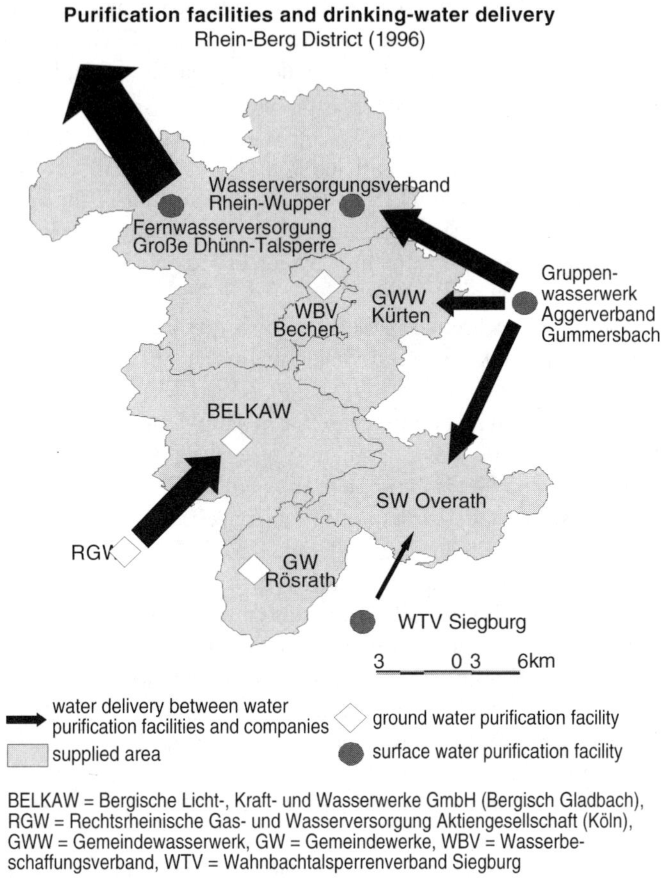

FIGURE 13.3 Purification facilities and drinking water delivery in Rhein-Berg district, Germany.

The local health department has detailed epidemiological data for the period 1988 through 1998, including information on the causative pathogen, date of onset, date of registration, other infected persons, travel, age, sex, connection to private or public water supply, etc. The data are address-based, and therefore allow for the construction of a high-resolution-point layer that constitutes an efficient basis for spatial analysis within the GIS when linked with exposure variables.

The distribution of cases of infection is extremely incomplete, even though this information is notifiable. The Robert Koch Institute (National Department for Infectious Diseases) estimates that less than 10% of all cases of infection are registered by the health departments.[21] Most often, cases of infection are notified by laboratories rather than by physicians.

Health insurance data, collected during 1991 and 1998, are coded according to the ninth revision of the International Classification of Disease (ICD). Of the reported cases of diarrhea, 99% are in the category ICD 009, which covers insufficiently diagnosed infections. The data include all kinds of pathogens causing enteritis, including *Salmonella* and *Shigella*. In addition, the data are only aggregated on the basis of 11 postcode areas and therefore are not very useful for spatial analysis. In fact, the two data sets are not very comparable. The insurance data show a high rate of diarrhea (1130 cases/100,000 subscribers/year) and confirm that the cases reported to the public health department (48 cases/100,000 inhabitants/year) under-represent the actual number of cases. It should be taken into account that the low value may be due in part to the fact that cases linked to journeys to foreign countries are removed from the database. In 1999, the mean incidence rate of enteritis in North Rhine-Westphalia was 111 cases/100,000 inhabitants, and in Germany as a whole, 135 cases/100,000 inhabitants.[22]

Once the coordinates of the address-based data of the local public health department were transferred to the GIS model, they could be displayed on screen. Each point object represents a case of enteritis. When one clicks on a point, a window appears that displays all available information on that case (causative pathogen, registration date, etc.).

An interactive query about the water supply is also possible. The sampling sites of the distribution network were integrated into the system and linked with the results of tests of water quality, which are provided by the TWDB and TEIS databases. The results of the water quality analysis can be used to make regional comparisons and trace temporal trends. The location of waterworks is connected to the attributes "water treatment," "water origin," and "quantity of water delivered to different areas."

The advantage of this GIS technique is that it affords quick access to important information. It can be used to monitor the links between water quality and gastrointestinal infections and to indicate the need for measures to be taken.

Before carrying out correlations between the water supply structures and the incidence rate, the spatial variation in disease rates was examined. Aggregating the epidemiological point data on the smallest administrative units yields choropleth maps of incidence.

Map B in Figure 13.4 shows the distribution of incidence rates by the location quotient, which compares observed rates with expected values under the theoretical assumption of equal distribution. The highest rates of illness are found in the southern districts. Values between 1.10 and 2.55 are found for the middle and south authority units. In contrast, rates below 1 are mainly found in the north.

The Poisson probability distribution was applied to detect high incidence rates. Areas with extreme values — with a probability level of 1 to 20% of occurrence by chance — were also detected in the south and in the middle of the study area (Figure 13.4, Map C). Two subdistricts seem to have the highest risk of infection. It should be recalled that in the southwest, drinking water is mainly derived from groundwater.

The spatial autocorrelation model (Moran I test) verified the spatial clustering of enteritis cases ($r = 0.28$, $p < 0.01$).

The spatial heterogeneity of enteritis can be shown using relatively simple graphical and statistical methods.

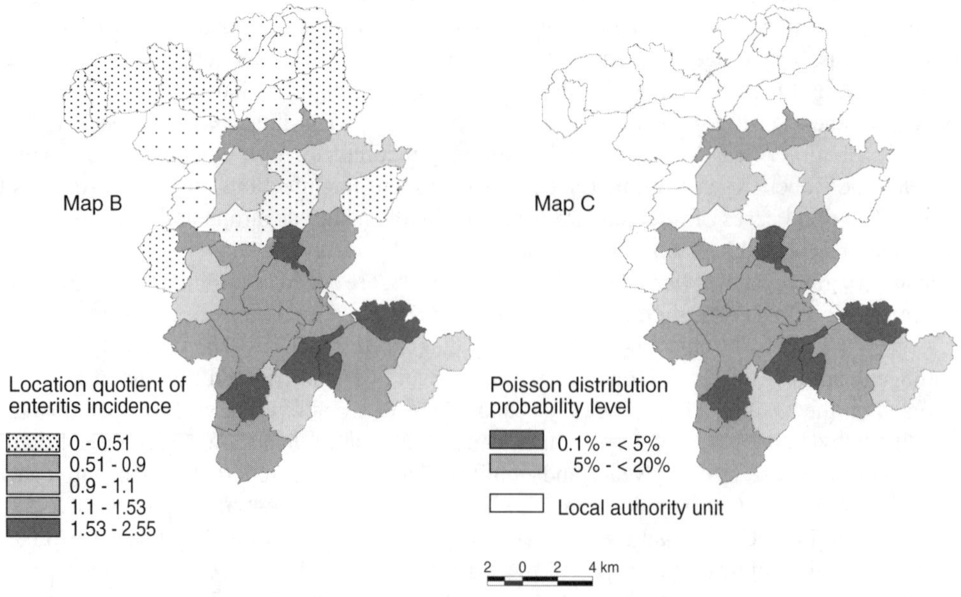

FIGURE 13.4 Spatial patterns of the enteritis incidence in the subdistricts of Rhein-Berg, Germany (1988–1998).

TABLE 13.1
Product–Moment Correlation of Water Supply Structures and Incidence of Enteritis

Independent variables	Enteritis Incidence y	Pearson's Correlation Coefficient r
% Surface water	x_1	–0.371[a]
% Groundwater	x_2	0.371*
% Private supply	x_3	–0.217
Mobility of people	x_4	0.087
Density of physicians	x_5	0.205

[a] Significant at a level of 5%.

The construction of an aggregate database makes it possible to investigate if the origin of drinking water has a significant statistical influence on the incidence of enteritis within a population. Therefore parameters have to be formulated which could represent the water supply structure in the different areas. The number of people supplied by dam or groundwater and the amount of public and private water supply per sub-district were evaluated.

In the study area there are many water supply companies serving different populations and covering areas of different sizes. In addition the boundaries of district and service areas sometimes overlap, so it is very difficult to determine the amount of water delivered per local authority unit.

The Pearson's product–moment correlation model was applied to analyze the association between the incidence of enteritis and the number of people supplied by surface- or groundwater. The coefficient of the correlation between these two parameters was –0.37 for surface supply (+0.37 for groundwater supply) (Table 13.1). The values are significant at the $P = 0.05$ level. The coefficient of the correlation between the variable "private wells" and the incidence rate revealed a weak association of $r = -0.217$ ($p > 0.05$).

It has to be recognized that a simple correlation calculation does not give a high degree of certainty. Many other factors can affect the variation in the incidence of disease, such as the mobility of people who leave their home districts for work or the density of physicians, which can affect the registration of disease. The most interesting value is the r value of –/+0.37 for the number of people served by surface- or groundwater supply and the disease rate.

This coefficient should be more meaningful if confounding variables are isolated. The partial correlation model was used to try to control for the parameters "private water supply," "mobility of people," and "density of physicians." The calculated r values are illustrated in Table 13.2. The

TABLE 13.2
Results of the Partial Correlation of the Influence of Surface Water Supply on the Variance in the Incidence of Enteritis

	Pearson's Partial Correlation Coefficient; Controlled Variables		
	Private Water Supply yx_1x_3	Mobility of People yx_1x_4	Density of Physicians yx_1x_5
r value incidence of enteritis and the percentage of surface water			
$yx_1 = -0.371$	–0.363	–0.379	–0.328
p =	0.02	0.015	0.037

partial correlation coefficient for the amount of surface water, isolated by the "mobility of people" (yx_1x_4), revealed a slightly higher r value (–0.38). The other partial coefficients show lower r values. The degree of yx_1 controlled by x_3 is –0.36 (private water supply) and that controlled by x_5 (density of physicians) is –0.33. These variables affect the residual variance of y, but in all cases the amount of surface water supply has a greater influence than the confounder. When this calculation is carried out for incidence rate and groundwater supply, the results yield the same but positive partial correlation coefficients, though this time the value is positive.

It is apparent that under existing water supply conditions in the Rhein-Berg district, the local authority subdistricts that are mainly supplied by surface water have a statistically significant lower incidence of enteritis. However, as the study is an ecological one, it was not possible to prove a causal relation at the level of individuals owing to the so-called ecological fallacy.[23]

13.4 DISCUSSION

This chapter presents methods for analyzing the distribution of gastrointestinal infections with respect to the supply of drinking water. The intention was to demonstrate the utility of a GIS in this context.

Recent research papers have quite successfully applied GIS to drinking water epidemiology in terms of assessment of the exposed population, ability to connect data sets to a map, calculation of new variables, and quick access to important information about the relation between the distribution of disease and the water supply.[7,24] The surveillance of waterborne disease requires a wide range of data sets, most often from different sources and of different sizes. The strength of the GIS is the capacity to handle large amounts of data in one system.[25]

It was pointed out that the quality and resolution of the available data do influence the functionality of the GIS. High resolution (appropriate area units, point data from address coordinates) increases the value of the analysis.

Policies to ensure protection of the individual's right to confidentiality sometimes make the collection of personal data very difficult.[26] However, the study revealed that the databases used to characterize the water supply and the distribution of gastrointestinal infections in the study area are of sufficient quantity and quality to operate a surveillance system using a GIS. The address-based data of the public health department can be displayed on screen and overlaid by the spatial data on the water supply (service areas, private wells, etc.). Rapid access to important attributes and the ability to create new maps and calculate new variables help to interpret data in spatial dimensions and may lead to further investigation.

The first step in developing a task-specific GIS project (the determination and the collection of the relevant databases) is the most time- and cost-consuming aspect. A drawback of the GIS might be the time required to integrate noncomputerized data into the system.[7] To reduce the costs and time required, existing databases should be used. In Northrhine-Westphalia the local public health departments are responsible for monitoring the quality of drinking water at the district level. Using the TEIS computer package, it is possible to run a centralized monitoring system at the state level (TWDB, the drinking water database of the state department of health).[27] Although this was very useful, some corrections had to be made before integrating the data into the TEIS.

The health departments are also responsible for the control of communicable diseases. Reporting is provided at local, state, and federal levels and the Robert Koch Institute publishes special health reports. In Rhein-Berg, data were stored in handwritten registers until 1999. Now, an electronic system has been put in place to provide a computerized database not only for basic health reports but also for the connection to a geographical information system.

A GIS-based surveillance system is only as good as the databases it integrates. Routine health data do not always give spatially referenced data sets at the required level of detail.[10] Systematic collection of data should start at the local level. Complete and accurate data processed using standard computerized tables and agreed variables should be the basis for the surveillance of water quality and waterborne diseases at the state and probably also at the national level.

Distributing the aggregated point data on the basis of smallest area units revealed choropleth maps of incidence. GIS functions can strongly support ecological studies comparing groups of aggregated data. They can help to generate hypotheses about the distribution and cause of disease.[4] The variation in incidence rates across regions can be analyzed using methods that are commonly used in medical geography. Location quotients, for example, are very useful for assessing the distribution of disease across regions. Probability mapping using the Poisson distribution was needed to identify units within the study area with significantly high or low disease rates.[16] The spatial auto-correlation calculated with the Moran I test revealed a positive coefficient. Use of the geostatistical methods made it possible to show spatial heterogeneity in the distribution of gastrointestinal infections in the Rhein-Berg district.

To analyze the hypothesis of spatial variation of disease rates due to different sources of drinking water, correlation methods were used. The Pearson's product–moment correlation statistic is often used in ecological studies. Exposed population groups were compared across spatial units.[16]

Parameters of the water supply, such as the number of people supplied by dam or groundwater, were correlated with the incidence of gastrointestinal infections. The results of the product–moment correlation coefficients show a positive linkage between the incidence of disease and the number of people served by groundwater. In other words, districts with large surface water supplies seem to have lower disease rates.

Correlation results may lead to biased interpretation owing to the ecological fallacy. It is advisable to analyze data on the basis of small geographic units to minimize misinterpretation.[23] For this reason, the correlation models were carried out on the smallest available local units (42 subdistricts).

In addition, potential confounders have to be taken into account.[4,23] The partial correlation model was applied to calculate the influence of the important confounders: mobility of people and density of physicians.[20] The partial correlation coefficients revealed that the variable "number of people supplied with surface- or groundwater" had the highest influence on the variance of the incidence of disease.

Our study showed that under the existing water supply conditions in the Rhein-Berg district, those local authority districts that are mainly supplied by surface water had a lower incidence of enteritis during the study period. Although surface water sources are generally more vulnerable to contamination than groundwater bodies, we assume that our results reflect the higher standards of water treatment in the large surface water companies.

Some factors are still missing in the correlation calculation, especially with regard to the HACCP concept. The differing supply systems in the 27 service areas make it extremely difficult to relate factors to the residential population. Therefore, parameters which characterize the distribution networks in detail (length, age, dead ends, material, and other distribution facilities)[13] could not be included in the current correlation model.

Whenever possible, potential confounders should be integrated in partial and multiple correlation analysis to reduce biases and to verify the preliminary results.

At present, the authors are carrying out a survey about drinking water consumption in Rhein-Berg. Evaluation of individuals' exposure to tap water will provide a more accurate assessment of the health risks due to drinking water in a given area.[28]

13.5 CONCLUSIONS

GIS provides a set of very powerful tools in the investigation of waterborne disease. Associations between geographically variant data, such as water supply source and illness, are very easily presented in a graphically clear fashion. Furthermore, any apparent association between disease incidence and water supply can be tested statistically within the GIS. Because GIS can also be used to detect clustering of cases of illness, they can play a extremely valuable role in the detection of outbreaks of potentially waterborne infectious disease and in their investigation once detected (see also Chapter 6).[29,30]

On the other hand, GISs are critically dependant on the quality of the primary data. As is discussed in many of the chapters in this book, the quality of infectious disease surveillance data is often quite poor. GISs may also require considerable effort to simply enter all the data into a computer readable form. This effort will also need to be continued, as the system is kept up-to-date as new data becomes available. Finally, as has been discussed, by their nature, GISs look at population level exposure rather than individual exposure, and as such, any apparent association may be due to bias from the "ecological paradox."

Nevertheless, GISs will contribute substantially to our understanding of the contribution of drinking water to human infectious disease. In order to realize the full potential of GIS technology in environmental health studies, interdisciplinary cooperation will be necessary.[4] Collaboration among researchers from different fields, including epidemiologists, medical geographers, biostatisticians, and environmental scientists, could lead to creative and practical GIS applications.

REFERENCES

1. Van den Berg, N., Geoinformations systeme in der Epidemiologie, *Kartographische Nachrichten*, 2, 52, 1997.
2. Curtis, A., Using a spatial filter and a geographic information system to improve rabies surveillance data, *Emerg. Infect. Dis.*, 5, 603, 1999.
3. Mott, K. et al, New geographical approaches to control some parasitic zoonoses, *Bull. WHO*, 73, 247, 1995.
4. Vine, M.F., Degnan, D., and Hanchette, C., Geographic information systems: their use in environmental epidemiological research, *Environ. Health Perspect.*, 106, 598, 1997.
5. World Health Organization (WHO), Geographical information systems (GIS): mapping for epidemiological surveillance, *Wkly. Epidemiol. Rec.*, 74, 281, 1999.
6. Aral, M.M. and Maslia, M.L., Evaluation of human exposure to contaminated water supplies using GIS and modelling, in *HydroGIS 96: Application of Geographic Information Systems in Hydrology and Water Resource Management,* Kovar, K. and Nachtnebel, H.P., Eds., Proceedings of the Vienna Conference, April 1996, *IAHS Publ.*, 235, 243, 1996.
7. Nuckols, J.R. et al., Evaluation of the use of a geographic information system in drinking water epidemiology, in *Assessing and Managing Health Risks from Drinking Water Contamination: Approaches and Applications*, Reichard, E. and Zapponi, G., Eds., *IAHS Publ.*, 233, 111, 1995.
8. Sweeny, M.W., Geographic information systems, *Water Environ. Res.*, 69, 420, 1997.
9. Goodchild, M.F., Communicating geographic information in a digital age, *Ann. Am. Geogr.*, 90, 344, 2000.
10. Twigg, L., Health-based geographical information systems: their potential examined in the light of existing data sources, *Soc. Sci. Med.*, 30, 143, 1990.
11. Lack, T., Water and health in Europe: an overview, *B.M.J.*, 318, 1678, 1999.
12. Kistemann, T., Trinkwasserinfektionen: Risiken in hochentwickelten Versorgungsstrukturen, *Geographische Rundschau*, 29, 210, 1997.
13. Havelaar, A.H., Application of HACCP to drinking water supply, *Food Contr.*, 5, 145, 1994.
14. Payment, P. et al., A prospective epidemiological study of gastrointestinal health effects due to the consumption of drinking water, *Int. J. Environ. Health Res.*, 7, 5, 1997.
15. Cliff, A.D. and Haggett, P., *Atlas of Disease Distribution: Analytical Approaches to Epidemiological Data*, Blackwell Publishers, Oxford, U.K., 1988.
16. Gesler, W., The use of spatial analysis in medical geography: a review, *Soc. Sci. Med.*, 23, 963, 1986.
17. Olsen, F., Martuzzi, M., and Elliott, P., Cluster analysis and disease mapping: why, when, and how? A step-by-step guide, *B.M.J.*, 313, 863, 1996.
18. Oden, N., Jaquez, G., and Grimson, R., Realistic power simulations compare point- and area-based disease cluster tests, *Stat. Med.*, 15, 783, 1996.

19. Bahrenberg, G., Giese, E., and Nipper, J., *Statistische Methoden in der Geographie: Univariate und Bivariate Statistik* (1), Teubner, Stuttgart, 1990,
20. Bahrenberg, G., Giese, E., and Nipper, J., *Statistische Methoden in der Geographie: Multivariate Statistik* (2), Teubner, Stuttgart, 1992.
21. Robert Koch Institute (RKI), Zur Situation bei wichtigen Infektionskrankheiten im Jahr 1998: Teil 1: Darminfektionen, *Epidemiologisches Bull.*, 15, 99, 1999.
22. Robert Koch-Institute (RKI), Wichtige Infektionskrankheiten in Deutschland — Zur Situation im Jahr 1999. Teil 1: Darminfektionen (Gastroenteritiden) — 1. Folge, *Epidemiologisches Bull.*, 23: 183, 2000.
23. Walter, S., The ecological method in the study of environmental health. II. Methodologic issues and feasibility, *Environ. Health Perspect.*, 94, 67, 1991.
24. North West Water (NWW), The use of geographical information systems (GIS) within NWW, *Water Health*, 26, 7, 1999.
25. Dunn, C., *GIS and Epidemiology*, The Association for Geographic Information (AGI), AGI Publishers, London, U.K., 1992.
26. Croner, C.M., Sperling, J., and Broome, F.R., Geographic information sytems (GIS): new perspectives in understanding human health and environmental relationships, *Stat. Med.*, 15, 1961, 1996.
27. Lacombe, M. and Fehr, R., Development of a comprehensive drinking water surveillance system, in *Environmental Health Surveillance: Results of an International Workshop, March 1997*, Fehr, R., Berger, J., and Ranft, U., Eds., University of Bielefeld, Landsberg, 1997.
28. Shimokura, G., Savitz, A.D., and Symanski, E., Assessment of water use for estimating exposure to tap water contaminants, *Environ. Health Perspect.*, 106, 55, 1998.
29. Bridgman, S. et al., Outbreak of cryptosporidiosis associated with a disinfected groundwater supply, *Epidemiol. Infect.*, 115, 555, 1995.
30. Hunter, P.R. and Quigley, C., Investigation of an outbreak of cryptosporidiosis associated with treated surface water finds limits to the value of case control studies, *Comm. Dis. Public Health*, 1, 234, 1998.

14 Time Series Analyses

Pascal Beaudeau

CONTENTS

14.1 Introduction....155
14.2 The Basic Method....156
14.2.1 Source Data....156
14.2.2 Statistical Analytical Methods....156
14.3 Avoiding False Correlations....157
14.3.1 Avoiding False Positive Correlation....157
14.3.1.1 Controlling for Confounders....157
14.3.1.2 Choosing the Time Step....157
14.3.1.3 Validating the Model....157
14.3.2 Avoiding False Negative Results....158
14.3.2.1 Determining the Statistical Power....158
14.3.2.2 Determining Whether the Population at Risk is Stable....158
14.3.2.3 Designing the Variables for Exposure....159
14.4 Measuring the Risk....161
14.4.1 Relative or Proportional Attributable Risk....161
14.4.2 Assessment of the Risk....161
14.5. Conclusions....162
14.6 Acknowledgments....162
References....162

14.1 INTRODUCTION

Time series analysis is the statistical analysis of a series of observations made at successive points in time. For waterborne disease, time series analysis has been mainly used to study effects on human health (such as hospital visits because of diarrhea) of water quality (such as turbidity). Time series studies (TSS) published on the epidemiology of environmental health are ecological studies. This means that the focus of study is a population rather than individuals. No information on the exposure of individuals or their health is entered into the model.

In the 1980s, the time series approach was widely used to study the epidemiology of air pollution. More recently, it has been introduced in the field of drinking water epidemiology.[1–5] The use of time series analyses for water and health has been delayed for several reasons, one being a relative lack of interest in water quality data by epidemiologists before the Milwaukee outbreak.[6]

0-8493-1259-0/03/$0.00+$1.50

14.2 THE BASIC METHOD

14.2.1 Source Data

The available indicators of health effects and exposure to pathogens are indirect. Sanitary indicators are restricted to short-term effects of some waterborne diseases, i.e., indicators of the symptoms of acute gastrointestinal illness (AGI). Daily counts of hospitalizations or outpatient visits,[1,3–5] emergency room visits,[1,3] physician billings,[1] and drug sales for AGI have been used to date.[2]

Currently, few indicators of water quality are suitable for continuous online measurement. Those available are not specific for pathogens or for fecal pollution but simply indicate the probability of pathogen occurrence in distributed water. Significant background events may be contamination of raw water, especially after rainfall, or transient treatment deficiencies. Suitable corresponding indicators are turbidity of raw water[1,2] and turbidity of filtered water[3–5] or disinfectant content in distributed water,[2] respectively. Turbidity (cloudiness) is caused by the presence in water of suspended particle matter (SPM) such as clay, silt, organic matter, microscopic organisms and mixed aggregates, flocculated or not flocculated. These particles cause light entering the water to be scattered to a degree that depends on their density, size, and nature. Turbidity is measured on the basis of this optical property and is usually reported in nephelometric turbidity units (NTU). There are few reliable data on the physical relationship between turbidity and microbial contamination.

14.2.2 Statistical Analytical Methods

TSSs use regression models that have two parts: the first expresses the "deterministic" relationship (linear or curvilinear) between exposure variable and health variable; the second expresses the stochastic pattern of the residual (that part of the variation in the health variable that is not explained by the variation in the covariates). The deterministic part includes three kinds of covariates: the past values of the target variable itself, the confounding variables, and the variables for exposure.

The best known model is the Auto-Regressive Integrated Moving Average with eXogenous inputs (ARIMAX) model promoted by Box and Jenkins.[8] It is linear and the residual is Gaussian. AR and MA terms stand for the inertia of the target variable over time. Schwartz managed to remove ARMA terms by thoroughly controlling the confounders, thus highlighting the true relationship between the variables for exposure and the variables for morbidity, i.e., the risk.[4] Others point out that autocorrelation in the morbidity process partly results from the intrinsic inertia of the process and may not be removed.[1,2]

The models used today may be categorized according to the shape of the deterministic relationship between the target variable and its covariates and to the type of the residual stochastic process (Table 14.1). Actually, the target variable is the number of cases of AGI. When these cases

TABLE 14.1
Statistical Models for Time Series Modeling

Residual Distribution	Shape of the Transfer Function: Linear	Nonlinear
Gaussian	ARIMAX	Artificial neural network
Poisson ($se^2 = m$)[1]	Poisson regression	
Poisson with overdispersion ($se^2 = k.m, k > 1$)[1]	Generalized linear model	Generalized additive model

[1] m: Average; se: Standard Error.

occur randomly, the underlying process is a Poisson process, but they often cluster in time, resulting in over-dispersion. For this reason, the general linear model or general additive model is often preferred to Poisson regression.[9,10]

14.3 AVOIDING FALSE CORRELATIONS

14.3.1 Avoiding False Positive Correlation

14.3.1.1 Controlling for Confounders

A great advantage of TSS is that potential confounders are restricted to those that vary over time. Even so, direct correlations between exposure variables and health variables cannot be assumed to be causal, as temporal confounding effects may still be present (such as trend, seasonal, and weekly patterns). These possible confounders have to be filtered out of the target series before computing cross-correlation. As well, other confounding variables, such as temperature, have to be controlled before introducing the exposure indicators into the model.

Of the possible confounders in water-related studies, seasonal variation is the most important. Some authors have addressed seasonal pattern as a sum of sine and cosine of time terms, according to Fourier's theorem. Year-to-year variations of the seasonal pattern affect both the range of the wave height and the location of the peak within the year. Under such conditions, the model requires additional parameters to adapt the sine function to specific yearly conditions. However, using these additional variables may risk over-fitting of the model, which may prevent the reproduction of any relationship identified between the exposure and outcome variables.

Nonparametric smoothing or moving average filtering are other ways of modeling the trend and the seasonal pattern.[2,4] The span of the moving average has to be long enough not to erase short-term effects. For instance, an approximate 100-day span removes the yearly rhythm but does not spoil the response of the target variable to pollution, even if it is delayed by 1 full month.

14.3.1.2 Choosing the Time Step

Availability of daily counts for sanitary indicators does not imply that a daily time step has to be used to model the underlying time process, as has been done in the field of air pollution. In order to identify the relevant time step, one has to take into account the expected delay in the response to water contamination, i.e., occurrence of turbidity-related cases of disease, and its dispersion (the two features being strongly linked). Thus, it is important to fit the time step to what is known about the possible delays in an effect. For example, there may be delays in the distribution of affected water through the system. There may also be delays due to the incubation period of a particular infection and the clinical progress of an illness before a sick individual seeks medical attention or buys medication. These delays vary from very short for most viruses and bacteria to potentially very long (up to 1 month) for protozoan parasites such as *Cryptosporidium*.

14.3.1.3 Validating the Model

Significant correlations shown in studies are selected among a batch of statistical trials that have been performed, i.e., N1 variables for health × N2 variables for exposure × N3 lags (allowed delays between exposure and outcome effects). Given the inflation in the number of trials, the probability threshold of significance should be adjusted according to the number of tests carried out. For instance, when testing 40 lags one by one (and assuming the independence of the tests), the threshold probability of the individual risk alpha has to be reduced to 0.001 in order to observe, by chance, one spuriously significant correlation in 40 or more, with a probability of 0.05.

Cross-validation gives strong evidence of the global consistency of the model. The most demanding way to carry out cross-validation is first to fit the model with one set of data (the so-called learning set) and then run the obtained model with another set (the testing set) in order to check the agreement between the expected and the observed outputs. Unfortunately, few models in regard to waterborne disease successfully pass this test. A less demanding way is to run the model with each data set and then compare the parameter values obtained. The relevant question is then: "Are the values of the coefficients consistent with each other and with prior knowledge?" rather than: "Do they differ significantly?"

14.3.2 Avoiding False Negative Results

14.3.2.1 Determining the Statistical Power

The power of the study depends on the level and the variability of exposure, the size of the population at risk, and its degree of susceptibility. In order to detect an average of one case of AGI a day, the minimum size of the population studied should be about 4000 when considering drug sales data, including over-the-counter sales, as the AGI incidence indicator;[2] 6000 when considering physician billing data; 40,000 when considering emergency home visit data; and 80,000 when considering data on hospital admissions.[1] The population sizes required explain the interest in a sensitive morbidity indicator.

14.3.2.2 Determining Whether the Population at Risk is Stable

Any stationary time process, i.e., a variable of time with a constant mean and a constant variance over time, can be modeled as an ARIMAX process.[8] Basically, the population at risk must be stable throughout the study period, e.g., seasonal inhabitants must not account for a large proportion of the whole population. This is why time series are not a convenient approach to assess the risk of infection due to recreational activities such as bathing or due to irregular events such as shellfish eating.

The behavioral constancy of the population is also a prerequisite. Though a high risk was expected, there was not a significant correlation between turbidity and antidiarrheal drug sales in rural areas around Le Havre, France where karstic water is distributed following simple chlorination. The lack of a positive outcome likely results from the relatively small population at risk (i.e., those continuing to drink tap water), because health authorities issue a warning when turbidity exceeds 2 NTU or cloudiness is detected by the naked eye above 5 to 10 NTU (Figure 14.1). People may react similarly when they experience an unusual taste of chlorine by-products, which may be related to a change in the microbial quality of raw water.

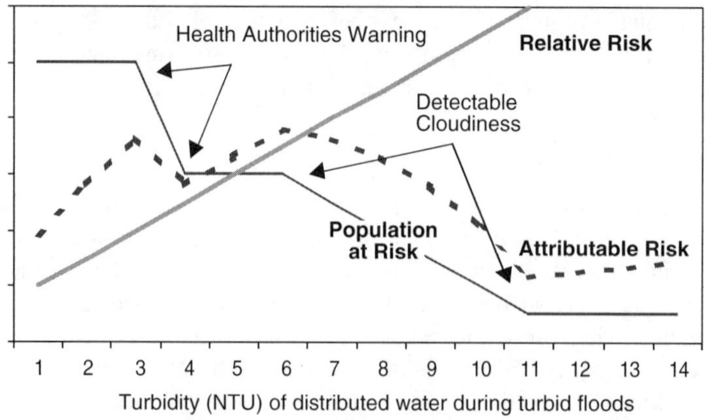

FIGURE 14.1 Hypothetical scheme of infectious waterborne risk in rural sectors of Eastern Normandy.

Given the gap between the need for a stationary process and the observed pattern of the process, additional information (e.g., on water consumption) may be introduced into the model in order to reduce the gap and, thus, achieve a stationary time process, i.e., one in which the residual behaves in a stationary manner. If no relevant information is available, the use of TSS may be compromised.

14.3.2.3 Designing the Variables for Exposure

It is not always possible to ascertain from which water treatment plant or which resource a particular area gets its water. The interconnection between distribution pipe networks and uncertainties about the flow of water may prevent tracking water from the plant to the taps. Consequently, it may be difficult to accurately define over time the area exposed to potentially contaminated water.

Additional treatment (coagulation and settling) may be applied at the plant during turbidity episodes. For instance, full treatment combining coagulation/settling and filtration may be set up at karstic springs when turbid floods occur, instead of relying on filtration alone as may be done during dry weather (Figure 14.2). This affects not only the level of turbidity but also the size and nature of suspended particles. In this case, the two types of turbidity have to be distinguished by splitting the original variable into a pair of specific variables.

The search for biological plausibility involves not only the possible interpretation of the results but also the design of the exposure indicators. For instance, hourly minima of free chlorine content better expresses the subsequent risk of AGI than the average over-the-time step, insofar as disinfection breakdowns are usually transient events (Figure 14.3).

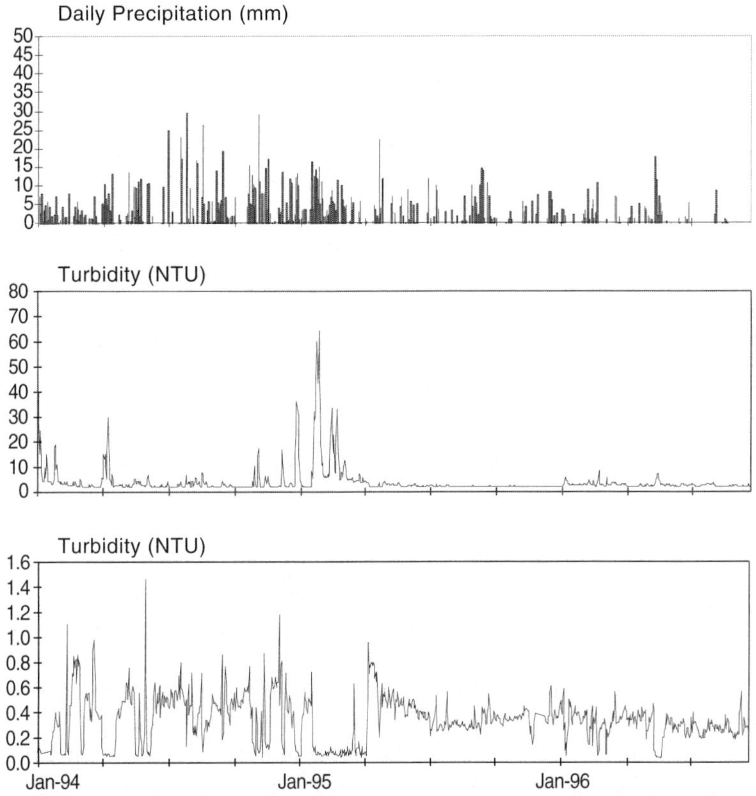

FIGURE 14.2 Precipitation, raw water turbidity, and treated water turbidity at a karstic spring in Eastern Normandy. The treatment alternates filtration and flocculation/settling + filtration, according to the level of the raw water turbidity.

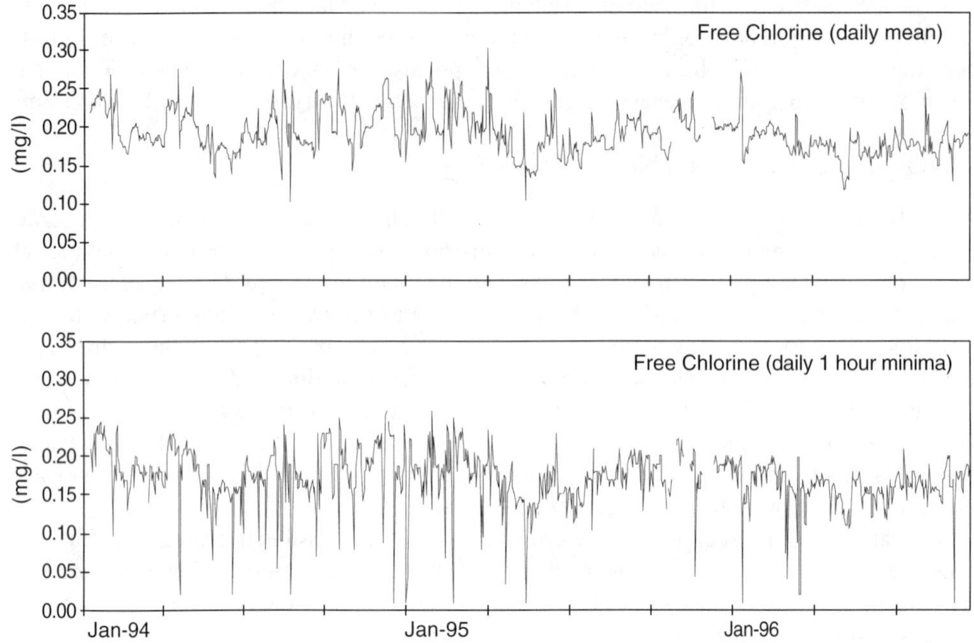

FIGURE 14.3 Free residual chlorine in finished water from a karstic spring in Eastern Normandy.

Turbidity raises the probability of pathogen occurrence in two quite independent ways. First, turbidity in raw water may result directly from the runoff of contaminated surfaces, the erosion of contaminated soils, the resuspension of contaminated sediments, or the overflow of sewage systems. Second, turbidity impairs disinfection efficiency and increases bioavailability of dissolved organic matter. Reduced disinfection and increased organic matter enhance bacterial regrowth in treated water downstream of the plant. Thus, turbidity is an indicator of raw water contamination and a measure of the impairment of water treatment. Use of turbidity as an exposure indicator remains a challenging task for epidemiologists. The nature of the turbidity — and, thus, its meaning in sanitary terms — may not only change from one type of water to another, but also from one site to another (depending on catchment basin features and treatment level) and over time for a given site.

Turbidity of water from karstic springs may occur without fecal bacteria being detectable in the water. Conversely, fecal burden may increase markedly, although the rise in turbidity is weak. The relationship is only statistical, depending on the dynamics of the system and on the size distribution of the particles.[7,11]

Some observations suggest that the first flush of runoff episodes picks up most of the microbial pollution deposited on soil or inside the karstic network. This means that the earliest stage of turbid flooding at karstic springs is more contaminated than the later stages. Thus, rises in the turbidity level can be more relevant than the absolute level for predicting adverse health effects. The improvement of the cross-correlation between the turbidity and the health indicator obtained by filtering out self-correlation from the turbidity series (i.e., removing the memory of the process) is consistent with these observations.[2]

Gregory[12] showed that the instant fluctuations of the turbidity signal provide some information on the size of the particles causing turbidity and suggested applying this finding to detecting the passage of parasites through the treatment line.

Progress towards a more accurate assessment of risk will come not only from reconsidering the information contained in the turbidity signal but also from combining external information with turbidity data (Figure 14.4). There is a special need for research on the relationship between the

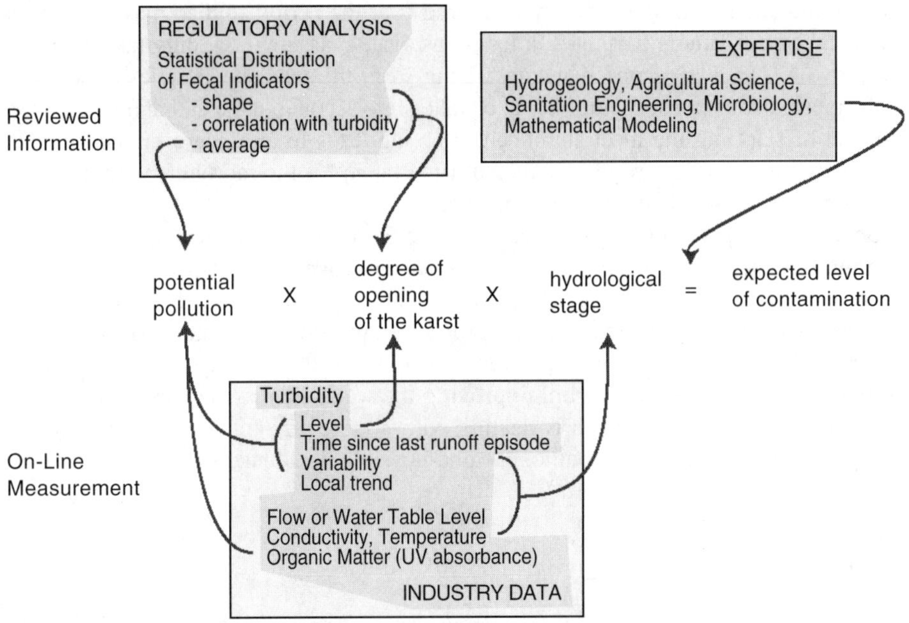

FIGURE 14.4 Assessment of the contamination of a raw karstic water. Available sources of relevant information.

state of the hydrological system, the amount and the nature of SPM, and the microbial burden (distinguishing parasites, viruses, and bacteria). The infective power of particle-associated or biofilm-embedded microbes is also an open question.

14.4 MEASURING THE RISK

For linear models, the coefficient of the exposure term is a risk expressed per conventional variation of this variable, e.g., a 1 NTU rise in turbidity or an interquartile variation of turbidity. For nonlinear modeling, the risk is a nonlinear function of the turbidity.

14.4.1 Relative or Proportional Attributable Risk

The type of risk revealed through TSS depends on the event considered for exposure. In the example of turbidity in tap water, the event considered is either the occurrence of turbidity at the tap, in which case the corresponding coefficient in a linear model is a relative risk (RR), or it is the consumption of the turbid water, and this coefficient may easily be reformulated as an attributable risk (AR). If one wants to look at RR associated with tap water consumption, the exposure to the vector of risk has to be known.

14.4.2 Assessment of the Risk

Assuming that long-term variations and auto-correlation have been filtered out of both the morbidity and the exposure variables, only the short-term variations of the variables are entered into the model. As a result, the cases of disease corresponding to seasonal variations or to the background level are not included in the risk assessment, even if linked to water quality. The risk of a false negative is the price to pay for avoiding a false positive correlation. In addition, if the filtered signal is flat, no risk will be detectable whatever the actual risk attributable to water.

The next step in the analysis is to assess the global AGI burden attributable to tap water from a TSS model of risk. If background turbidity is not contaminated by pathogens, applying a linear dose-response function to all the turbidity measured over the period studied may overestimate the disease burden. Some authors have used a less conservative assumption, only taking into account turbidity above 1 NTU.[1] A second question arising from the published studies concerns the lag times of the morbidity response to turbidity to be taken into account in the global impact assessment. The approach of selecting the most significant time lag leads to an underestimated impact.[1] The reason for not considering the whole significant time range for the morbidity response, including potential secondary causes, is not clearly documented.

Although TSS is very useful and effective, it is only a rough statistical approach to studying the epidemiology of gastrointestinal disease. Concept-driven models, such as compartment dynamic models,[13] can describe the epidemiology more accurately. TSS cannot estimate the indirect benefits such as the decreasing excretion or environmental contamination, but only the direct impact of pathogens to human transfer in drinking water. Thus, it could severely underestimate the benefit to be expected from improving the water treatment. The difficulty of implementing the concept-driven approach is dealing with a large amount of parameters to be fitted, considering the multiple species of pathogens and possible health status for people (susceptible, infected, ill, immune).

14.5. CONCLUSIONS

TSS is a powerful tool for estimating the endemic risk of waterborne gastroenteritis. However, to be effective, the time series approach requires a stable population at risk (i.e., the population that drinks tap water), a good overlap of the geographical areas of exposure and morbidity measured, and short-term changes in water quality. Insofar as the data used for exposure assessment are collected at the plant, microbial contamination must be present in the water when leaving the plant, i.e., it must not be due to contamination within the distribution network. The gap between this ideal and the actual situation results in an increasing probability of nonconclusive TSS outcomes.

The main drawback of this approach is the lack of any clear relationship between indicator data and specific pathogens. Since the nature of the turbidity and its pathogen content depend both on the raw water quality and treatment, it will be difficult to compare studies as long as the studies are conducted under various conditions. Specific studies should address the biological plausibility of the relationship between turbidity and human health effects in order to improve the power of this approach to predict the likelihood of pathogen occurrence.

The advantage of the time series approach mainly rests on its low cost, which may be lower than an intervention study by a factor of 10. Furthermore, by basing the risk assessment directly on water industry data, a time series approach can be helpful in the dialog between public health staff and water suppliers, especially for risk management.

14.6 ACKNOWLEDGMENTS

The author wishes to thank Claire Sourceau, Alain Le Tertre, and Pierre Payment for their assistance in writing this chapter.

REFERENCES

1. Aramini, J. et al., *Drinking Water Quality and Health Care Utilization for Gastrointestinal Illness in Greater Vancouver*, Report of Health Canada, University of Guelph and Vancouver/Richmond Health Board, 2000.
2. Beaudeau, P. et al., A time series study of anti-diarrheal drug sales and tap-water quality, *Int. J. Environ. Health Res.*, 9, 293, 1999.

3. Morris, R.D. et al., Temporal variation in drinking water turbidity and diagnosed gastroenteritis in Milwaukee, *Amer. J. Public Health,* 86, 237, 1996.
4. Schwartz, J., Levine, R., and Hodge, K., Drinking water turbidity and pediatric hospital use for gastrointestinal illness in Philadelphia, *Epidemiology,* 8, 615, 1997.
5. Schwartz, J., Levine, R., and Goldstein, R., Drinking water turbidity and gastrointestinal illness in the elderly of Philadelphia, *J. Epidemiol. Comm. Health,* 54, 45, 2000.
6. MacKenzie, W.R. et al., A massive outbreak in Milwaukee of *Cryptosporidium* infection transmitted through the public water supply, *N. Engl. J. Med.,* 331, 161, 1994.
7. Atteia, O. and Kozel, R., Particle size distributions in waters from a karstic aquifer: from particles to colloids, *J. Hydrol.,* 201, 102, 1997.
8. Box, G.E.P. and Jenkins, G.M., *Times Series Analysis, Forecasting and Control,* Holden-Day Publishers, San Francisco, 1976.
9. McCullagh, P. and Nelder, J.A., *Generalized Linear Model,* Chapman and Hall, London, 1983.
10. Hastie, T.J. and Tibshirani, R.J., *Generalized Additive Model,* Chapman and Hall, London, 1990.
11. Nebbache, S. et al., Health risks and transport processes associated with suspended particulate matter in a karst aquifer in the chalk of Haute-Normandie (France), *J. Hydrol,* accepted.
12. Gregory, J., *Cryptosporidium* in water: treatment and monitoring methods, *Filtra. Sep.,* 283, May 1994.
13. Eisenberg, J.N.S. et al., An analysis of cryptosporidiosis outbreak based on a dynamic model of the infection process, *Epidemiology,* 9, 255, 1998.

15 Seroepidemiology

Floyd J. Frost, Tim Muller, Twila Kunde, Gunther Craun, and Rebecca Calderon

CONTENTS

15.1 INTRODUCTION

ELISA and Western blot assays have been used to detect serological responses to *Cryptosporidium* antigens.[1–16] A Western blot assay that uses a miniblot was developed by the Lovelace Clinic Foundation (LCF) with funding from the U.S. Environmental Protection Agency (EPA). This miniblot assay has been used to conduct a range of serological surveys of populations in the U.S.[5,6,10–12,14] and elsewhere.[3,4,13,15,16] The serological surveys have provided prevalence estimates of prior *Cryptosporidium* infections. This report summarizes the findings of analyses conducted at a single laboratory for 20 serological surveys in 16 different cities located in the U.S., Canada, Australia, Russia, and Italy.

A motivation for conducting these surveys was the frequent detection of *Cryptosporidium* oocysts in source and treated drinking waters in the U.S. and elsewhere.[17–21] In some cases, enhanced enteric disease surveillance has been initiated following detection of oocysts in the drinking water.[17,21] These disease surveillance studies have prompted laboratories and physicians to collect data on clinically diagnosed cryptosporidiosis or occurrences of symptoms compatible with cryptosporidiosis. However, the studies did not detect elevated rates of infection or of symptoms compatible with infection at the time of oocyst detection. Illness rates were not higher than in similar cities where no oocysts were detected in the drinking water.[17,20,21]

Reasons for not finding an elevated risk of cryptosporidiosis in exposed communities are unclear.[20] A prior study suggested low rates of drinking water-attributable infections (e.g., 1/1000 per year) together with difficulties in diagnosing and reporting cases of cryptosporidiosis probably accounts for low rates of detectable disease.[22] It is possible that many oocysts detected in drinking water are not viable or infectious for humans. Moreover, *Cryptosporidium* infections may not result in overt or clinically detectable illness for a substantial proportion of the population. If people are regularly exposed to drinking water with low concentrations of oocysts, the risk of symptomatic illness or the severity of illness from infection may be reduced because of protective immunity.[1,2,12,23] Since surveillance systems for *Cryptosporidium* infections generally focus on the occurrence of clinically detected disease (cryptosporidiosis), little information is available on endemic levels of infection.

0-8493-1259-0/03/$0.00+$1.50

Estimating the risks of infection and understanding risk factors for illness among those infected are critical to understanding the etiology of this disease and the public health importance of various environmental factors responsible for the transmission of *Cryptosporidium*. Even during cryptosporidiosis outbreaks, studies suggest that illness may occur in only a small proportion of the people infected.[4–6,10,11] Unfortunately, little is known about the incidence of *Cryptosporidium* infection or cryptosporidiosis in non-outbreak situations.

Since *Cryptosporidium* infection elicits a serological response in most infected humans,[1,9,10] surveys for the presence of this response have been used to estimate the prevalence of prior *Cryptosporidium* infection in populations.[11–16] Other studies have tracked serological responses in people intentionally or unintentionally exposed to *Cryptosporidium* oocysts.[1,8] Most recent studies have focused on responses to a 15/17-kDa and a 27-kDa antigen group.[1–16] Serological responses to these two markers appear to be specific for *Cryptosporidium* infection.[1,9,10] Infection usually elicits a serological response to these antigen groups[1,9,10] that peaks 4 to 6 weeks after infection.[9,10] The 15/17-kDa marker declines to baseline levels observed prior to the infection in 4 to 6 months after infection,[9,10] while the 27-kDa marker remains elevated for 6 to 12 months.[9,10] Responses detected by ELISA tests based on all *Cryptosporidium* antigens tend to be both less sensitive and specific than responses detected for the two markers by the Western miniblot assay.[5,8]

15.2 METHODS

Results are reported from 13 different studies, several of which included multiple locations. Sera were frequently obtained from surplus sera of blood donors or diagnostic testing. This occurs when, because of initial test results, not all of the multiple tubes of sera obtained for safety testing or diagnostic work are needed. In most studies, sera were obtained from selected participants or volunteers. None of the sera provided to the Lovelace Clinic Foundation included personal identifiers, but in several studies, information was obtained about water exposures and other risk factors. These 13 studies are described below.

Study 1 — A cryptosporidiosis outbreak occurred in Jackson County, OR in January to June 1992. Sera were collected from 504 residents at or near the time of the outbreak and up to 6 months after the outbreak.[5,6]

Study 2 — Seventy-eight sera were obtained from Milwaukee, WI residents prior to a 1993 outbreak and were tested for the occurrence of serological responses to infection. These were surplus sera from routinely conducted blood tests that had not been discarded.

Study 3 — A paired city study was conducted in two central Midwest cities in the U.S. One city gets its drinking water from a major river system and the water is treated with conventional filtration and chlorination. The other city is also located adjacent to a major river, but obtains its drinking water from a high-quality groundwater source. Blood donors were recruited from local volunteer blood banks (462 from the surface-water city and 503 from the groundwater city). In Tables 15.1 and 15.2, these are designated **SW2** and **GW2**. The sera were obtained between May and August 1996.[11,12]

Study 4 — In the spring of 1995, a year prior to the study, sera from 107 volunteer blood donors from the same surface-water city and 51 paid blood donors from the same groundwater city were obtained and tested for serological responses to the two antigen groups. These surveys were conducted to obtain a preliminary estimate of the prevalence of response to infection in the two cities. In the same tables, these surveys are designated **SW1** and **GW1**.

Study 5 — In 1994, Las Vegas was the site of a cryptosporidiosis outbreak that may have been waterborne, and a serosurvey was conducted in 1996 to determine if there was evidence of ongoing elevated risks of *Cryptosporidium* infection. The survey included 200 Las Vegas, NV and 200 Albuquerque, NM blood donors. Albuquerque residents were surveyed as a comparison population because Albuquerque uses a high-quality groundwater source for drinking water and, like Las Vegas, is a large city located in the desert Southwest.[14]

TABLE 15.1
Serological Responses to 15/17-kDa Antigen as a Percent of Positive Control Responses for Surfacewater (SW) or Groundwater (GW) Systems

Site	Samples	Detectable Response (%)	%> 10%	%> 20%	%> 30%	%> 40%
		Surfacewater — U.S.				
SW3	186	72.6	71.1	64.0	58.6	52.7
Las Vegas (SW)	201	49.8	46.8	41.8	36.3	29.9
Las Vegas 1 (SW)	36	41.7	38.9	27.8	25.0	16.7
SW1	107	50.5	40.2	28.0	18.7	17.7
SW2	502	45.2	41.4	30.7	25.3	19.9
Milwaukee (SW)	78	35.9	26.9	18.0	12.8	12.8
Medford (SW)	504	68.3	57.9	46.4	36.7	28.6
		Canada				
B.C. — Rural (GW)	273	18.0	15.4	12.8	9.5	7.7
B.C. — City (SW)	874	30.4	29.2	22.7	17.5	14.3
Payment (SW)	278	81.8	78.1	65.8	50.7	37.1
		Australia				
Sydney (SW)	104	56.7	50.1	36.5	30.8	24.0
Melbourne (SW)	104	61.5	46.2	38.5	34.6	27.9
Melbourne AIDS cases (SW)	298	53.0	49.0	36.2	28.2	22.5
		Other				
Russia (SW)	108	67.6	67.6	61.1	50.0	44.4
Italy (SW)	150	84.0	76.0	66.0	56.0	44.7
		Groundwater — U.S.				
Albuquerque (GW)	201	36.3	34.3	25.3	18.9	11.9
GW1	51	47.1	25.5	15.7	13.7	9.8
GW2	503	26.0	24.1	17.1	12.5	9.3
GW3	120	70.0	68.3	58.3	43.3	38.3
GW4	120	39.2	38.3	34.2	24.2	19.2

Study 6 — Thirty-six surplus sera were obtained from a Las Vegas sexually transmitted disease clinic. These sera were obtained in 1992 and 1993, prior to the 1994 Las Vegas *Cryptosporidium* outbreak. The purpose of the study was to determine if serological responses were less frequent or less intense in Las Vegas prior to the 1994 outbreak. These sera are designated as Las Vegas 1 in Tables 15.1 and 15.2.

Study 7 — A second paired city serological study was conducted in the U.S. Midwest. The data reported here include sera from 186 individuals residing in a city that obtains drinking water from a heavily contaminated river water source. The water is chlorinated and filtered using conventional filtration. This population is designated as **SW3.** Sera were also collected from residents of two communities in the same state that obtain drinking water from a high-quality groundwater source. These drinking water supplies are chlorinated but not filtered. These two communities are designated as **GW3** and **GW4**. Sera were collected in the summer of 1999.

Study 8 — A cross-sectional serosurvey was conducted among 232 homosexual or bisexual males infected with human immunodeficiency virus (HIV) in Melbourne, Australia. The study was conducted from March to July 1997 and was restricted to people living in Melbourne that year and

TABLE 15.2
Serological Responses to 27-kDa Antigen as a Percent of Positive Control Responses for Surfacewater (SW) or Groundwater (GW) Systems

Site	Samples	Detectable Response (%)	%>10%	%>20%	%>30%	%>40%
			Surfacewater — U.S.			
SW3	186	81.2	75.3	66.1	53.8	44.1
Las Vegas (SW)	201	55.2	43.8	36.3	31.8	28.9
Las Vegas 1 (SW)	36	36.1	25.0	25.0	25.0	16.7
SW1	107	49.5	37.4	30.8	25.2	20.6
SW2	502	47.6	38.9	25.7	16.3	12.6
Milwaukee (SW)	78	37.2	25.6	21.8	9.0	3.9
Medford (SW)	504	68.5	60.5	54.4	49.2	46.8
			Canada			
B.C. — Town (GW)	273	33.7	25.6	18.3	10.6	9.5
B.C. — City (SW)	874	35.6	29.1	22.2	17.4	13.6
Payment (SW)	278	83.1	68.4	49.3	38.1	27.7
			Australia			
Sydney (SW)	104	60.6	43.3	30.8	24.0	16.4
Melbourne (SW)	104	65.4	48.1	33.7	23.1	17.3
Melbourne AIDS cases (SW)	298	67.1	59.7	45.0	31.9	21.8
			Other			
Russia (SW)	108	88.9	77.8	65.7	50.9	38.0
Italy (SW)	150	69.3	54.0	38.0	30.0	22.7
			Groundwater — U.S.			
Albuquerque (GW)	201	50.8	38.3	26.4	20.9	15.4
GW1	51	58.8	52.9	41.2	33.3	29.4
GW2	503	35.6	27.0	18.1	12.5	8.8
GW3	120	82.5	68.3	53.3	42.5	33.3
GW4	120	65.8	49.2	36.7	25.0	17.5

who obtained drinking water from the Melbourne Water Corporation. All were men who had sex with other men or sex with men and women.[13,27]

Study 9 — In response to detection of *Cryptosporidium* oocysts in the Sydney, Australia water supply, a serosurvey of 104 blood donors from Sydney and 104 from Melbourne was conducted in October and November 1998. The purpose of the study was to determine if Sydney blood donors had more common or more intense responses to the 15/17-kDa and 27-kDa markers.[3]

Study 10 — A serosurvey of 100 blood donors residing in a northern Italian city was conducted in 1998. Another 50 blood donors were added to the study in 1999. The purpose of the study was to estimate the seroprevalence in a southern European population without many reports of cryptosporidiosis which had not experienced a cryptosporidiosis outbreak.[15]

Study 11 — Two surveys were conducted using sera routinely collected for rubella screening in British Columbia, Canada.[28] A total of 874 sera were collected from a large southwest B.C. city that uses filtered surfacewater from a protected watershed. A total of 273 sera were collected from rural parts of the province that obtain drinking water from groundwater sources. The results presented are for laboratory work done at LCF or for laboratory work done using the authors' positive control sera and imaged at LCF.

Study 12 — In 1989, a prospective epidemiological study was conducted in the Province of Quebec, Canada to assess the health effects of the consumption of tap water.[29] The study included people who later were assigned to one of two groups that were either provided or not provided a reverse osmosis filtration device on their tap. Baseline sera for 278 individuals were collected for this analysis.

Study 13 — One hundred sera were obtained from adult residents of Cherepovets, Russia.[30] Fifty of the participants were recruited by a random household survey while the other 50 were blood donors at a local blood bank. Sera were collected from June to December 1999.

15.2.1 Western Blot Procedures

Sera were analyzed by immunoblot to measure IgG serological response to the 15/17- and 27-kDa antigen groups. The methods have been described elsewhere.[11–16] The intensities of the serological responses to the 15/17- and 27-kDa antigen groups were digitally analyzed by an IS-2000 Digital Imaging System (Alpha Innotech). The image is captured using a high performance CCD camera and the system calculates the pixel density of the manually selected band of the immunoblot. This allows the intensity of the serological response on the immunoblot to be quantified. Due to limited resources, it was not possible to blind the microbiologist to the origin of the samples. However, use of the computer to measure detection and the intensity of responses minimizes the risk of introducing operator bias.

15.2.2 Statistical Analysis

The IgG results for each specimen were standardized by taking the ratio of the response intensity for the unknown sample to the response intensity of a positive control serum contained on each blot. The IgG positive control serum was obtained from individuals with a strong serological response to both antigens, approximating the intensity of responses observed from several individuals with laboratory confirmed cryptosporidiosis. The same positive control serum was used for all blots. An extensive quality control effort was conducted analyzing replicate samples.[10] The correlation between the intensity of serological response for replicate analyses ranged from 0.92 for the 15/17-kDa marker to 0.84 for the 27-kDa marker. Lacking a standard for a positive serological response, five alternative intensity levels, measured as a percent of the positive control, were used to define a positive serological response (>0%, >10%, >20%, >30%, >40%).

15.3 RESULTS

The intensities of serological responses for the 15/17-kDa and 27-kDa antigen groups are presented in Table 15.1 and Table 15.2, respectively. The percentage of the samples with a response greater than 0%, 10%, 20%, 30%, and 40% of the positive control are presented for each site. Statistically, significant differences were detected between sites ($p<0.001$). One site had as few as 18% of the samples with a detectable response to the 15/17-kDa antigen, while for another site 84% of the sera tested had a detectable response. Interestingly, the two sites with among the highest fraction of responses to the 15/17-kDa antigen group included a U.S. Midwest city served by a surfacewater system and a Midwest system that uses groundwater. However, residents of this groundwater city had considerable exposure to farm animals and this may have contributed to their high seroprevalence to the *Cryptosporidium* markers. For the 27-kDa antigen the range was almost as large. In two systems (one surfacewater unfiltered and one groundwater), only 37% of the sera had a detectable response to the 27-kDa antigen. However, in samples from Cherepovets, Russia, and Quebec, Canada, 86 to 89% had a detectable response to the 27-kDa antigen group.

TABLE 15.3
Results of Paired City Comparisons (Surfacewater [SW] or Groundwater [GW] Systems) — Response as a Percent of Positive Control Responses for the 15/17-kDa Antigen Group

Site	Samples	Detectable Response (%)	%≥10% Positive Control	%>20% Positive Control	%>30% Positive Control	%>40% Positive Control
Las Vegas (SW)	201	49.8	46.8	41.8	36.3	29.9
Albuquerque (GW)	201	36.3	34.3	25.3	18.9	11.9
B.C. — City (SW)	874	30.4	29.2	22.7	17.5	14.3
B.C. — Rural (GW)	273	18.0	15.4	12.8	9.5	7.7
SW2	502	45.2	41.4	30.7	25.3	19.9
GW2	503	26.0	24.1	17.1	12.5	9.3
SW3	186	72.6	71.1	64.0	58.6	52.7
GW3	120	70.0	68.3	58.3	43.3	38.3
GW4	120	39.2	38.3	34.2	24.2	19.2

Statistically, significant differences were not detected for the results of surveys conducted in Australia. The Melbourne AIDS cohort had slightly more intense responses than blood donors from either Melbourne or Sydney, but the differences were not statistically significant. The three Canadian surveys found very different responses, most likely related to the extent of contamination of the water source. The cohort from Quebec receives water from a major river with sewage and agricultural discharges; 78% had a response to the 15/17-kDa antigen group and 86% had a response to the 27-kDa antigen group. In British Columbia, the population receives water from remote reservoirs with no sewage discharges; only 15 to 29% of the subjects from B.C. responded to the 15/17-kDa antigen group and 37% responded to the 27-kDa antigen group.

In contrast to the Canadian surveys, the two European sites had different responses for the15/17-kD and the 27-kDa antigen group. A higher fraction of the Italian group had a response to the 15/17-kDa antigen group than did the Russian group ($p = 0.14$). However, a lower fraction of the Italian group had a response to the 27-kDa antigen (71 vs. 89%) ($p<0.001$).

For these surveys, the comparisons remained stable for each of the different definitions of a positive response (>0%, >10%, >20%, >30%, or 40% of the positive control). For the four paired-city studies, the results for the 15/17-kDa antigen group are presented in Table 15.3. In each case, the surface water city had a higher prevalence of responses at every intensity level; however, not all of the differences were statistically significant. As stated earlier, the GW3 site was a farming community with considerable animal exposure. These exposures may have contributed to the apparent high level of prior infections for participants from this site.

The statistical testing shows some interesting insights into the differences in the frequency and intensity of responses between the two antigen groups for the different paired-city combinations. Table 15.4 shows differences between the four paired-city tests. In all four studies, the surface water city had evidence for more intense response to both antigen groups; however, the differences in responses to the 15/17-kDa antigen group were more consistent. In each study, all definitions of a positive response were statistically significant for the 15/17-kDa antigen group for residents of the surface water city. The 27-kDa marker has a longer duration of response, and this may be the reason consistent differences were not found for this marker between the surface water and groundwater city residents.

15.4 CONCLUSIONS

As was previously reported, these surveys suggest that populations using surface water-derived drinking water treated with conventional filtration and chlorination and meeting all water quality standards may

TABLE 15.4
Comparisons of Surface- vs. Groundwater Sources — Significance Level under Different Definitions of a Positive Response

Intensity as a Percent of Positive Control Intensity	MW1 p-value	MW2 p-value	Las Vegas/Albuquerque p-value	British Columbia p-value
15/17-kDa				
Detectable response	0.001	0.001	0.001	0.001
10% positive control	0.001	0.001	0.001	0.001
20% positive control	0.001	0.001	0.002	0.002
30% positive control	0.001	0.001	0.004	0.004
40% positive control	0.001	0.001	0.013	0.013
27-kDa				
Detectable	0.001	0.301	0.841	0.901
10% positive control	0.001	0.132	0.424	0.617
20% positive control	0.001	0.001	0.361	0.306
30% positive control	0.001	0.001	0.018	0.176
40% positive control	0.001	0.001	0.013	0.008

have an increased risk of waterborne *Cryptosporidium* infection. However, very large differences in seroprevalence have been observed between cities and even between cities that use groundwater sources that are unlikely to be contaminated with *Cryptosporidium* oocysts. These findings suggest that although surface water-derived drinking water appears to be a risk factor for *Cryptosporidium* infection, other factors varying geographically are likely to significantly influence the risk of infection.

The findings of these serological studies suggest that endemic *Cryptosporidium* infections may commonly occur in many cities in North America, Europe, and Australia. Between 18 and 84% of subjects tested had evidence of prior *Cryptosporidium* infection based on responses to the 15/17-kDa antigen group. Between 34 and 89% have been infected based on responses to the 27-kDa antigen group. Therefore, *Cryptosporidium* infections may be relatively common in diverse areas of the world. Based on prior studies, the authors believe that most of these infections may be asymptomatic or very mild and self-limiting.[11,12]

These surveys focused on infection defined as a positive serological response rather than excretion of oocysts or illness. This definition of infection differs from that used in prior *Cryptosporidium* research, which defined infection as detection of oocysts in the stool[24] or illness consistent with cryptosporidiosis.[25–26]

There are advantages and disadvantages of each definition of infection. An advantage of using serological responses rather than oocyst excretion or illness is that it may be less influenced by immune responses from prior infections that may reduce the occurrence or severity of cryptosporidiosis or the excretion of oocysts.[2,4,9,10,23] Unfortunately, the detection of a response provides little information on when the infection may have occurred. Additional research is needed to better understand the relationships between immune response, oocyst excretion, and illness.

Although these surveys suggest that *Cryptosporidium* infections occur commonly, additional information is needed on the frequency of illness from infection and about risk factors for illness from infection. It is possible that although the general population may not be at elevated risks of illness from infection, certain subpopulations may be at elevated risk. For example, travelers, young children, and people with compromised immune systems may be at risk of illness even though the general population shows little or no evidence of elevated risk of illness. Whether this is a significant public health issue is uncertain and needs to be further elucidated with additional serological studies, clinical studies, and epidemiologic studies on endemic diarrheal disease.

REFERENCES

1. Moss, D.M. et al., The antibody response to 27-, 17- and 15-kDa *Cryptosporidium* antigens following experimental infection in humans, *J. Infect. Dis.,* 178, 827, 1998.
2. Frost, F.J. and Craun, G.F., Serological response to human *Cryptosporidium* infection, *Infect. Immun.,* 66, 4008, 1998.
3. Frost, F.J. et al., Serological evaluation of *Cryptosporidium* oocyst findings in the water supply for Sydney, Australia, *Int. J. Environ. Health Res.*, 10, 35, 2000.
4. Frost, F.J. et al., Serological analysis of a cryptosporidiosis epidemic, *Int. J. Epidemiol.,* 29, 376, 2000.
5. Frost, F.J. et al., Comparisons of ELISA and Western blot assays for detection of *Cryptosporidium* antibody, *Epidemiol. Infect.,* 121, 205, 1998.
6. Frost, F.J. et al., A two-year follow-up of antibody to *Cryptosporidium* in Jackson County, Oregon following an outbreak of waterborne disease, *Epidemiol. Infect.,* 121, 213, 1998.
7. Moss, D.M et al., Kinetic and isotypic analysis of specific immunoglobulins for crew members with cryptosporidiosis on a U.S. Coast Guard cutter, *J. Eukaryotic Micro.,* 41, 52S, 1994.
8. Moss, D.M. et al., Enzyme-linked immunoelectrotransfer blot analysis of a cryptosporidiosis outbreak on a U.S. Coast Guard cutter, *Am. J. Trop. Med. Hyg.,* 51, 110, 1998.
9. Priest, J.W. et al., Enzyme immunoassay detection of antigen-specific immunoglobulin G antibodies in longitudinal serum samples from human cryptosporidiosis patients, *Clin. Diagn. Lab. Immunol.,* 8, 415, 2001.
10. Muller, T.B. et al., Serological responses to *Cryptosporidium* infection, *Infect. Immun.,* 69, 1974, 2001.
11. Frost, F.J., Two-city *Cryptosporidium* study, American Water Works Association Research Foundation, *Drinking Water Res.,* 8, 6, 2, 1998.
12. Frost, F.J. et al., Serological evidence of endemic waterborne *Cryptosporidium* infections, *Ann. Epid.,* in press.
13. Friedman, N.D. et al., One year follow up of antibodies to *Cryptosporidium* among individuals with HIV infection, *Venereology,* 14, 21, 2001.
14. Frost, F.J. et al., Paired city *Cryptosporidium* serosurvey in the southwest USA, *Epidemiol. Infect.,* 126, 301, 2001.
15. Frost, F.J. et al., Serological evidence of *Cryptosporidium* infection in southern Europe, *Eur. J. Epidemiol.,* 16, 385, 2000.
16. Caputo, C. et al., Determinants of antibodies to *Cryptosporidium* infection among individuals infected with HIV, *Epidemiol. Infect.,* 122, 291, 1998.
17. McClellan, P., First Interim Report, Possible Causes of Contamination, Sydney Water Inquiry, New South Wales Premier's Department, August 1998. (http://www.premiers.nsw.gov.au/pubs.htm)
18. Lisle, J.T. and Rose, J.B., *Cryptosporidium* contamination of water in the USA and UK, a mini-review, *J. Water SRT-Aqua,* 44, 1003, 1995.
19. Rose, J.B.N., Gerba, C.P., and Jakubowski, W., Survey of potable water supplies for *Cryptosporidium* and *Giardia, Envir. Sci. Technol.,* 25, 1393, 1991.
20. Craun, G.F. et al., Waterborne outbreaks of cryptosporidiosis, *J. Am. Water Works Assoc.,* 90, 81, 1998.
21. Dawson, A., *Cryptosporidium* surveillance: isolation from human stools and water supplies, in *Proceedings of a Workshop on* Cryptosporidium *in Water Supplies*, Dawson, A. and Lloyd, A., Eds., Her Majesty's Stationary Office, London, 1994.
22. Perz, J.F., Ennever, F.K, and LeBlancq, S.M., *Cryptosporidium* in tap water: comparison of predicted risks of observed levels of disease, *Am. J. Epidemiol.,* 147, 289, 1998.
23. Frost, F.J. et al., So many oocysts, so few outbreaks, *J. Am. Water Works Assoc.,* 89(12), 8, 1997.
24. Okhuysen, P.C. et al., Susceptibility and serological response of healthy adults to re-infection with *Cryptosporidium parvum, Infect. Immun.,* 66, 441, 1998.
25. DuPont, H.L. et al., The infectivity of *Cryptosporidium parvum* in healthy volunteers, *N. Engl. J. Med.,* 332, 855, 1995.
26. Chappel, C.L. et al., *Cryptosporidium parvum*: intensity of infection and excretion patterns in healthy volunteers, *J. Infect. Dis.,* 173, 232, 1996.
27. Caputo, C. et al., Determinants of antibodies to *Cryptosporidium* infection among individuals infected with HIV, *Epidemiol. Infect.,* 122, 291, 1998.

28. Isaac-Renton, J. et al., Epidemic and endemic seroprevalence of antibodies to *Cryptosporidium* and *Giardia* in residents of three communities with different drinking water supplies, *Am. J. Trop. Med. Hyg.*, 60, 578, 1999.
29. Payment, P. et al., A randomized trial to evaluate the risk of gastrointestinal disease due to the consumption of drinking water meeting currently accepted microbiological standards, *Am. J. Public Health,* 81, 702, 1991.
30. Egorov, A. et al., Serological evidence of *Cryptosporidium* infections in a Russian city and evaluation of risk factors for infection, *Eur. J. Epidemiol.*, in press.

16 Case–Control Studies

Brent Robertson, Christopher K. Fairley, Jim Black, and Martha Sinclair

CONTENTS

16.1 Introduction....175
16.2 Investigation of Endemic Waterborne Disease....176
16.3 Selection of Epidemiological Study Designs....176
16.3.1 Case–Control Studies....177
16.3.1.1 Key Pathogens....177
16.3.1.2 Study Area for Case–Control Studies....177
16.3.1.3 Measuring Drinking Water Consumption....178
16.3.1.4 Definition and Recruitment of Cases....178
16.3.1.5 Definition and Recruitment of Controls....179
16.3.1.5.1 Optimal Recruitment Method for Controls....179
16.3.1.5.2 Matching of Controls to Cases....180
16.3.1.6 Questionnaire and Database....180
16.4 Conclusions....181
References....181

16.1 INTRODUCTION

Outbreaks of waterborne disease provide ample evidence of the capacity of waterborne pathogens to cause illness in consumers of contaminated drinking water. Such events can have severe health effects and major economic impacts on an individual community; however, they are quite rare in comparison to the large number of water supplies that operate without apparent health problems.

In recent years, questions have been raised about the possible involvement of waterborne pathogens in endemic disease, particularly gastroenteritis, even in supplies that meet conventional microbiological water quality criteria. Endemic gastroenteritis refers to the amount of illness that occurs continually at variable "background" levels in a community. Outbreaks appear as sudden dramatic increases in illness rates over this background rate, but the overall burden of illness and economic impact of endemic disease is much greater than the effect of outbreaks.

Estimation of the prevalence of gastroenteritis at the community level is difficult since most cases involve mild, short-term illness that does not normally come to the attention of medical authorities. A number of recent epidemiological studies suggest that the prevalence of gastroenteritis in developed nations is around 0.7 episodes per person per year.[1,2] On this basis, it can be estimated that in the U.S. during 1993 waterborne gastroenteritis from recognized outbreaks accounted for less than 0.25% of all gastroenteritis despite the occurrence of over 400,000 cases of illness from the Milwaukee *Cryptosporidium* outbreak.[3] Therefore, if pathogens in drinking water are indeed responsible for a significant fraction of endemic gastroenteritis, this may represent a substantial and potentially avoidable health burden to the community.

0-8493-1259-0/03/$0.00+$1.50

The pathogens which contribute to endemic gastroenteritis may be transmitted by several routes, including drinking water, recreational water, food and beverages, person-to-person contact, animal-to-person contact, and indirectly through contamination of the environment with human or animal fecal material. Therefore, the identification of the relative contribution of different transmission routes to overall rates of gastrointestinal illness, or to illness caused by any individual pathogen, is difficult and requires specific epidemiological studies.

16.2 INVESTIGATION OF ENDEMIC WATERBORNE DISEASE

A number of approaches have been adopted to address the question of endemic waterborne disease including randomized intervention trials, seroprevalence surveys, and ecological studies. For some individual pathogens, the methodology of quantitative microbial risk assessment has also been applied to estimate the potential disease burden.

To date, epidemiological studies of endemic waterborne disease have given conflicting results and the question remains unresolved. It is possible that significant amounts of endemic disease may exist in some water supplies but not others because of differences in pathogen content that are not apparent from conventional measures of microbiological water quality. Current methods of assessing microbiological water quality rely on the detection of indicator bacteria such as *Escherichia coli* or fecal coliforms. These indicators are regarded as providing a good indication of potential risks from bacterial enteric pathogens, but correlate less well with risks from viruses, and rather poorly with risks from protozoa.[4,5] No alternative indicators suitable for routine use have yet been identified for viruses and protozoa, and direct measurement of individual pathogens is considered impractical from a technical perspective and ineffective for the protection of public health.[6]

16.3 SELECTION OF EPIDEMIOLOGICAL STUDY DESIGNS

In order to determine the optimal approach to investigating the role of waterborne transmission for enteric pathogens, the strengths and weaknesses of different epidemiological study designs must be considered. The strongest design suitable for the individual purpose should be used to ensure that the best possible quality of evidence will be obtained.

The randomized double-blinded trial design is acknowledged as being the strongest epidemiological design that can be applied to the study of human disease. This type of study involves the use of one or more interventions, which are expected to affect disease rates, and are assigned to randomly selected groups of participants. The assignment of the interventions is not known to the participants or the researchers until after completion of the trial in order to minimize potential sources of bias. Often one group will receive a sham or placebo intervention, which is expected to have no effect but which acts as a control representing the normal disease rate for comparison purposes. Such studies are common in pharmaceutical research but have seldom been used in the area of environmental epidemiology. As the design requires comparison of disease rates between the different intervention groups, it is most suitable for situations where the health outcome is fairly common and can be expected to occur in a substantial proportion of subjects in the control group during the observation period.

A study of this design was recently undertaken in Melbourne, Australia to investigate the issue of waterborne endemic gastroenteritis.[1] This city of 3.4 million people is served by a surface-water supply drawn from protected forest catchments, and the water receives minimal treatment in the form of chlorination before being distributed to consumers. The Melbourne Water Quality Study involved 600 families (2800 people) who were randomly assigned to receive either a functional water treatment unit that removed microorganisms or a sham water treatment unit that had no effect. Thus, the intervention involved a reduction in presumed exposure to waterborne pathogens in the test group compared to the control. The families recorded details of their health for a period of 15 months.

Comparison of the two groups at the end of the study showed no difference in the rate of gastroenteritis (rate ratio = 0.99, 95% CI 0.85–1.15), indicating that waterborne pathogens did not make a significant contribution to community gastroenteritis in Melbourne. The results also showed no difference in the nature of gastroenteritis episodes as measured by the duration of symptoms or use of healthcare services.

While this study design is appropriate for the investigation of the possible impact of collective waterborne pathogens on rates of community gastroenteritis, consideration of the frequency of individual pathogens demonstrates that a different strategy is required to characterize the role of waterborne transmission. For example, of 795 fecal specimens submitted by participants from the Melbourne Water Quality Study, only 13 were positive for *Cryptosporidium parvum* and 20 for *Giardia lamblia*. These low numbers indicate how a randomized, controlled trial is unlikely to have the statistical power to address the contribution of specific pathogens. Thus, a different type of study design is necessary to examine these risks.

16.3.1 Case–Control Studies

Case–control studies are a useful adjunct to randomized controlled trials in the assessment of pathogen-specific waterborne disease, particularly when the disease in question is uncommon or rare. This is because a case–control study selects a group of participants on the basis of having a particular disease (i.e., cases) and compares them to a selected group of participants who don't (i.e., controls). The proportions of cases and controls who have exposure to drinking water are then compared and deductions can then be made about whether or not drinking water is a risk factor. Although limited to the examination of only one disease, a case–control study has the advantage of being able to examine multiple exposures at the one time so that the relative contribution of each can be estimated.

16.3.1.1 Key Pathogens

The issue of what pathogen to study is determined by individual circumstances. The Melbourne Water Quality Study described earlier was supplemented by case–control studies examining cryptosporidiosis. This pathogen was selected because it has been responsible for numerous waterborne outbreaks worldwide, it is resistant to routine chlorination, and it is a devastating disease in the immunocompromised. It has also been a source of summer and autumn epidemics in several Australian states affecting mainly children.[7–10] Surveys of Melbourne pathology laboratories have indicated that approximately 1% of fecal specimens submitted for microbiological analysis are positive for the parasite *C. parvum*.[11] Using an estimated 0.7 episodes of gastroenteritis per person per year and a Melbourne population of 3.4 million people, there would be about 2.4 million cases of gastroenteritis from all causes each year, of which about 24,000 may be attributable to *C. parvum*. If drinking water did account for a proportion of this disease, then this fraction may be potentially preventable.

16.3.1.2 Study Area for Case–Control Studies

The choice of study area is again determined by individual circumstances. The Australian case–control studies were undertaken in metropolitan Melbourne and Adelaide, with each city representing a different end of the water quality spectrum. As discussed earlier, the people of Melbourne are served by a lightly chlorinated water supply that is principally drawn from highly protected catchment areas, where public access, farming, and recreational activity is not allowed. In contrast, Adelaide is a city of 1.1 million people, who are served by a water supply drawn from the River Murray and supplemented by local open catchment areas. All of these water sources are affected by residential and agricultural development and provide a relatively poor quality source water. The water supply undergoes full conventional treatment (flocculation, sedimentation, filtration) and chlorination prior to consumption. Residents in each study area are provided with drinking water of relatively uniform aesthetics (i.e., taste, odor, color) and conventional measures of microbiological quality, which ensures that results aren't biased by regional differences in consumption.

16.3.1.3 Measuring Drinking Water Consumption

One of the methodological limitations of case–control studies is recall bias of exposures, particularly when reliant on human memory. The measurement of drinking water intake by participants is based on self-reported estimates. Not surprisingly, these estimates have only moderate validity and reliability.[12] Self-reported estimates are likely to result in random error, which would have the effect of underestimating the association between drinking water and disease. However, biased over-reporting of estimates is possible for cases who suspect that drinking water is responsible for their illness. Such a situation is likely to occur if publicity which links the disease in question to drinking water is heightened at the time a study is conducted.

Both the random error in drinking water estimates and the potential recall bias of cases emphasize the caution required in attributing disease to drinking water. This is particularly important when the association is not strong, with many epidemiologists concerned about observational studies with odds ratios of less than three, even when accurate measurements of exposure are possible.[13]

It is useful to estimate the proportion of the study population exposed to drinking water. For the Melbourne and Adelaide case–control studies, approximately 80 and 60% of participants, respectively, consumed unboiled drinking water. Power calculations, therefore, were based on these figures. The *usual* drinking water consumption of cases and controls was requested in standard glasses per day. *Usual* patterns were requested because the volume of water consumed over the incubation period was unlikely to be recalled accurately, and because increased volumes of fluid were likely to be consumed over the duration of the diarrheal illness for cases which could have biased results.[14] A reminder was given to include water put into cordials, juices, and other drinks. Participants' drinking water exposure was collected as numerical data according to the number of glasses consumed per day, with data analysis performed in two ways: (1) according to those who consumed any water compared to no plain water, and (2) as a dose–response relationship to see if those who consumed increasing amounts of water were more likely to develop cryptosporidiosis.

16.3.1.4 Definition and Recruitment of Cases

One of the fundamental issues to be considered in a case–control study is the definition of a case. Diagnostic criteria using clinical details and tests that are highly specific and sensitive are preferable to prevent cases from being misclassified. For the Melbourne and Adelaide case–control studies, a case had to have gastrointestinal symptoms including either diarrhea or vomiting, in addition to pathology laboratory confirmation of *C. parvum* oocysts in a fecal specimen. Because laboratory confirmation was sought, this meant that those recruited would have disease from the more severe end of the clinical spectrum. Thus, cases could only be identified if they had gone through the following processes:

- A visit to their doctor
- Having their doctor request a fecal specimen
- Submitting at least one fecal specimen
- Having the parasite identified by a pathology laboratory, some of which applied selective criteria to testing fecal specimens

The issues that determined the method of case recruitment were ensuring the rapid recruitment of all cases occurring in the general community, going through the appropriate and legally correct institutional channels, and patient–doctor confidentiality. The recruitment process involved Melbourne and Adelaide pathology laboratories sending reports of all newly diagnosed cases of cryptosporidiosis to their respective health departments, which in turn sent a facsimile of the pathology report to the Department of Epidemiology and Preventive Medicine (DEPM), the institute from which the case–control studies were conducted. To ensure all cases were recruited, cryptosporidiosis bulletins were sent to organizations to remind them of the study. Cases were contacted by telephone, which provided rapid recruitment. This was important to maximize the accurate recall of exposures being examined. On making contact with the case, the interviewer would code the call according to its outcome, e.g., agreed to participate, refused to participate, etc. Speed was tempered by the time constraints of going through both legally appropriate government health departments and private pathology laboratories. The preservation of confidentiality between the patient and the doctor was also considered very important, so doctors were contacted before speaking to patients. The doctor was given the option of contacting the case directly to seek consent to participate in the study or having the research assistant do it on their behalf. To maximize patient autonomy, the former option was preferred. As an incentive and to thank participants for a completed questionnaire, each was sent instant lottery tickets. According to interviewers, this was unnecessary as most would have been willing to participate without an incentive.

16.3.1.5 Definition and Recruitment of Controls

Just as it is very important to clearly define a case, the same principle also applies to controls who should be free of the disease being studied. The control definition for the Melbourne and Adelaide case–control studies was the same as the case definition, with the exception of trying to ensure that controls truly didn't have symptomatic disease. Prior to administering a questionnaire, the authors therefore ensured controls were free from gastrointestinal symptoms, including diarrhea and vomiting. The option of excluding controls who had been exposed to *C. parvum* but were not symptomatic according to a fecal specimen or serology was also considered. This would have required potential controls to submit a fecal specimen and/or blood for analysis, which could have reduced participation rates. A case and control definition reliant upon symptoms rather than exposure was chosen because it was considered more relevant.

16.3.1.5.1 Optimal Recruitment Method for Controls

Just as cases were recruited from the general population, controls also had to be randomly recruited from the general population. Telephone recruitment using an electronic white pages (EWP) residential telephone directory was used for this purpose.[15] High levels of telephone coverage are needed in designated study areas using this methodology to avoid noncoverage selection bias.[16] In Australia there are very high percentages of telephone coverage in households (97.5%).[17] EWP is reported to have the following advantages:[18,19]

- Lower cost
- Simple to administer
- Increased likelihood of contacting valid residential telephone numbers
- Increased response rates because of introductory letters that could easily be sent to households prior to the first telephone call (because name and address of household occupants are recorded)

It is also reported to have the following disadvantages:[18,19]

- Exclusion of unlisted (silent) telephone numbers
- Calling outdated telephone numbers
- Not calling numbers issued since the EWP publication date

EWP has been criticized particularly because it includes only households with a telephone number listed in a directory, so that unlisted (silent) numbers are excluded. Research indicates that minimal bias is introduced in an Australian context, in part because of low levels of unlisted numbers.[19,20] To increase the participation rate of controls, an introductory letter was sent to each household prior to telephone contact being made.[21]

Options other than EWP for telephone recruitment include random digit dialing (RDD) and commercially available lists.[18] RDD has the advantage of including both listed and unlisted (silent) telephone numbers, but it is technically difficult to administer and can have a lower response rate.[19]

16.3.1.5.2 Matching of Controls to Cases

Controls need to be recruited in a timely fashion. This is an important study design feature to ensure the period of recall is similar for both cases and controls. This task is made more difficult by a matched study where controls are matched to cases according to specified criteria. The Melbourne and Adelaide case–control studies matched controls to cases according to age and sex. This proved more difficult than expected particularly for those 12 years old or less. To address this difficulty, a large database of potential controls was created in advance of cases. To establish this database, additional research assistants were employed to recruit controls over the winter and spring periods. This was a time of year when the number of cases was typically low, so resources could be primarily directed towards this task. All willing household members were added to the database with address, age, and sex recorded. This subsequently allowed cases from all age brackets to be rapidly and completely matched according to the specified ratio of one case to four controls.

After a case had the questionnaire administered, the names of four random potential controls (of the same sex and age bracket) were automatically generated from our database. The household of the potential control was then telephoned and the interviewer would code the call according to its outcome. Only one control from each household was matched to each case, and the control was then retained in the database of potential controls for possible selection at a later time. Controls were retained to prevent possible bias by their exclusion from the database. As for cases, controls were also sent instant lottery tickets as an incentive to participate and to thank them for completing a questionnaire. Interviewers again said this was unnecessary, as most would have been willing to participate without an incentive.

16.3.1.6 Questionnaire and Database

A method of questionnaire administration was needed to record participant responses. It needed to be timely, inexpensive, and combine easily with telephone recruitment. A computer-assisted telephone questionnaire (CATQ) was suitable for this task.[22,23] Other less satisfactory options included self-administration of a questionnaire sent through the mail or a face-to-face questionnaire.

Although the main objective of our study was to examine drinking water as a risk factor for cryptosporidiosis, the opportunity was also taken to examine other risk factors. To ensure that the most relevant risk factors were inquired into, the questionnaire was a synthesis of previously used questionnaires from published studies examining cryptosporidiosis. Relevant local and overseas investigators were contacted to obtain previously used questionnaires. To ensure the reliability, relevance, and comprehensibility of the questionnaire, it underwent several revisions overseen by a collaborating committee who met several times prior to the final version. The questionnaire was also piloted prior to its actual use.

Microsoft® Access was used to generate the on-screen computer questionnaire with an accompanying database.[24] It had the advantages of direct data entry, automated skips of irrelevant questions, prevention of missing values, built-in warnings to prevent responses that fall outside the acceptable range, and the scheduling of telephone call-backs. It was also able to generate automated reports and analyses over the course of the study. Such information can be sent to relevant health departments to inform them of disease clusters occurring in place and time, so that immediate action can be taken to prevent an outbreak of disease. It has the disadvantages of needing a database manager on-site, cost, programming skills, and irretrievable typing errors.[22,23]

16.4 CONCLUSIONS

Endemic gastroenteritis is likely to account for considerably more disease than that caused by outbreaks. Waterborne disease has been mainly studied in relation to outbreaks, but if drinking water makes a substantial contribution to the background rate of gastroenteritis, then this represents a large, potentially preventable source of disease. Although a number of approaches have been adopted to examine endemic disease, no epidemiological study is perfect in reassuring the public that there is no disease. Combined studies are likely to be most useful. Randomized controlled trials are useful in examining disease caused by several pathogens, but when a specific disease is uncommon or rare, these study designs usually lack the necessary statistical power to establish disease causation. In this instance, a case–control study is then suitable. After deciding upon the key pathogen to study, one of the most important issues to consider is the method of subject recruitment. Telephone recruitment is likely to be suitable for most developed countries, but not necessarily for developing countries that have lower levels of telephone coverage. The other important issue to consider, particularly with a matched case–control study, is having a database of willing controls to draw upon to ensure that cases are rapidly matched. A well-conducted case–control study, with recognition of its limitations, can provide important information about the relative contribution of drinking water to pathogen-specific disease.

REFERENCES

1. Hellard, M.E. et al., A randomized blinded controlled trial investigating the gastrointestinal health effects of drinking water quality, *Environ. Health Perspect.,* 109, 773, 2001.
2. Payment, P. et al., A randomized trial to evaluate the risk of gastrointestinal disease due to consumption of drinking water meeting current microbiological standards, *Am. J. Public Health,* 81, 703, 1991.
3. Kramer, M.H. et al., Surveillance for Waterborne-Disease Outbreaks — United States, 1993–94. *MMWR,* 45(SS-1), 1, 1996.
4. Craun, G.F., Berger, P.S., and Calderon, R.L., Coliform bacteria and waterborne disease outbreaks, *JAWWA,* 89, 96, 1997.
5. Sobsey, M.D., Inactivation of health-related microorganisms in water by disinfection processes, *Water Sci. Tech.,* 21, 179, 1989.
6. Allen, M.J., Clancy, J.L., and Rice, E.W., The plain, hard truth about pathogen monitoring, *JAWWA,* 92, 64, 2000.
7. Tzipori, S. et al., Cryptosporidiosis in hospital patients with gastroenteritis, *Am. J. Trop. Med. Hyg.,* 3, 931, 1983.
8 van Leeuwen, P., Lawrence, A., and Hansman, D., An outbreak of cryptosporidial infection amongst children in Adelaide, *Med. J. Aust.,* 154, 708, 1991.
9. Veitch, M.G.K., Cryptosporidiosis in Victoria: an important illness of autumn?, *Aust. N.Z. J. Med.,* 26, 621, 1996.
10. Veitch, M.G.K., *Victorian Cryptosporidiosis Surveillance Bulletin Number 5,* (Final Report), University of Melbourne, Australia, 1996.
11. Hellard, M.E. and Fairley, C.K., Gastroenteritis in Australia: who, what, where, and how much?, *Aust. N.Z. J. Med.,* 27, 147, 1997.
12. Robertson, B. et al., How well does a telephone questionnaire measure drinking water intake?, *Aust. N.Z. J. Public Health,* 24, 619, 2000.
13. Taubes, G., Epidemiology faces its limits, *Science,* 269, (14 July), 164, 1995.
14. Casemore, D.P., Wright, S.E., and Coop, R.L., Cryptosporidiosis — human and animal epidemiology, in *Cryptosporidium and Cryptosporidiosis,* Fayer, R., Ed., CRC Press, Boca Raton, FL, 1997, 65.
15. Australia on Disc: Dependable Database Data P/L, Sydney, NSW, Australia, November 1997.

16. Wacholder, S. et al., Selection of controls in case–control studies. II. Types of controls, *Am. J. Epidemiol.,* 135, 1029, 1992.
17. Australian Bureau of Statistics, (ABS 1998), Household Use of Information Technology, Canberra, 1999.
18. Lepkowski, J.M., Telephone sampling methods in the United States, in *Telephone Survey Methodology,* Groves, R.M. et al., Eds., John Wiley & Sons, New York, 1988, 73.
19. Wilson, D.H. et al., Random digit dialing and electronic white pages samples compared: demographic profiles and health estimates, *Aust. N.Z. J. Public Health,* 23, 627, 1999.
20. Taylor, A.N., Wilson, D.H, and Wakefield, M., Differences in health estimates using telephone and door-to-door survey methods — a hypothetical exercise, *Aust. N.Z. J. Public Health,* 22, 223, 1998.
21. Robertson, B. et al., The effect of an introductory letter on participation rates using telephone recruitment, *Aust. N.Z. J. Public Health,* 24, 552, 2000.
22. Abramson, J.H., Interviews and self-administered questionnaires, in *Survey Methods in Community Medicine: Epidemiological Studies Programme Evaluation Clinical Trials,* Churchill Livingstone, Edinburgh, 1990, 165.
23. Watson, E.K. et al., Conducting regional health surveys using a computer-assisted telephone interviewing method, *Aust. J. Public Health,* 19, 508, 1995.
24. Microsoft® Access 97: Microsoft 97®.

17 Prospective Epidemiological Studies

Denis Zmirou and Leila Gofti-Laroche

CONTENTS

17.1 INTRODUCTION

Identification and investigation of disease outbreaks can provide valuable information about causes of failures in water treatment or distribution systems. Also, it may give some indication of the relative importance of different microbial or chemical agents of concern for water and health authorities. However, it is recognized that most of the burden related to poor drinking water quality takes the form of sporadic/endemic disease cases whose active and, even more, passive surveillance is of poor sensitivity.[1] Low levels of disease in the community are hardly detected. Moreover, investigation of outbreaks may be misleading when assessing the main causes of burden. One reason is that the agents responsible for epidemic cases may differ, in terms of both nature and virulence, from those involved in the occurrence of sporadic cases. Furthermore, data on outbreaks tend to overestimate the relative importance of longer lasting or more severe conditions, and may also overemphasise illnesses that predominantly affect particularly susceptible subjects. [2,3]

In this setting, prospective epidemiological studies are useful means of evaluating the impact of endemic waterborne diseases, to complete the picture of the relative susceptibility of subgroups within the general population and to assess the association between water quality and disease rates.

17.2 KEY ISSUES FOR EPIDEMIOLOGICAL DESIGN

The following characteristics of exposure to waterborne hazards and of associated conditions may have important implications when designing epidemiological studies.

Exposure is a time variable — While most epidemiological studies are designed in relation to geographical differences of water quality, time is often overlooked. Even in well-designed water systems, it is impossible to fully guarantee that no infectious microorganism will ever be present along the whole chain. Sources of water contamination are many (see Chapters 9 and 10), and each

0-8493-1259-0/03/$0.00+$1.50

may exhibit distinct time patterns that should be accounted for in prospective studies. Poor raw water quality is the critical point and often presents some seasonality in relation to rainfall. In addition, unpredictable failures at the water treatment plant may occur. The distribution system is sensitive to small accidents or water pressure variations that allow intrusion of microorganisms or organic matter into the pipes. Finally, contamination of storage tanks and of home plumbing may show other time patterns. In such circumstances, determining the contributing roles of the different sources that can lead to infection and disease is extremely challenging.[4]

Species of pathogens are many — In order to assess the risk, conventional exposure characterization relies heavily on the traditional bacterial indicators, which provide only limited information.[5,6] Bacterial indicators of fecal pollution have made a substantial contribution to water quality throughout the past century, and still do so, but waterborne outbreaks often occur in absence of bacterial indicators.[1,7–9] Because novel analytical methods are now available, efforts should be made to search for additional microbial indicators that could better predict the risk associated with pathogens that resist the usual disinfection treatments. It is clear, however, that it is impossible to measure routinely all potential pathogens, even using the most recent analytical techniques, nor is it necessary.

Health outcomes of infection are uncommon — Hence, their exploration demands large population samples. Prospective studies in Europe and North America that allowed quantification of rates of acute gastrointestinal conditions provide similar figures, about 0.5 to 2.0 cases/person/year, according to age and to case definition.[4,5,10–14] Outbreaks are also rare events, at least those large enough to be detected by existing surveillance systems (see Chapters 3 and 12). Health effects associated with water microbiological quality are not specific and could well be confused with infection transmitted by food, aerosols, or by person-to-person contact. As a consequence, one should carefully select study populations such that exposure subgroups are as similar as possible for these potential confounding factors. Finally, the health outcomes are not often severe. It follows that most studies on waterborne infectious diseases have ascertained cases through declaration of subjects, which raises the issue of differential reporting according to perceived or true risks. In Western countries, proportions of affected subjects who seek care from medical professionals range from 5 to 10,[14,15] and are usually greater among susceptible categories.[2,15] The alteration of daily activities due to acute disease or school absenteeism may be more sensitive health indicators, but they lack specificity.

17.3 SOME FEATURES OF PROSPECTIVE EPIDEMIOLOGICAL STUDIES

17.3.1 Population Selection And Participation Maintenance

The characteristics of the study population obviously depend upon the study objectives. One question relates to whether one wants to assess disease rates within susceptible subgroups, such as the very young, the elderly, the immunocompromised (including specific segments such as HIV patients or subjects with home dialysis). In theory, this is of great interest in order to quantify the degree of susceptibility — increases in rates, in disease severity, and/or duration — and thus to give insight into the additional level of security required to protect fragile populations. However, studies in these target populations pose serious ethical challenges in addition to problems associated with sample size considerations.[16] Much can be learned from more empirical evidence, e.g., the observation that most subjects affected during the 1994 Las Vegas outbreak pertained to the immunocompromised segment of the population.[7] To the authors' knowledge, published prospective studies on water quality have restricted the susceptible subjects to children, who exhibit greater disease rates.[4,5,10,13,14]

Another question relates to the population selection procedure. This issue is of special importance since prospective studies on water quality and health are usually long term. Because disease

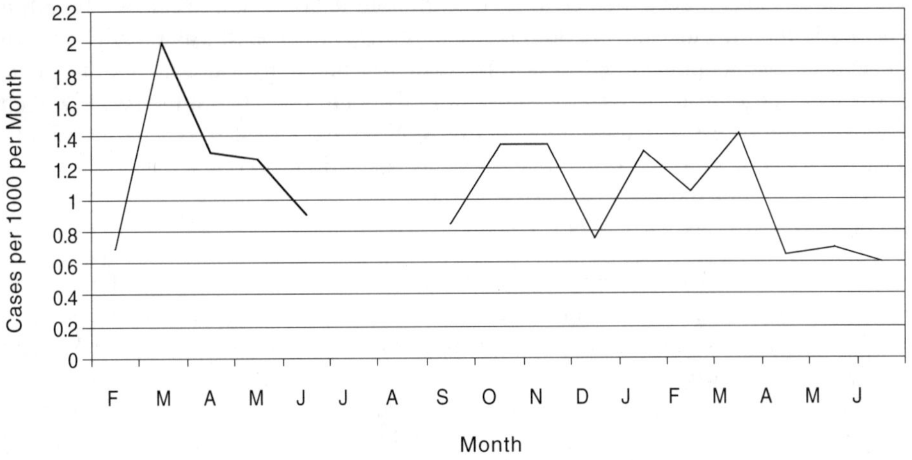

FIGURE 17.1 Time trend of acute digestive conditions incidence rates among children in a prospective study.

rates are low, and in order to demonstrate seasonal variations, prospective studies last months, often a year or more. Hence, epidemiologists, who most often depend on case reporting by study subjects, are faced with the risk of falling participation. Figure 17.1 illustrates this phenomenon in the setting of a prospective study conducted among school children who were asked to complete a symptoms diary under the guidance of their teacher during a 14-month study period.[5] Although care was taken to secure against differential declaration according to water quality across school classes, the data show evidence of a downward trend of disease rates along time, which combines the effects of seasonal variations of disease rates and decreasing participation.

Random selection procedures within the population of interest provide disease rate estimates that are less prone to selection bias. However, when study subjects are requested to undertake demanding tasks, in terms of time or effort, some degree of selection occurs, however careful the epidemiologist may be; this is known as the "Hawthorne effect."[17,18] In such cases, it may be advisable to call for volunteers, insofar as their characteristics match the study selection criteria. When the main study objective is to assess the relationship between water quality and disease rates, population representation is less critical than exhaustivity of case enumeration. In this setting, the prospective design results in a panel-type study in which study participants are asked to notify, by any relevant means, occurrence of acute conditions along time. It is of paramount importance to plan beforehand to maintain a good level of participation along the course of the study; if care has not been taken to remotivate the panel periodically, subjects will tend to *under*declare morbidity after some time. The reverse also may be true. It has often been shown that subjects tend to *over*declare disease occurrence at the beginning of their participation in prospective studies in an effort to be as helpful as possible. Provision should be made, when relevant, for discarding data from the first 2 or 3 weeks of participation in studies that typically last several months.

Sample size determination depends on whether the study is aimed primarily at comparing risks throughout the entire study period or according to multiple calendar segments. Conventional formulae for sample size computation are based on incidence rates in the least exposed (or referent) group, the magnitude of the expected rate ratio or ratios, power and type1 error considerations, and sample size ratio or ratios across study subgroups. One may also want to investigate the incidence of episodes with a given number of concomitant symptomatic subjects (i.e., outbreaks with, say, at least k cases).

If α is the expected number of diseased persons occurring in a population of size N on a given day, and assuming it follows a Poisson distribution, then the probability, P, of observing k cases is: $P_k = e^{-\alpha}.\alpha\ k/k!$. The probability of having more than k cases in that population is $P_{+}k = 1-\Sigma P_k$.

The probability, P, that n episodes occur, each with more than k cases, occur in a time frame t (t = number of days during the study period) is $P = [1-(1-P_{+k})^t]^n$, under the assumption that episodes are independent, i.e., not influenced by phenomena such as immunity acquisition. This is equivalent to the power $p_{1\text{-}\beta}$ of a prospective study whose objective is to find, during the period t, n episodes of size greater than k cases in a population of size N. N can be estimated backwards, for a required $p_{1\text{-}\beta}$value, when one has an idea of the rate of disease $\alpha/t.N$ in this population.

17.3.2 Case Definition and Ascertainment

Acute gastrointestinal (GI) conditions are an ill-defined clinical entity whose definition may vary across subjects. With a view to reducing misclassification and sources of differential bias in disease enumeration, it is important to define in a standardized manner what is to be reported and counted. One may want to optimize sensitivity and utilize a large definition that will encompass any acute GI condition or ancillary (e.g., abdominal pain). Specificity of such a definition is poor, however. Following Cabelli et al.'s paper on recreational water quality,[19] most authors have defined "highly credible gastrointestinal (HCGI) conditions" as including at least "vomiting or liquid diarrhea; or loose stools or nausea with abdominal pain," so as to derive greater relative risks between exposure groups.[13] This more specific definition comes at the price of sensitivity loss. In the recent EMIRA study, a broader definition of "general acute GI conditions" yielded six times greater rates of disease than the stricter HCGI definition.[20] It is prudent, in such circumstances, to accommodate different definitions of cases, and to do some sensitivity analysis in order to check whether the study results are influenced by the more or less stringent definition of cases.

Reporting of GI conditions by participating subjects is the most common approach for case ascertainment.[4–6,10–14,20] This information can be retrieved through periodic visits or, more easily, telephone calls to the study participants. It can also be collected in school settings, contingent upon active participation of teachers, whereby students (children, in most cases) are asked to complete daily logs. Since morbidity is generally mild, it can easily be overlooked or forgotten; therefore, absence of systematic stimulation of case reporting by the study coordinator would invariably result in loss of sensitivity. Active reporting is indeed much more efficient than passive declaration and prevents shrinking of case reports. In the EMIRA study, for example, a panel of 176 households was asked to complete a diary with all acute GI conditions to be reported for all members of the family. Each weekday, a study assistant called a small number (20%) of all households to retrieve retrospectively the information for the previous week, thus checking on disease incidence of the whole panel once each week unit. By the end of the 210 days of follow-up, information was collected on 92,492 person-days.[20]

As exemplified in the previous section, one may be interested in identifying aggregate cases, which is a form of sporadic events.[21] In the EMIRA study, such mild episodes were investigated. The operational definition of an outbreak was "occurrence during the past 48 hours of at least two cases" — provided they did not involve the same family. Due to the sampling procedure that allowed collection of daily information on 20% of the panel, these two cases were related to a daily set of about 210 subjects. Blindness is a difficult issue. Because reporting is very sensitive to subjective factors, it is important to organize the study such that participants and investigators are not in a situation where information bias may occur. Ideally, subjects in the investigated community should not know or think that they pertain to an *exposed* or *unexposed* group, otherwise differential reporting may occur. In the Melbourne study of the gastrointestinal health effects of drinking water quality, participants' houses were equipped with active or sham treatment devices.[10] Other studies have been recently funded and are under way under the Safe Drinking Water Act by the Centers for Disease Control and Prevention and the U.S. Environmental Protection Agency, to assess the feasibility of water intervention trials blinding participants to group assignment. In the EMIRA study, the assistant who made the daily calls to the panelists was unaware of the results of the parallel water microbial quality surveillance.

17.3.3 Exposure Assessment

Exposure assessment is a critical issue in all epidemiological studies. It is especially so in the drinking water setting.[22] In individual-type (i.e., not ecological) studies, control of random misclassification is achieved by greater statistical power. Power loss can result from two main types of measurement errors: classic error and Berkson error. The former refers to typical situations where exposure and effect assessment are both at the individual level. In this situation, random errors lead to bias, which, in most cases, attenuate the regression coefficient. This is a rare situation in water-quality studies. Rather, they are semi-individual studies where the Berkson type of error occurs.[23] This applies when exposure is assigned on a group level. In prospective studies on water quality, exposure of subjects is inferred from water quality monitoring that takes place at a given point on the distribution system and covers all subjects served by the same water source, while health status is ascertained on an individual level (hence, the "semi-individual" concept). It was shown that random Berkson error does not lead to biased association estimates, provided that the common exposure value correctly represents the average group exposure and that the standard error of the mean exposure is constant across exposure groups.[24] However, since true individual exposures vary about the assigned common value, this error leads to larger confidence intervals of measures of association, and thus to power loss.[24] Perfect personal data are unattainable to date because, unlike air pollution studies, there are no personal samplers that can be used in epidemiological studies on water microbial quality. However, one should make efforts to estimate personal exposure as closely as possible. One obvious way is to account for the amount of water that subjects drink throughout the study period. Since this might be time- and space-dependent, prospective studies should include investigation of water consumption within the surveyed population. In the EMIRA study, average water consumption within the ninth decile was 2.8 times greater than in the first decile, age being the most important predictor of water consumption.[25] Also, mobility of study participants should be accounted for, when relevant. At work, at school, or when traveling, subjects may drink water whose origin and quality differs from that which is monitored within the study, thus yielding some additional exposure misclassification. Some rules as to subjects' selection procedures, or regarding whether to keep in the study participants who exhibit an appreciable amount of "unknown" water quality consumption, should be stated *a priori*. In the second Laval study, subjects were asked to take with them wherever they went a bottle with the same type of water that they were assigned.[4]

Water quality is often variable with time, as suggested above. As a result, one should pay a great deal of attention to this time dependence. Repetitive water sampling and analysis is recommended but is expensive, especially when dealing with novel analytical techniques used to evaluate exposure to other microbial agents than bacterial indicators. Continuous monitoring is possible with indirect indexes of water quality such as turbidity[26] or epifluorescence assays. In the future, DNA chips might become a means to assess exposure with a speed and sensitivity that is impossible today. In the EMIRA study, one local "sentinel" in the area of each of the four different supplies studied was responsible for taking daily samples of 4.5 liters of tap water throughout the whole study period and storing them in the refrigerator for 3 days (or 5 days if the weekend intervened), so that a technician could collect the set of bottles in the event of an outbreak (see the corresponding operational definition above).

Chapters 7 and 8 deal in depth with issues related to microbial analyses. Using bacterial indicators to characterize microbial quality may result in some degree of misclassification, because various pathogens which are important causes of outbreaks and possibly endemic diseases (e.g., protozoa or viruses other than enteroviruses) are poorly represented by bacterial indicators. Novel analytical techniques are increasingly used in epidemiological studies to explore the roles of specific viral or parasitic pathogens. Even so, these also have limitations, especially in relation to issues such as recovery rates and germ viability and infectivity.[20,27,28]

17.3.4 Data Analysis

Prospective studies with repetitive health and/or exposure measurement over time typically require data analyses that allow the time dependence of these key variables to be taken into account. Longitudinal data analysis techniques (e.g., GEE models or Poisson regression with time-dependent variables) may be used. In some instances, the repetition of measurements over time is separated by long periods of time (e.g., several weeks), which alleviates the degree of time correlation within subjects, thus allowing usage of more classical statistical analyses resting on the hypothesis that observations are independent.

The case crossover technique is becoming increasingly popular and has been used in air pollution epidemiology because it can deal effectively with transient effects. It is also appropriate for water quality prospective studies.[29,30] It is a paired case–control design nested within a follow-up study where the exposure experience of the study cases, before or after the subject became a case, can be used as a control period. Consider a study with monthly water quality monitoring. Dealing with variable water quality over time, it would be possible to assign to each case the water quality data the month just before and/or after a given subject exhibited a GI condition (i.e., became a case) as the paired control period. Consideration should be given to the maximum lag between the closest water sample and the occurrence of the case, such that one can be confident as to how valid this sample characterizes the water quality at the time of exposure of the case (e.g., 3 days? 1 week?). There is no published quality epidemiological analysis to date that has followed this rationale, but it might well come soon. One limitation of this design could be when infection results in effective immunity.[21]

17.4 CONCLUSIONS

Prospective epidemiological studies may be suitable tools for assessment of the health impact of water quality, which might be especially fruitful in relation to revisiting and complementing the paradigm of microbial indicators and exploring new indicators of treatment efficacy and water quality. Because they are demanding in resources, few examples of prospective studies exist to date. They may be useful for hazard identification, however. Risk assessment approaches are increasingly popular as a scientific rationale for risk management, in the areas of both microbial and chemical hazards. Now, most data used in risk assessment are based on experimental data, stemming from animal studies, seldom on human control studies, and warrant validation with observational data. There is still a need for real-life epidemiological studies to confirm these experimental studies because the conditions of survival and of virulence of germs in the natural environment may differ substantially from that of the same species that are artificially bred, and also because the general population includes susceptible subgroups whose risks might not be well evaluated by experimental data.

Hence, one should use all the pieces of information that can be gained, starting from germ prevalence studies, experiments, clinical studies, outbreak investigation and surveillance, and also epidemiological studies, in order to assess the new waterborne risks.

REFERENCES

1. Frost, F.J., Craun, G.F., and Calderon, R.L., Waterborne disease surveillance, *JAWWA*, 88(9) 66, 1996.
2. Gerba, C.P., Rose, J.B., and Haas, C.N., Sensitive populations: who is at the greatest risk?, *Int. J. Food Microbiol.*, 30, 113, 1996.
3. Steiner, T.S., Thielman, N.M., and Guerrant, R.L., Protozoal agents: what are the dangers for the public water supply?, *Ann. Rev. Med.*, 48, 329, 1997.
4. Payment, P. et al., A prospective epidemiological study of gastrointestinal health effect due to the consumption of drinking water, *Int. J. Environ. Health Res.*, 7, 5, 1997.

5. Ferley, J.P. et al., Etude longitudinale des risques liés à la consommation d'eaux non conformes aux normes bactériologiques, *Rev. Epidémiol. Santé Publique,* 34, 89, 1986.
6. Raina, P.S. et al. The relationship between *E. coli* indicator bacteria in well water and gastrointestinal illnesses in rural families, *Can. J. Public Health*, 90, 172, 1999.
7. Goldstein, S.T. et al., Cryptosporidiosis: an outbreak associated with drinking water despite state-of-the art water treatment, *Ann. Intern. Med.,* 124, 459, 1996.
8. MacKenzie, W.R. et al., A massive outbreak in Milwaukee of *Cryptosporidium* infection transmitted through the public water supply, *N. Eng. J. Med.,* 331, 161, 1994.
9. Rose, J.B., Environmental ecology of *Cryptosporidium* and public health implications, *Ann. Rev. Pub. Health*, 18, 135, 1997.
10. Hellard, M.E. et al., A randomized blinded controlled trial investigating the gastrointestinal health effects of drinking water quality, *Environ. Health Perspect.,* 109, 773, 2001.
11. Hoogenboom-Verdegaal, A.M.M. et al., Community-based study of the incidence of gastrointestinal diseases in The Netherlands, *Epidemiol. Infect.,* 112, 481, 1994.
12. Monto, A.S. and Koopman, S., The Tecumseh study. XI. Occurrence of acute enteric illness in the community, *Am. J. Epidemiol.*, 112, 323, 1980.
13. Payment, P. et al., A randomized trial to evaluate the risk of gastrointestinal disease due to the consumption of drinking water meeting current microbiological standards, *Am. J. Pub. Health*, 81, 703, 1991.
14. Zmirou, D. et al., Residual health risk after simple chlorine treatment of drinking water in small community systems., *Eur. J. Pub. Health*, 5, 75, 1995.
15. Perz, J.F., Ennever, F.K., and Le Blancq, S.M., *Cryptosporidium* in tap water. Comparison of predicted risks with observed levels of disease, *Am. J. Epidemiol.,* 147, 289, 1998.
16. Balbus, J., Parkin, R., and Embrey, M., Susceptibility in microbial risk assessment: definitions and research needs, *Environ. Health Perspect.*, 108, 901, 2000.
17. Grufferman, S., Complexity and the Hawthorne effect in community trials, *Epidemiology*, 10, 209, 1999.
18. Oglesby, L. et al., Personal exposure assessment studies may suffer from exposure-relevant selection bias, *J. Expo. Anal. Environ. Epidemiol.*, 10, 1, 2000.
19. Cabelli, V.J. et al., Swimming-associated gastroenteritis and water quality, *Am. J. Epidemiol.*, 115, 606, 1982.
20. Gofti-Laroche, L. et al., A new analytical tool to assess health risks associated with the virological quality of drinking water (EMIRA study), *Water Sci. Technol.*, 43, 39, 2001.
21. Frost, F.J. et al., Serological evidence of *Cryptosporidium* infections in southern Europe, *Eur. J. Epidemiol.*, 16, 385, 2000.
22. Armstrong, B.K., White, E., and Saracci, R., *Principles of Exposure Measurement in Epidemiology*, Oxford University Press, Oxford, U.K., 1995.
23. Künzli, N. and Tager, I.B., The semi-individual study in air pollution epidemiology: a valid design as compared to ecologic studies, *Environ. Health Perspect.,* 105, 1078, 1997.
24. Steenland, K. and Deddens, J.A., Design and analysis of studies in environmental epidemiology, in *Topics in Environmental Epidemiology*, Steeland, K. and Savitz, D.A., Eds., Oxford University Press, Oxford, U.K., 1997, 9.
25. Gofti-Laroche, L. et al., Description de la consommation d'eau de boisson en France a l'usage des épidémiologistes et évaluateurs du risque (étude E.MI.R.A.), *Rev. Epidémiol. Santé Pub.,* in press.
26. Schwartz, J. and Levin, R., Drinking water turbidity and health, *Epidemiology*, 10, 86, 1999.
27. Smith, H.V. and Rose, J.B., Waterborne cryptosporidiosis: current status, *Parasitol. Today*, 14, 14, 1998.
28. Häfliger, D., Hübner, Ph., and Lüthy, J., Outbreak of viral gastroenteritis due to sewage-contaminated drinking water, *Int. J. Food Microbiol.*, 54, 123, 2000.
29. Maclure, M., The case-crossover design: a method for studying transient effects on the risk of acute events, *Am. J. Epidemiol.,* 133, 144, 1991.
30. Lee, J.T. and Schwartz, J., Reanalysis of the effect of air pollution on daily mortality in Seoul, Korea: a case-crossover design, *Environ. Health Perspect.,* 107, 633, 1999.

18 Intervention Studies

Pierre Payment and Paul R. Hunter

CONTENTS

18.1 Introduction......191
18.2 Objectives of Intervention Studies......192
 18.2.1 Natural Conditions......192
 18.2.2 Uncontrolled Conditions......192
 18.2.3 Controlled Conditions......193
18.3 Designs of Intervention Studies......193
 18.3.1 Description......193
 18.3.2 A Case Study......194
  18.3.2.1 Hypothesis......194
  18.3.2.2 Outcome and Sample Size......194
  18.3.2.3 Intervention......194
  18.3.2.4 Area Water Treatment Plant......195
  18.3.2.5 Selection Criteria, Enrollment, and Randomization......195
  18.3.2.6 Surveys......195
  18.3.2.7 Analysis of Data and Results......195
  18.3.2.8 Discussion......195
18.4 Conclusions......196
References......196

18.1 INTRODUCTION

Until recently, intervention studies were rarely used to evaluate the level of endemic waterborne illness in populations. They were mostly used to monitor the effects of a new or improved water supply on the health of a population or to demonstrate the effectiveness of various sanitation procedures. In developing countries, intervention studies provided data on the reduction of various diseases in the population and the value of water treatment or availability to reduce waterborne diseases. However, results were often confounded by other factors linked to the overall sanitation and cultural habits of the populations studied. The true effect played by the water route is interlinked with these other factors, and any interpretation needs to be carefully validated. As water quality improves, it becomes more and more difficult to design and implement intervention studies that will not be subject to criticism and do not require a large number of followers.

The studies performed by one of the authors in 1988–1989 and 1993–1994 in Canada, using randomized intervention trials, led the way to similar studies.[1–4] It was discomforting to many that significant proportions of nonoutbreak-related gastroenteritis in communities served by state-of-the-art water treatment facilities might be waterborne. In the 1993–1994 study, a representative sample of 1400 families was selected and randomly allocated into four groups: tap water, tap water from a continuously purged tap, bottled plant water, and purified bottled water. The data suggest that 14 to 40% of the gastrointestinal illnesses are attributable to tap water that meets current

0-8493-1259-0/03/$0.00+$1.50

standards. The study has shaken consumer confidence and has spurred a flurry of research activity. The U.S. Centers for Disease Control and Prevention (CDCP) together with the U.S. Environmental Protection Agency (EPA) have recently announced that a significant amount of resources have been set aside to repeat the Canadian study in multiple sites across the U.S.[5]

Following the example of the Payment studies in Canada, the Australians and Americans have repeated these prospective intervention studies.[5–8] The Australian study reported no health effects due to unfiltered clean surface waters.[6] However, initial results of the first of several ongoing American studies appear to confirm the Canadian studies.[7] This chapter introduces the different types of intervention studies and uses the experience gained in the Canadian study to describe in more detail the design of randomized controlled intervention trials.

18.2 OBJECTIVES OF INTERVENTION STUDIES

In the drinking water-related field, the main objective of intervention studies is to assess the effect of a public health intervention. These studies can be performed under natural conditions (i.e., accidental trials), under uncontrolled conditions (i.e., public measures, such as the introduction of a new water treatment plant), or under controlled conditions (i.e., clinical trials or field studies).

18.2.1 Natural Conditions

Intervention studies performed under natural conditions are often the result of accidents, and the researchers have little control over the nature of the intervention. Since it is an accident, there is nothing that can be planned but it is possible to sort out exposed from non-exposed subjects and to assess the level of exposure to a contaminant (e.g., level of bacteria in contaminated water or food). The exposure and the distribution of subjects will be independent from the researcher, and bias on the part of the analysis can be prevented by maintaining the level of exposure.

Quasi-experimental (non-randomization) interventions are similar because they make use of historical data to compare past treatment to new treatment. For example, studies that have demonstrated that drinking bottled water or using point-of-use devices are protective during outbreaks of waterborne disease provide strong supportive evidence of the role of drinking tap water in the outbreak.[9–11] The problem with such studies is that the choice of whether or not to use a particular intervention is not uniformly distributed in society. For example, it may be that only wealthier sections of society drink mainly bottled water, and so any disease associated with deprivation may be negatively associated with bottled water consumption. Bottled water consumption in this case is a confounding variable. Furthermore, because these studies tend to be undertaken in outbreak situations, they provide little evidence of the value of intervention in a nonoutbreak situation.

18.2.2 Uncontrolled Conditions

The introduction and application of public health measures can be considered as intervention studies. Examples of these measures are vaccination to decrease disease incidence, mosquito control program to reduce vector-borne diseases, and sanitation programs. In regard to drinking water, interventions may include the building of a new water treatment plant or implementation of an additional stage in water treatment such as filtration. For some public health interventions, such as immunizations, not all subjects receive the intervention (through personal choice or because they are not in the target group). Drinking water interventions tend to apply to everyone in the population receiving water from a particular treatment plant.

Numerous examples of such studies exist in developing nations.[12–15] However, relatively few such studies have been reported to date in Western nations. One recently published study used seroprevalence to *Cryptosporidium* (see Chapter 17) to investigate the impact of adding a filtration step to a water treatment plant that previously only used chlorination.[16] This particular study showed no decline in antibody levels in a student population. Other studies are under way in the U.S.[17]

The main problem with these types of studies is determining the most appropriate control population. There are basically two options for water supply interventions. The first is the historical control, the same population before the intervention. The second control is the neighboring population control, a similar community that has not yet received the benefit of the particular public health intervention. Both these approaches can suffer from significant bias and confounding effects. Infectious diseases vary from time to time and place to place for a number of factors that have nothing to do with water supply. Disentangling these factors from the impact of water supply can be very difficult and may be impossible. An unidentified outbreak of food poisoning in either group during a study could substantially bias the results one way or another.

The other problem with these studies is that they do not measure exposure in individuals but in groups, and as such, suffer from the ecological paradox.

18.2.3 Controlled Conditions

The classical clinical trials and field studies as performed today allow for simultaneous comparison enabling researchers to test a hypothesis and compare a predefined outcome in a group of individuals. The researcher chooses comparable subjects and creates two or more groups of subjects who are exposed to various interventions. One potential source of bias is that if people know to which subgroup they belong, they may be more or less likely to say that they suffer the outcome measure. In order to minimize these effects, subjects may be blinded. Blinding may be simple (the subjects do not know to which group they belong but observers and investigators do), double (subjects and observers are blinded), or triple (subjects, observers, and investigators are blinded). Confounders (variables that are unrelated to the hypothesis under investigation, but which can directly or indirectly influence the outcome) are another group of factors that need to be considered. As we see below, most studies will gather data on any factors that can affect the outcome of the study.

18.3 DESIGNS OF INTERVENTION STUDIES

18.3.1 Description

Most studies are randomized experimental studies, but some can be non-randomized. The advantages of randomization are that it facilitates statistical analysis, provides an unbiased distribution of confounders, and blinding is more likely to be possible. The main disadvantage is that they are expensive, they can be quite long for observations that are not frequent, and they are subject to volunteer bias (the volunteers may not be representative of the general population).

Non-randomized studies enable the investigator to do a simultaneous comparison of events in paired subjects, to compare standardized series, and to compare different groups with different treatments or identical groups with different treatments. However, subjects may choose their own intervention.

During observational cohort studies, two existing populations are compared. For example, in a water study which assumes differences in water quality and some level of continuity in time, the researcher compares rate of disease in the two populations over a specific period of time.

During interventional cohort studies, the level of exposure to water can be modulated in randomized individuals from a population. The type of intervention may vary but include the use of bottled water, point-of-use device, or point-of-entry device.

In all types of studies, group selection must be representative and some level of blindness might be required. A crossover design is often used, where the group (subject to the chosen intervention) is swapped with the initial control group after a predetermined period. All subjects serve as their own controls and error variance is reduced, thus reducing sample size. All subjects receive treatment, which is an ethical consideration. Statistical tests assume randomization can be used and blindness can be maintained. The main disadvantage is that they are more costly due to a longer period of observation which may be needed. Also, there may be biases if a primary exposure to infection in the first half of the study reduces the probability of infection in the second half.

Most intervention studies involving water are a compromise between the following factors:

- Study design that reduces bias
- Willingness of sufficient subjects to participate
- Willingness of subjects to comply with the restrictions placed upon them, especially in relation to water consumption outside of the home
- Risk to subjects from exposure to contaminated water
- Risk of no treatment (illness, death)
- Ethical considerations, such as the need to obtain biological samples
- Time required
- Cost

18.3.2 A Case Study

This section presents the background and the choices that had to be made before Payment's first intervention study was initiated.[1] This study was a randomized clinical trial to evaluate the risk of gastrointestinal disease due to the consumption of drinking water meeting currently accepted microbiological standards.

18.3.2.1 Hypothesis

The authors wanted to test the hypothesis that drinking water meeting the water standards applicable at the time in Canada was safe and not contributing to disease in the population studied. The hypothesis was that pathogens from the water could infect the population. Microorganisms would have had to be present in river water in order to show that the waterworks had eliminated those contaminants. If the river water had not contained pathogens, the demonstration would not have been convincing.

18.3.2.2 Outcome and Sample Size

Gastrointestinal illness was chosen as the outcome because this was known to be of sufficiently high incidence to enable the observations to take place in a manageable period of time. After discussion with Canadian and American authorities, it was determined that if less than 5% of the observed illnesses were due to tap water, this would be acceptable. A sample size calculation was then done and it was determined that we needed 300 children between the ages of 5 and 12 in each group. The children were chosen as the index because of their higher level of gastrointestinal illness (about 1.6/person/year), which enabled the study to be completed in 18 months.

18.3.2.3 Intervention

Cost effectiveness of various interventions were compared including the use of point-of-use filters, bottled water, and treatment changes. Finally, we selected a point-of-use domestic reverse-osmosis unit that would remove all contaminants from drinking water and could be quality controlled using simple conductivity measurement. These units were installed under the kitchen sink and a small tap on the counter provided rapid access to the purified water.

A sham filter was not used because previous studies had demonstrated that it was very difficult to prevent participants from identifying the type of unit installed. This particular aspect has been resolved in the recent Australian and American studies and blindness should not be an issue anymore. Epidemiologically, the lack of blinding was a weak point, but it was felt to be acceptable for such a long study period using a highly critical definition of disease.

18.3.2.4 Area Water Treatment Plant

The area under study was served by a single water treatment plant (non-confounder) and the river water used was known to be contaminated by human sewage (exposure). This was a well-operated plant that met or exceeded national and provincial regulation requirements.

18.3.2.5 Selection Criteria, Enrollment, and Randomization

All families were required to be French-Canadian (minimizing the language issue and potential bias from ethnic diversity), consist of at least one child 2 to 12 years of age, usually drink tap water, own their dwellings (for legal reasons, such as the installation of a filter), and, finally, be willing to participate.

For the selection of families with children, the authors were able to access a government database (a child-support program) and then were able to use phone calls to assess eligibility. Once contacted, if the family met all criteria, they were enrolled and randomized to one of the groups: filter or no filter. A plumber then installed and tested the reverse-osmosis unit in the filter group families.

18.3.2.6 Surveys

The information was collected in a diary to record symptoms on the day of their occurrence (to minimize recall bias). A call was placed to the family respondent every 2 weeks to obtain data recorded, and the diary was returned to us for cross-checking every 6 months. Water consumption surveys were conducted on four occasions to assess the level of exposure during four different time periods.

18.3.2.7 Analysis of Data and Results

The two outcome variables were gastrointestinal episodes (GI) and a more strict, highly credible gastrointestinal illness (HCGI). An episode was defined as being separated by at least 6 consecutive days without symptoms. All results were analyzed by group, age, gender, informant status, geographical location, and water consumption. Statistical methods used were Poisson regression with correction for clustering (intrafamilial transmission being highly probable).

The group that did *not* have a filter was the control group (no intervention). The hypothesis being tested was that there would not be a significant difference in the group with the filter. To our surprise, a very significant difference of 35% less HCGI was observed in the intervention group. Details can be found in several publications.[1–4]

18.3.2.8 Discussion

This study was the first to really address the level of waterborne endemic illness in a population consuming water considered of a very high standard.

The elegance of this intervention trial was that the populations differed by a single parameter, i.e., the presence of a reverse-osmosis filter. The measure of the proof was high, but it still remained to be repeated. The authors' second study in 1993–94[2,4] provided a similar answer using a different design: bottled water was used and blindness of participants was obtained. Similar studies are being conducted in several countries using this basic design that was demonstrated to be feasible and cost effective.

18.4 CONCLUSIONS

Intervention studies are effective tools to evaluate the level of preventable waterborne illness in a population, but such studies need to be very carefully designed to exclude bias and confounders. Intervention studies are more expensive than other types of studies, but they provide data invaluable to the public health community and to water industry risk managers.[1]

Finally, prospective randomized studies are probably the most desirable epidemiological design. They are less subject to bias from possible confounding factors and, especially if blinded, should not be subject to recall bias in the same way that other methods discussed elsewhere in this book might be. Unlike some of the other types of intervention study described above, they do not suffer from the ecological paradox because they measure exposure in individuals and are less likely to suffer from biases due to temporal and geographical variations in disease not related to water treatment. The retrospective studies of interventions done as part of outbreaks do not give much useful information regarding the epidemiology of sporadic disease, but can give valuable additional evidence as to the cause of outbreaks.

REFERENCES

1. Payment, P. et al., A randomized trial to evaluate the risk of gastrointestinal disease due to the consumption of drinking water meeting currently accepted microbiological standards, *Am. J. Public Health,* 81, 703, 1991.
2. Payment, P. et al., A prospective epidemiological study of gastrointestinal health effects due to the consumption of drinking water, *Int. J. Environ. Health Res.,* 7, 5, 1997.
3. Payment, P., Epidemiology of endemic gastrointestinal and respiratory diseases — incidence, fraction attributable to tap water and costs to society, *Water Sci. Technol.,* 35, 7, 1997.
4. Payment, P. et al., *An Epidemiological Study of Gastrointestinal Health Effects of Drinking Water*, AWWA Research Foundation, Denver, CO, 2000.
5. Hayward, K., Science supports a national estimate, *Water,* 21 (December), 12, 2000.
6. Hellard, M.E. et al., A randomized blinded controlled trial investigating the gastrointestinal health affects of drinking water quality, *Environ. Health Perspect.,* 109, 773, 2001.
7. Colford, J. M. et al., Participant blinding and gastrointestinal illness in a randomized, controlled trial of an in-home drinking water intervention, *Emerg. Infect. Dis*., 8, 29, 2002.
8. Hunter, P.R. et al., Waterborne diseases, *Emerg. Infect. Dis.,* 7, 544, 2001.
9. Joseph, C. et al. Cryptosporidiosis in the Isle of Thanet: an outbreak associated with local drinking water, *Epidemiol. Infect.*, 107, 509, 1991.
10. Cardenas, V. et al., Waterborne cholera in Riohacha, Columbia, 1992, *Bull. Pan Am. Health Org*., 27, 313, 1993.
11. Addis, D.G. et al., Reduction of risk of watery diarrhea with point-of-use water filters during a massive outbreak of waterborne *Cryptosporidium* infection in Milwaukee, Wisconsin, 1993, *Am. J. Trop. Med. Hyg*., 54, 549, 1996.
12. Conroy, R.M. et al., Solar disinfection of drinking water protects against cholera in children under 6 years of age, *Arch. Dis. Childhood*, 85, 293, 2001.
13. VanDerslice, J. and Briscoe, J., Environmental interventions in developing countries: interactions and their implications, *Am. J. Epidemiol.,* 141, 135, 1995.
14. Esrey, S.A. et al., Effects of improved water supply and sanitation on ascariasis, diarrhoea, dracunculiasis, hookworm infection schistosomiasis, and trachoma, *Bull. World Health Org*., 69, 609, 1991.
15. Gross, R. et al., The impact of improved water supply and sanitation facilities on diarrhea and intestinal parasites: a Brazilian experience with children in two low-income urban communities, *Rev. Saude Publica*, 23, 214, 1989.
16. Frost, F.J. et al., A serological survey of college students for antibody to *Cryptosporidium* before and after the introduction of a new water filtration plant, *Epidemiol. Infect.* 125, 87, 2000.
17. Calderon, R. and Craun, G., Community intervention study for estimation of endemic waterborne disease, *Epidemiology*, 11, 414, 2000.

19 Prospective Studies of Endemic Waterborne Disease in Developing Countries

Christine L. Moe

CONTENTS

19.1 INTRODUCTION

In this, the final chapter of the book, we focus on studies conducted within the developing world. Most of the discussion in earlier chapters has focused on water and health problems and investigation appropriate for developed nations. However, concentrating only on developed nations, one will miss the major part of the disease burden related to drinking water globally. Any waterborne disease epidemiologist who wishes his or her work to have the biggest impact on health must look to work in the developing nations. In many ways, the methods described earlier in this book are all applicable in the setting of the developing world. However, as will be discussed later, work in developing nations generates a number of additional problems and complexities over and above those experienced by researchers in the industrialized nations. But before discussing study design, we first consider the issue of the waterborne disease burden in developing nations and some of the aspects of water supplies in these countries.

19.2 GLOBAL BURDEN OF WATERBORNE DISEASE

From a global perspective, waterborne disease is one of the major health problems in the developing world, especially for young children. Developing countries often have poor water supplies and limited resources for water treatment and distribution. This situation is aggravated by concurrent problems with inadequate sanitation that result in fecal contamination of surface- and groundwater.

0-8493-1259-0/03/$0.00+$1.50

TABLE 19.1
Global Burden of Diarrheal Diseases in Children < 5 Years[2,33,34]

Region	Pop. <5 (millions)	Episodes Per Child Per Year: Snyder & Merson 1982	IOM 1986	Bern & Glass 1994	Annual Cases (millions)
Africa	89.8	2.2	5	2.5	197–450
Asia	351.0	2.2	3	2.3	772–1053
Latin America	62.5	2.2	4	3.9	137–250
Total					1106–1753

The World Health Organization (WHO) currently estimates that 1.1 billion people worldwide lack access to improved water supplies and 2.4 billion do not have access to proper sanitation facilities.[1] Under these circumstances, water supplies can become a very efficient means of transmitting enteric infections within and between communities. Several estimates have been made of global pediatric morbidity associated with diarrheal disease. The most recent estimate by Bern and Glass,[2] based on numerous studies of diarrheal disease, suggests that the number of diarrhea episodes per child per year ranges from 2.3 in Asia to 3.9 in Africa (Table 19.1).

The magnitude of the overall disease burden associated with pediatric diarrhea, estimated to be between 1106 and 1753 million cases per year, is staggering, and the proportion of this disease that is directly or indirectly associated with poor water quality and inadequate water quantity is difficult to determine. A closer examination of data from 22 longitudinal studies of diarrhea incidence in Africa, Asia, and Latin America indicates that the highest disease rates are in children 6 to 11 months of age. This vulnerable time in a child's life is when water and weaning foods are introduced into the child's diet. At this time, levels of maternal antibodies are declining as the child's immune system begins to produce its own antibodies. Also, the child is crawling and coming into contact with floors as well as objects that are frequently introduced into the child's mouth. Thus, multiple transmission routes of infectious agents are responsible for this disease burden.

In addition to diarrheal disease, other water-related diseases pose significant health risks in the developing world. Typhoid fever continues to be a major problem in many parts of the world, with an estimated 17 million cases and 600,000 deaths occurring each year.[3] *Helicobacter pylori*, associated with peptic and duodenal ulcers and stomach cancer, may be transmitted via contaminated drinking water or produce washed or irrigated with contaminated water. Diagnostic surveys suggest that over two-thirds of the world's population is infected with this organism.[4] Dracunculiasis (Guinea Worm infection) is a crippling health problem endemic in 13 sub-Saharan African countries. Infection occurs from ingestion of water contaminated with larvae of the parasite *Dracunculus medinensis*. Recent eradication efforts have dramatically reduced the burden of disease from approximately 422,000 cases in 1992 to an estimated 90,000 cases in 1999.[5] This disease affects the ability of infected adults to work, and thus impacts agricultural activity and food supply. Although not associated with drinking water, schistosomiasis may, on a global scale, be the greatest water-related disease problem in the developing world, with over 200 million people infected and 20 million seriously ill. This disease is endemic in 76 developing countries and is spread by contact with water containing a life stage of the schistosome worm that penetrates the skin and then initiates infection.[6] The large number of eggs produced by the worm causes damage to the liver, intestines, lungs, and bladder of the host.

19.3 WATER SUPPLIES IN DEVELOPING COUNTRIES

Several important differences that exist between water supplies and living conditions in developing countries compared to industrialized countries should be considered in designing studies of waterborne disease in developing countries.

1. There is a wide spectrum of drinking water sources used in developing countries. Many of these water sources are unprotected, often have high levels of fecal contamination, and are used with little or no treatment. The microbiological quality of these water sources can be quite poor. "Fecal" or thermotolerant coliform concentrations in drinking water sources have been reported up to 100,000 per 100 ml (Table 19.2). However, the WHO guidelines for drinking-water quality recommend that no thermotolerant coliform bacteria be detectable in any 100-ml sample.[7] Piped water supplies in developing countries are also vulnerable to contamination due to illegal connections and pressure loss.
2. In tropical areas, ambient water temperatures are warmer (typically around 30°C) than waters in temperate climates. Traditional measures of microbiological water quality, such as total or fecal coliform indicator bacteria, may not be appropriate for tropical source waters because of higher ambient temperature and nutrient loads in the water.
3. Many households do not have a water tap or pump within the house or compound. Water is collected and transported in a variety of vessels. Transport and storage of water in contaminated vessels has been shown to be a source of water contamination.[8,9]
4. Fecal pathogens are transmitted by multiple routes due to poor sanitation, food hygiene, and personal hygiene. These routes are closely linked to waterborne transmission and make it difficult to assess the risk of disease associated solely with drinking water. Often, both inadequate water quality and water quantity contribute to waterborne disease.

TABLE 19.2
Reported Microbiological Quality of Domestic Water Sources in Developing Countries

Country	Water Source	Fecal Coliforms per 100 ml
Gambia	Open, hand-dug wells	Up to 100,000
Nigeria	Open, hand-dug wells	200–580
Philippines	Open dug wells	190[a]
Uganda	Hand-dug wells	8–200
Tanzania	Open wells	343
Tanzania	Protected wells	7
Lesotho	Unprotected springs	900
Lesotho	Protected springs	200
Philippines	Springs	72[a]
Philippines	Boreholes	3[a]
Philippines	Municipal piped water	3[a]
Philippines	Community piped water	178[a]

[a] Geometric mean fecal coliform concentration per 100 ml.

Source: Extracted from Feachem, R.G. et al., *Sanitation and Disease: Health Aspects of Excreta and Wastewater Management*, John Wiley & Sons, Chichester, U.K.,1983, and Moe, C.L., An evaluation of four bacterial indicators of risk of diarrheal disease from tropical drinking waters in the Philippines, Ph.D. thesis, University of North Carolina, Chapel Hill, 1989.

These issues and how they affect specific aspects of study design and implementation will be examined in greater detail in the following sections.

19.4 STUDIES OF ENDEMIC WATERBORNE DISEASE

The study of endemic waterborne disease is very complex, regardless of whether the setting is an industrialized country or a developing country. Because of the multiple factors involved in waterborne transmission of enteric diseases, successful studies of the relationship between water supply and various health outcomes require a multidisciplinary team of investigators with expertise in water engineering, hydrology, anthropology, sociology, infectious disease epidemiology, water microbiology, clinical microbiology, nutrition, health education, health behavior, and biostatistics. Since the early 1960s, many studies of waterborne diseases in developing countries have been carried out. Many evaluations of the impact of improved water supply on health were conducted during the International Drinking Water Supply and Sanitation Decade (1981–1990) when research and development efforts focused on how to implement effective water and sanitation interventions in developing countries.

Most of these studies used a prospective cohort design to examine differences in health between communities or households that received a water intervention and those that did not. The intervention was typically either a new, "improved" water supply, some type of treatment to an existing community water supply, or treatment of water within the household. Subjects with exposure to different water sources were recruited into the study and observed for a period of time. In some studies, all the subjects lived within the same community but used different water sources. In other studies, subjects were recruited from different communities that had different water sources. Exposure to water quality and/or water quantity was assessed by determining the water source used by each study subject and sometimes by actually measuring microbiological water quality by laboratory analyses and measuring water use by means of a household interview. Health effects were monitored over the follow-up period and comparisons were made between subjects exposed to different water sources. Health outcomes were compared between the households or communities with the intervention vs. the households or communities without the intervention. In some studies, health outcomes were compared within a single community before and after implementation of a water supply intervention.

For example, a typical study of endemic waterborne disease in a developing country may recruit households in two communities: one community that uses untreated spring water as its water supply and another nearby community that has a new communal borehole with disinfection. Diarrheal disease incidence may be measured by weekly household interview, and diarrheal rates between the two communities would be compared to determine whether the households in the community with the treated water supply had a lower incidence of diarrheal disease than households in the community that drank untreated spring water. In this example, one would expect that the use of an "improved" treated water source would result in a reduction of diarrheal disease. However, several large studies that have evaluated expensive water intervention projects in Bangladesh, Guatemala, and elsewhere could not demonstrate a health benefit associated with a water supply intervention.[10,11] Is this failure to detect a health benefit due to methodological problems with the study or to the effects of other transmission routes of infectious agents that somehow mask the benefit of an improved water supply? Investigators in this field have debated whether improved water is a necessary but not sufficient condition for a beneficial impact on health.

19.5 METHODOLOGICAL PROBLEMS WITH STUDIES OF ENDEMIC WATERBORNE DISEASE

Blum and Feachem, Esrey, and others critically reviewed studies of waterborne disease in developing countries and cited common methodological problems.[12–14] These can be grouped into four main categories: (1) problems with overall study design, (2) problems with exposure assessment, (3) problems measuring health outcomes, and (4) problems with analytical approaches. These are discussed in more detail below.

19.5.1 Study Design Problems

Epidemiological study design usually starts with consideration of the sample size needed to detect a statistically significant difference between the incidence or prevalence rate of the health outcome of interest among households or communities using different water supplies. Sample size calculations are based on some *a priori* knowledge of the baseline illness rate in the study population using the traditional water supply and deciding what degree of illness reduction attributable to an improved water supply the study should be able to detect. This decision depends on the health outcome measure that is chosen and the length of follow-up period that the study population is monitored. Less common health outcomes require a larger sample size and a longer study period in order to be able to measure a meaningful difference between different exposure groups. Economic resources often limit sample size and duration, and many studies have suffered from inadequate sample size and follow-up length to detect possible subtle differences in health outcomes that may be due to water supply.

The lack of adequate and/or appropriate control observations is a serious problem in many studies. Typically, an appropriate control population is one that is similar to the "exposed" or "intervention" population in every respect except for water supply. Without such a control population, it is difficult to measure the impact of water supply on the health outcome of interest. Some studies have compared health outcomes between households or communities that have different water supplies but also have demographic or socioeconomic differences that may contribute to observed differences in health outcomes.

Confounders are factors that are related to both the health outcome and the exposure of interest. Because there are multiple transmission routes of enteric pathogens, factors other than water supply may explain observed differences in health outcomes between two study groups. In the previous example of the community drinking spring water vs. the community drinking treated borehole water, it is possible that the community with the borehole also had better sanitation, better nutrition, or higher household income. These factors may affect likelihood of exposure or susceptibility to enteric pathogens. In order to measure the disease burden associated with water supply, it is necessary to control for the effect of confounding factors in the study design stage through selection of an appropriate comparison community or by measuring these factors in the study and controlling for their effect during data analyses.

19.5.2 Exposure Assessment

A surprising shortcoming in many studies is the failure to observe and record actual use of water supply. Many studies assume that a household uses the closest water source or the intervention water supply as the drinking water source. Some households may not use the closest water supply because of taste preferences, family ownership, or social taboos. In Bangladesh, boreholes provided as an intervention by development agencies were not used for drinking water by some households because people did not like the taste of the groundwater.[15] Different water supplies may be used for different purposes, and the drinking water supply may be different from the water source used for bathing or laundry. It also can be a mistake to assume that children drink the same water as adults.[15] Parents may provide treated water or water with a better taste or warmer temperature for young children. Older children may drink from whatever water source is most accessible rather than the usual household drinking water source. In some settings, it may be critical to actually observe water-use patterns rather than rely on information from questionnaires or interviews, because actual water use may differ from reported water use.[15]

What is perhaps most surprising is the inadequate measurement of water quality that has been used by many studies of waterborne disease. Many studies of waterborne disease do not actually measure microbiological water quality but use types of water source as a surrogate for water quality or assume, sometimes mistakenly, that the intervention water supply provides higher quality water than a traditional source. While this seems to be a logical assumption on the surface, type of water supply is not an accurate predictor of water quality. A study of microbiological water quality in the Philippines observed that boreholes generally provided higher quality water than a piped water supply that was provided as an intervention in one community.[16] The quality of water provided by traditional water supplies can vary considerably. Reported water quality of hand-dug wells in different countries in Africa ranges from 100,000 fecal coliforms per 100 ml in Gambia to 200–580 fecal coliforms per 100 ml in Nigeria to 8–200 fecal coliforms per 100 ml in Uganda (Table 19.2).[17]

Among the studies that do include microbiological analyses of water quality, many studies, especially older ones, used inadequate indicators of microbiological water quality and/or poor laboratory methods. Most studies measured total or fecal coliform concentrations in water. While these are standard indicators of microbiological water quality in many temperate climates, they have serious shortcomings. Both total and fecal coliforms are groups of bacteria that are defined by reactions in specified test media and incubation conditions. The fecal coliform test includes incubation at 44.5°C as a means to promote detection of enteric organisms, but both total and fecal coliforms include microorganisms of nonfecal origin. Therefore, the term "thermotolerant coliform" is more accurate than "fecal coliform." These indicators may not work well in tropical waters because of the higher ambient temperature and nutrient loads. Tropical waters frequently have ambient temperatures around 30°C. These higher ambient water temperatures foster the growth of thermotolerant aquatic microorganisms that are well adapted to the higher temperatures used to detect thermotolerant coliforms during water analyses. Some investigators have reported problems with false positive results due to naturally occurring thermotolerant coliforms in the aquatic environment.[18] Others have reported extra-enteral regrowth of indicator organisms in warm, nutrient-rich waters that results in falsely inflated estimates of fecal contamination.[18] In addition, the growth of thermotolerant, nonfecal microorganisms in the test media can make it difficult to detect and enumerate the target indicator organism. More recent studies report greater success with measuring *Escherichia coli* as an indicator of tropical drinking water quality.[16,19] This is a more fecal specific indicator, and the detection method allows the laboratory to distinguish the target organism from interfering background growth.[20,21]

Assessment of the microbiological quality of source water can be complicated by high variability of source water quality, especially in water sources impacted by runoff during rainfall. In the rainy season, increased run-off entering surface water supplies may bring increased fecal contamination and result in a degradation of water quality. Alternatively, water quality may improve during the rainy season due to increased dilution of fecal contamination in the water source and may degrade during periods of drought due to the concentration of fecal contamination in smaller volumes of water. Groundwater quality also can be affected by precipitation and flooding. Some water sources with low average *E. coli* concentrations may have occasional high peaks of contamination that may be missed if water sampling is infrequent or only for a short study period. Wright noted extreme seasonal variation in fecal indicator concentrations in a variety of water sources used in Sierra Leone.[22] For accurate exposure classification of a water source, investigators should consider the average and peak concentrations of a sufficient number of samples collected over an extended time period. Generally, unprotected water sources need to be tested more frequently than protected sources. However, even water quality in piped water supplies in developing countries can experience considerable temporal and geographic variability. Water distribution systems can have local peaks of contamination from illegal connections and power outages that result in negative pressure and an influx of contaminated water or sewage.

Depending on the study setting, exposure assessment may also involve measuring household water quality. The quality of water stored in the household can be significantly different from the quality at the source. It is important to determine whether the study households practice any form of water treatment. Some families may treat household drinking water by boiling, filtration, chlorination, alum precipitation, or exposure to sunlight. Transport and storage of water in contaminated vessels has been shown to be a cause of water contamination.[8,9] Also, abstraction of water from storage vessels by dipping involves hand contact that may result in degradation of water quality. Contamination of water at the source poses a different health risk than contamination of stored water in the household. Because source water contamination may originate outside of the family or community, contaminated source water can introduce new pathogens into a household or community. In contrast, household contamination of stored water is likely to involve pathogens that are already within the household that are probably also being transmitted via other routes in the household. Other household members may be exposed to these pathogens by other routes of transmission or may already have immunity. Studies that have examined household water quality and source water quality have reported conflicting findings on the impact of household water contamination on health.[9,23,19]

19.5.3 Health Outcome Measurements

Diarrhea morbidity is the most common health outcome considered in studies of waterborne disease. One common weakness with this outcome is that many studies rely on self-reported illness from the study participants. Often, it can be difficult to define an "episode of diarrheal disease" because of age, diet, or cultural factors. Also, diarrhea incidence or prevalence is usually measured by periodic household interviews where study participants are asked to recall their personal illness history and/or the illness history of their children and other members of their household since the time of the last interview. The longer the recall time, the greater the opportunity for error in disease reporting, especially in households with many children and illiterate caregivers.

Some studies have examined infections from specific pathogens such as *Shigella* spp., *Vibrio cholera* or the carriage rate of intestinal parasites such as *Ascaris*. Information on specific pathogens can be useful in some circumstances when considering the impact of specific environmental interventions on specific populations or age groups. For example, communities where zoonotic infections are responsible for a high proportion of diarrheal disease may need to focus on protection of water supplies from contamination by animal feces and better control of human exposure to animal feces near the household. The prevalence of pediatric rotavirus infection may not be affected by an improved water supply because of person-to-person and respiratory transmission of rotavirus infection.

Anthropometric measures, such as weight-for-height, height-for-age, weight-for-age, and assessment of nutritional status have been used in several studies of the impact of water quality and availability on child health.[13,24–26] These can be sensitive indicators of nutritional deficiencies, helminth infections, and the cumulative effect of repeated diarrheal episodes on child growth. Low height-for-age indicates chronic nutritional problems and possibly the contribution of diarrheal disease. Low weight-for-height indicates the effect of acute nutritional problems and recent diarrheal disease. Low weight-for-age can indicate either chronic or acute problems or both.[13]

19.5.4 Analytical Approaches

Analysis of the complex data from studies of water and health typically require multivariate regression techniques to control for the effects of potentially confounding variables related to community, household (e.g., income, family size, type of sanitary facility, presence of soap), maternal (e.g., age, education), and child (e.g., age, sex) characteristics. Many regression models (e.g., logistic, proportional odds) assume that each of the observations is independent. Because the number of episodes experienced by a single individual over time or among individuals living together in a household are not likely to be independent events, additional analytical approaches are needed to adjust for individual and family clustering such as Poisson regression or generalized estimating equations.[27]

The analytical approach also must examine the potential for interaction between exposure and covariates, such as child age or season. A significant interaction indicates that a covariate, such as child age, modifies the effect of water supply on the risk of diarrheal disease. Failure to perform age-specific analysis of morbidity may miss the effects of a water intervention on specific subgroups of the study population. The rates of many health outcomes vary by age. Some of this difference is due to biological differences in host susceptibility for different age groups. Also, different age groups have different water use patterns and different risks from other exposures. Children under 5 years of age have higher rates of diarrheal disease and different environmental exposures than older children and adults.

Seasonal effects on morbidity and exposure also should be considered in the analysis. In most parts of the world, diarrheal disease has distinct seasonal peaks that must be considered in studies of the association between diarrhea and water supply. Water use patterns may change depending on the season. Families may switch their water source during periods of drought. Frequency of recreational water contact also will vary by season. Source water quality can change dramatically by season depending on the type of water source and its vulnerability to contamination.

19.6 THE EFFECT OF OTHER TRANSMISSION ROUTES ON STUDIES OF WATERBORNE DISEASE

Even a well-designed and well-conducted study of endemic waterborne disease in a developing country may not be able to detect an association between water supply and health because the water-related route of transmission may be only one of several paths through which humans are exposed to enteric pathogens. In some communities, waterborne transmission may be less important than person-to-person transmission or foodborne transmission of pathogens. However, water availability and water quality is often closely linked (directly and indirectly) with person-to-person transmission and transmission via food or fomites, so that it is extremely difficult to examine the independent effect of water supply on health. An insightful paper by Briscoe suggested that the effect of improvements in water quality should not be evaluated by the reduction in disease due to water supply improvements alone.[28] He further argued that such improvements should be evaluated by "the degree to which the improvement in water quality affects the health effects of other (simultaneous or subsequent) essential changes in environmental conditions or personal health practices." A study by Esrey provides evidence of this complex web of transmission routes and points out the need to look at the effect of more than one intervention.[13] Using data from multi-country surveys of water, sanitation, and health, Esrey examined the impact of improved water supplies on communities with different levels of sanitation and concluded that improved sanitation was necessary in order to see any health benefits from improved water supplies.

19.7 CONCLUSIONS

Despite methodological problems and budget limitations, the body of evidence from studies of endemic waterborne disease indicates that improvements in water supply can improve health, especially child health, in developing countries. In a review of 144 studies of the effects of improved water supply and sanitation on health, Esrey et al. concluded that improvements in water quality were associated with a 17% median reduction of diarrhea morbidity.[29] Improvements in water quality and quantity were associated with a 16% reduction and improvements in sanitation were associated with a 22% median reduction of diarrhea. The magnitude of disease reduction associated with improved water depends on the role of other transmission routes and the degree and frequency of contamination of the unimproved water supply. The study by Moe et al. in a variety of urban and rural communities in the Philippines observed that only grossly contaminated water with > 1000 *E. coli* per 100 ml was associated with significantly increased prevalence of diarrheal disease in children under 2 years of age.[16] However, a recent household water treatment study in urban Bangladesh observed that low to moderate average *E. coli* concentrations in tap water were associated with increased risk of diarrhea in a slum area with poor sanitation.[19]

In a recent review of domestic hygiene and diarrheal disease, Curtis and colleagues concluded that the multiple transmission routes of enteric pathogens (person-to-person, waterborne, foodborne, fly-borne, and contact with animal feces) could be most effectively controlled by interventions focused in two domains:[30]

1. Improved excreta disposal to protect water supplies
2. Effective handwashing after stool contact to reduce person-to-person and foodborne transmission within the household

A third approach, the introduction of improved water storage vessels and the treatment of stored household water with a chlorine solution, mixed oxidants, or exposure to solar radiation, has recently emerged as a promising intervention that does not require extensive financial resources or community organization. These interim techniques can provide improved water quality on a household level until sufficient resources can be garnered to improve the water supply on a community level. Furthermore, interventions that target household water quality offer the opportunity to evaluate the impact of water quality on health in a variety of environments. Studies of household water treatment in rural Kenya, periurban Bolivia, and urban Bangladesh have demonstrated 9, 44, and 46% reductions, respectively, of endemic diarrheal disease in pediatric populations.[19,31,32]

Given the limited financial resources available for development and the growing population without adequate water and sanitation, it is critical that environmental interventions be designed and implemented to provide the maximum health benefit with limited resources. These studies and future studies of endemic waterborne disease in developing countries can provide valuable information on the design and implementation of successful water and sanitation interventions that will improve health for the more than 1 billion people in the world who currently live without the most basic needs for life — sufficient quantities of clean water and safe sanitation.

REFERENCES

1. WHO, Global Water Supply and Sanitation Assessment, 2000, http://www.who.int/water_sanitation_health/Globassessment/Glassessment1.pdf.
2. Bern, C. and Glass, R.I., Impact of diarrheal diseases worldwide, in *Viral Infections of the Gastrointestinal Tract,* Kapikian, A.Z., Ed., Marcel Dekker, New York, 1994, 1.
3. World Health Organization, WHO Fact Sheet N149: Typhoid Fever, 1997, http://www.who.int/inf-fs/en/fact149.html.
4. Centers for Disease Control, *Helicobacter pylori* fact sheet for health care providers, 1998, http://www.cdc.gov/ulcer/hpfacts.PDF.
5. World Health Organization, Dracunculiasis: recent epidemiological data, 1999, http://www.who.int/ctd/dracun/epidemio.htm.
6. World Health Organization, Schistosomiasis: the disease, http://www.who.int/ctd/schisto/disease.htm
7. World Health Organization, Bacteriological quality of drinking water, http://www.who.int/water_sanitation_health/GDWQ/Summary_tables/Tab1.htm).
8. Han, A.M. et al., Contamination of drinking water during collection and storage, *Trop. Geogr. Med.*, 41, 138, 1989.
9. Roberts, L. et al., Keeping clean water clean in a Malawi refugee camp: a randomized intervention trial, *Bull. World Health Organ.*, 79, 280, 2001.

10. Shiffman, M.A. et al., Field studies on water sanitation and health education in relation to health status in Central America, *Prog. Water Technol.*, 11, 143, 1978.
11. Levine, R.J. et al., Failure of sanitary wells to protect against cholera and other diarrhoeas in Bangladesh, *Lancet*, 2, 86, 1976.
12. Blum, D. and Feachem, R.G., Measuring the impact of water supply and sanitation investments on diarrhoeal diseases: problems of methodology, *Int. J. Epidemiol.*, 12, 357, 1983.
13. Esrey, S.A., Water, waste, and well-being: a multicountry study, *Am. J. Epidemiol.*, 143, 608, 1996.
14. McJunkin, F.E., *Water and Human Health*, Agency for International Development, Washington, D.C., 1982.
15. Briscoe, J., The role of water supply in improving health in poor countries (with special reference to Bangla Desh), *Am. J. Clin. Nutr.*, 31, 2100, 1978.
16. Moe, C.L. et al., Bacterial indicators of risk of diarrhoeal disease from drinking-water in the Philippines, *Bull. World Health Organ.*, 69, 305, 1991.
17. Feachem, R.G. et al., *Sanitation and Disease: Health Aspects of Excreta and Wastewater Management*, John Wiley & Sons, Chichester, U.K., 1983.
18. Hazen, T.C., Fecal coliforms as indicators in tropical waters: a review., *Toxic. Assess.*, 3, 461, 1988.
19. Handzel, T., The effect of improved drinking water quality on the risk of diarrhea disease in an urban slum of Dhaka, Bangladesh: a home chlorination intervention trial., Ph.D. dissertation, University of North Carolina, Chapel Hill, 1998.
20. Dufour, A.P. et al., Membrane filter method for enumerating *Escherichia coli*, *Appl. Environ. Microbiol.*, 41, 1152, 1981.
21. Mates, A. and Shaffer, M., Membrane filtration differentiation of *E. coli* from coliforms in the examination of water, *J. Appl. Bacteriol.*, 67, 343, 1989.
22. Wright, R.C., The seasonality of bacterial quality of water in a tropical developing country (Sierra Leone), *J. Hyg. (Lond).*, 96, 75, 1986.
23. Vanderslice, J. and Briscoe, J., All coliforms are not created equal: a comparison of the effects of water source and in-house contamination on infantile diarrheal disease, *Water Resour. Res.*, 29, p. 1983, 1993.
24. Hebert, J. R., Effects of water quality and water quantity on nutritional status: findings from a south Indian community, *Bull. World Health Organ.*, 63, 145, 1985.
25. Esrey, S.A. et al., The complementary effect of latrines and increased water usage on the growth of infants in rural Lesotho, *Am. J. Epidemiol.*, 135, 659, 1992.
26. Cheung, Y.B., The impact of water supplies and sanitation on growth in Chinese children, *J. R. Soc. Health*, 119, 89, 1999.
27. Liang, K.Y. and Zeger, S.L., Longitudinal data analysis using generalized models, *Biometrika*, 73, 13, 1986.
28. Briscoe, J., Intervention studies and the definition of dominant transmission routes, *Am. J. Epidemiol.*, 120, 449, 1984.
29. Esrey, S.A. et al., Effects of improved water supply and sanitation on ascariasis, diarrhoea, dracunculiasis, hookworm infection, schistosomiasis, and trachoma, *Bull. World Health Organ.*, 69, 609, 1991.
30. Curtis, V. et al., Domestic hygiene and diarrhoea — pinpointing the problem, *Trop. Med. Int. Health*, 5, 22, 2000.
31. Conroy, R.M. et al., Solar disinfection of drinking water and diarrhoea in Masai children: a controlled field trial, *Lancet*, 348, 1695, 1996.
32. Quick, R.E. et al., Diarrhoea prevention in Bolivia through point-of-use water treatment and safe storage: a promising new strategy, *Epidemiol. Infect.*, 122, 83, 1999.
33. Snyder, J. D. and Merson, M.H., The magnitude of the global problem of acute diarrhoeal disease: a review of active surveillance data, *Bull. World Health Organ.*, 60, 605, 1982.
34. Institute of Medicine, *New Vaccine Development: Establishing Priorities*, National Academy Press, Washington, D.C., 1986.
35. Moe, C.L., An evaluation of four bacterial indicators of risk of diarrheal disease from tropical drinking waters in the Philippines, Ph.D. thesis, University of North Carolina, Chapel Hill, 1989.

Index

A

Absenteeism, surveillance of, 68
Acceptability, of surveillance systems, 9–10
Accidental trials, intervention studies as, 192
Acquired immunodeficiency syndrome (AIDS)
  cryptosporidiosis and, 92, 167–168, 170
  as surveillance target, 6, 17–18
  as susceptibility factor, 184
Action thresholds, in outbreak detection, 69–70, 72
Adenoviruses
  Germany surveillance of, 145
  in United States outbreaks, 113
Age
  as cryptosporidiosis factor, 171
  distribution from routine surveillance, 134–135
  as study design factor, 184–185, 195
    in developing countries, 198, 201, 203–204
Agriculture ministry, as outbreak control team member, 56
Aluminum sulfate (alum), for water treatment, 102–103, 119
Analysis
  in intervention studies, 195
  longitudinal, 188, 198
  in outbreak investigations, 61–63
    bias in, 63
    case selection and controls, 62
    data design options, 61–62
    sample size and power, 62–63
  in prospective epidemiological studies, 188
    for developing countries, 201, 203–204
  real time, of health and technical data, 21–23, 125, 138
  in sporadic disease investigations, 145–146, 150–151
  in surveillance systems, 7
    with integrated system, 21–23, 144, 150
    need for improvement, 38, 144
  time series, *see* Time series analysis
  of trends, *see* Trend analysis
Anthropometric measures, for child health assessment, 203
Antidiarrheal medications, over-the-counter sales surveillance of, 19, 35, 69
ArcView® software, for geostatistical analysis, 145–146
Artificial neural networks
  drawbacks of, 75
  forecasting with, 76
  origin and function of, 74–75
  for outbreak detection, 73–76
  practical applications of, 76
  training of, 74–76
Ascertainment
  of cases, in prospective studies, 186
  as surveillance component, 138–139
Attributable risk (AR), in time series analysis, 161–162
Auramine phenol test, for fecal screening, 132–133
Australia
  endemic disease studies in, 176–177, 186
  intervention studies in, 192, 195
Austrobilharzia variglandis, in United States outbreaks, 113
Authority, *see* Statutory authority
Autocorrelation
  in geographical information systems, 145–146, 148, 151
  in time series analysis, 161
AutoRegressive filters (AR), in outbreak detection, 73, 76, 156
Auto-Regressive Integrated Moving Average model (ARIMA), in outbreak detection, 73, 156
Auto-Regressive Integrated Moving Average with eXogenous inputs (ARIMAX), in time series studies, 156, 158

B

Backpropagation of errors, in outbreak detection, 74–75
Back-siphonage, as contamination source, 108, 115
Bacteria tests, for water quality, 176, 184, 187
  in developing countries, 199, 202
  sensitivity of, 32
Bathing activities, United States outbreaks associated with, 112–114, 116
Behavioral constancy, of population, in time series analysis, 158–159
Bias
  in case-control studies, 178, 180
  in intervention studies, 193–196
  in outbreak investigations, 63
  in prospective studies, 185
Biomarkers, in seroepidemiology, 166
Bioterrorism, national surveillance of, 17, 37
Blinded trials
  of endemic disease, 186
    double, 176–177
  of interventions, 193–196
Boil water devices, surveillance of, 36
Boil water notices, with investigations, 60–61
Bottled water
  in intervention studies, 192–193, 195
  use in Sweden, 32–33

C

Caliciviruses
  outbreak investigations of

case study, 82–84
diagnostic principles, 80–82
introduction, 79–80
risk assessment, 84
surveillance of, 84
Campylobacter spp.
fecal testing for, 133
Germany surveillance of, 145
local surveillance of, 18
reported outbreaks of, 37
United Kingdom surveillance of, 26–27
age distribution from, 134
data on, 133–134
Canada, intervention studies in, 191–192, 194–195
Case ascertainment, in prospective studies, 186
Case-control studies, 175–182
combined designs of, 176–177, 181, 188
of endemic waterborne disease
advantages of, 177
bias in, 178, 180
case definition, 178
case recruitment, 178–179
conclusions from, 181
control definition, 179
control recruitment, 179–180
database construction, 180–181
designs for, 176–181
drinking water consumption measurement, 178
introduction, 175–176
in investigations, 176
key pathogen selection, 177
matching controls to cases, 180
questionnaires for, 180–181
study area for, 177–178
in outbreak investigations, 61–62
conflicting results from, 176
sample size and power in, 62–63
selection and control of, 62
Case crossover analysis, in prospective study, 188
Case definitions
in case-control studies, 178
in outbreak investigations, 57–58
Case investigations, *see* Investigation(s)
Case recruitment, in case-control studies, 178–179
Centers for Disease Control, U.S. (USCDC)
classification definitions of, 16
as collaborative surveillance system, 28
data transmission to, 1, 17
water intervention trials, 186, 192
Centralization, of data, in international surveillance, 43
Centrist model, of international surveillance, 43–44
Chemical poisoning outbreaks
criteria for, 30
in United States, 107–109, 111, 113–114
Chemicals, for water treatment, 27, 35
case study of, 102–103
resistance to, 87
Chlorination
in karstic springs, 158–160
organism resistance to, 87, 116, 170–171
outbreaks and, 27, 35, 112–113
Cholera, WHO surveillance of, 43–44, 203
Choropleth maps of incidence, in geographical information systems, 148, 151
Classification(s)
of initial notification reports, 16
of waterborne outbreaks, 30–31
Climate change, national surveillance of, 37
Clinical laboratories, *see* Laboratory(ies)
Clinical trials, intervention studies as, 192–193
Cloudiness, of water, *see* Turbidity
Cluster identification
of *Cryptosporidium* spp., in United Kingdom, 135–136
by geographical information systems, 145–146, 152
globally, 204
integrated system for, 21–23
by local surveillance systems, 14, 16, 18
in outbreak detection, 69–70
in time series studies, 157
Coagulation, in water treatment process, 101–103
Coefficients, of correlation, in geographical information systems, 149–150
Cohort studies
of interventions, 193, 200
in outbreak investigations, 62
serological, of cryptosporidiosis, 170
Coliforms
analysis of
as collaborative surveillance system, 28–29
global perspectives, 202
standards for, 21, 110, 114
outbreaks associated with, in United States, 110–111, 114–116
total rule for, 110, 114, 116
as water quality indicator, 176
in developing countries, 199, 202
WHO guidelines for, 199
Collaboration, *see* International surveillance
Combined study designs, 176–177, 181, 188
Communicable disease control, consultants in, 14, 26
Communicable Disease Report (CDR), 7
Communicable Disease Surveillance Center (CDSC), 26, 44
outbreak detection by, 70, 72
Communicable Disease Weekly (PHLS), 26
Community drinking water, *see* Municipal drinking water
Compartment dynamic models, for epidemiology, 162
Competence, *see also* Education; Training
local, for investigations, 37–38, 43–44
Completeness, as local surveillance flaw, 17–18
Computer-assisted telephone questionnaires (CATQ), on endemic disease, 180–181
Computer programs
for case-control studies, 180–181
for geographic surveillance, *see* Geographical information systems (GIS)
for outbreak detection, *see* Artificial neural networks
Concept-driven models, of epidemiology, 162
Confidentiality, as surveillance barrier, 38, 42–43, 150
Confirmation, in outbreak investigations, 54, 56, 58
Confounders
in global studies, 201

in intervention studies, 191, 195–196
in time series analysis, 156–157
controlling for, 157
Consultants in communicable disease control (CCDCs), 14, 26, 122
Consumption, of drinking water, measurement with studies, 178, 195, 200
Contamination, *see* Water contamination
Control measures
in case-control studies, 179
in global studies, 201
in intervention studies, 193–195
with outbreak investigations
additional, 54, 63–64
initial, 54, 60–61
Control recruitment, in case-control studies, 179–180
Control team, *see* Outbreak control team (OCT)
Convention on the Protection and Use of Transboundary Watercourses and International Lakes (1992), 4
Copper poisoning, 108
Correlation methods
in geographical information systems, 145–146, 148, 151
partial, 149–151
in time series analysis, 156–157
avoiding false, 157–161
validation of, 157–158
Cost, of surveillance systems, 10
Cost effectiveness, of intervention studies, 194–196
Council of State and Territorial Epidemiologists
classification definitions of, 16
as collaborative surveillance system, 28
Covariates, in time series studies, 156
Cross-connections, as contamination source, 30, 108, 115
Crossover analysis, of cases, in prospective study, 188
Cross-sectional serosurvey, on cryptosporidiosis, 167–168
Cross-validation, in time series analysis, 157–158
Cryptosporidiosis, *see Cryptosporidium* spp.
Cryptosporidium spp.
in Australia studies, 176–177
case-control studies of, 175–180
disease risks with, 165–166, 171
fecal testing for, 88, 132–133
food poisoning from, 90–91
HIV infection and, 92, 167–168, 170
immunodeficiency and, 92–93
infection definitions, 171
microbiology of, 87–93
epidemiological applications, 87, 89–92
future prospects for, 92–93
genotypic differences, 92
geographic variation and travel, 91–92
HIV infection, 92
introduction, 87
method development, 88–89
outbreak associations, 90–91
sample testing, 89
species distribution, 89–90
taxonomy and nomenclature of, 92
reported outbreaks of, 37
serological responses to, 165–166
study conclusions, 170–171
study methods, 166–169
study results, 169–170
surface water treatment and, 170–171
surveillance of, 15–16, 18–19, 31
United Kingdom outbreaks, 119–126
analytical investigation of, 62–63
conclusions from, 125
control measures for, 64
descriptive epidemiology of, 58–59, 89
early regulations applicability to, 122
early regulatory framework, 120–121
genetic investigation of, 88–92
introduction, 119
new regulations, 124–125
surveillance-based, 38, 136
Torbay, 122–124
United Kingdom surveillance of, 26, 132–140
age distribution, 134–135
clusters, 135–136
outbreak surveillance, 27, 136
regional variations, 137–139
screening, 132–133
seasonality, 137
surveillance data, 133–134
typing, 134
value of, 138–140
United States outbreaks, 108, 111–112, 114–116
engineering investigation of, 97, 101–103
water testing for, 90–91, 93, 165
Cumulative sum chart (CUSUM), in outbreak detection, 71–72
Cyclospora spp., surveillance of, 34

D

Data and data set, surveillance-based, 6, *see also* Surveillance and surveillance systems
Database(s)
for endemic disease studies, 180–181
for geographical information systems, 144, 148–150
for local surveillance systems, 17
Data collection
geographic, *see* Geographical information systems (GIS)
in outbreak investigations, 57–58
decisions based on inadequate, 61
in surveillance, 43, 131–132, 150
Data control, in international surveillance, 43–44
Data dissemination
of geographically aggregated data, 151
by local surveillance systems, 15
Data flow, in surveillance system design, 6–7
Data integration, in surveillance systems
development of, 21–23
as flaw in local, 18
geographic, 144, 150
Data interpretation, *see* Analysis
Data presentation

in geographical information systems, 145–146
in outbreak investigations, 57–59
Data reporting
case classification with, 16
in international surveillance, 42–46
in local surveillance systems
flaws of, 17–18
requirements of, 16–17, 132
of United Kingdom, 14
of United States, 17–18
in national surveillance systems, 132
of Sweden, 33–34, 37
of United Kingdom, 26
of United States, 29–31
statutory, 17, 38
three-tiered system for, 16–17
variance of, 2
Data transmission, to USCDC, 1, 17
Declaration, in outbreak investigations, 54, 56–57
Description, in outbreak investigations, 54, 57–59
Descriptive epidemiology, in outbreak investigations, 57–59
Detection, *see* Outbreak detection
Deterministic relationship, in time series studies, 156
Developing countries
prospective studies in, 197–206
age factor, 198, 201, 203–204
analytical approaches, 201, 203–204
conclusions from, 204–205
exposure assessment, 200–201
global perspective of, 197–198
health outcome measures, 200–201, 203
introduction, 197
methodological problems with, 200–204
overview, 200
study design problems, 201
transmission routes effect on, 204–205
water supplies and, 199–200
water contamination in, 197, 199, 202–205
water quality testing in, 199, 202, 204–205
water treatment in, 199–201, 203, 205
Diapers, water contamination from, 114, 116
Diarrhea, *see* Gastrointestinal illness
Disease risk
with *Cryptosporidium,* 165–166, 171
determining acceptable, 5
factors of, *see* Risk factors
Disinfection process
in karstic springs, 158–160
as pathogen barrier, 98
resistance to, 116
turbidity and, 160
as water treatment, 101–103, 114
Distribution system/process
contamination of, United States outbreaks associated with, 108–109, 114–115
as pathogen barrier, 98
DNA chip, for water quality testing, 22
DNA extraction, for cryptosporidiosis identification, 88–89
Dose response relationship, in waterborne disease outbreaks, 63
Double-blinded trials, of endemic disease, 176–177
case-control studies with, 177–181
Dracunculiasis, as global problem, 198
Drinking water
bottled, *see* Bottled water
community, *see* Municipal drinking water
contamination case studies of, 98–103, 175–176
measuring consumption for, 178
in developing countries, 197–200
prospective study designs for, 200–205
in Germany, 144–150
intervention studies of, 191–196
multiple barrier concept of, 98
outbreaks associated with
in United Kingdom, 119–125
in United States, 29–31, 106–111
prospective study designs, 200–205
seroepidemiology of, 165–173
Drinking Water Inspectorate (DWI), of United Kingdom
authority of, 120–121, 124
in Tobray outbreak, 123–124

E

Ecological fallacy, 150–151
Ecological paradox, 193, 196
Economy of scale, for national surveillance systems, 39
Education
in national surveillance systems, improvement strategies for, 37–39
as pathogen barrier, 98
Electronic communications
in international surveillance, 17–18, 46
in local surveillance systems, 17–18
for surveillance, 2, 17, 45
Electron microscopy, for Norwalk-like virus identification, 80–81
ELISA-type reaction
for cryptosporidiosis identification, 165
for Norwalk-like virus identification, 82
E-mail systems, *see* Electronic communications
Emerging disease(s), national surveillance of, 37
EMIRA study, 186
Endemic disease, *see also* specific organism, e.g., *Cryptosporidium* spp.
definition of, 175
epidemiological study designs for, 176–196
in developing countries, 200–205
serological, 165–171
gastrointestinal, *see* Gastrointestinal illness
global burden of, 197–198
pathogen transmission with, 175–176, 198
in developing countries, 204–205
prevalence of, 175, 181
Engineering investigations, 97–103
discussion on, 103
expediency as basis of, 103
introduction, 97–98
multiple barrier concept, 98
United States case studies, 98–103

Gideon, Missouri, 98–99
Karl Meyer Hall, 100–101
Milwaukee, Wisconsin, 101–103
England, *see* United Kingdom (U.K.)
Enrollment, in intervention studies, 195
Enter-Net System, 42–43
Environmental and Public Health Committee, of Sweden, 33
Environmental evidence, in outbreak investigations, 61
Environmental Health Protection Board, of Sweden, 33
Environmental health specialist, as outbreak control team member, 56, 122
Environmental Protection Agency, U.S. (EPA)
on coliform limit, 110, 114, 116
as collaborative surveillance system, 28–29, 106
in Gideon, Missouri outbreak investigation, 99
recreational water testing and, 116
on seroepidemiology, 165
water intervention trials, 186, 192
in Wisconsin outbreak investigation, 101
Environmental sampling, in national surveillance
improvement strategies for, 38
of Sweden, 33
of United Kingdom, 26
of United States, 29
Environmental sources, of infections, 33
Environmental Systems Research Institute (ESRI), spatial data presentation by, 145–146
Epidemic(s)
data presentation techniques, 58–59
international surveillance of, 41–42
Epidemiologist, as outbreak control team member, 56
Epidemiology and epidemiologic data
descriptive, 57–59
in national surveillance systems
analytical improvement of, 38
of Sweden, 33, 36–37
of United States, 29–31
representativeness of, 9, 31–32
in outbreak investigations, 57–58
analytic designs, 61–63
bias in, 63
case selection and controls, 62
sample size and power, 62–63
serological, *see* Seroepidemiology
as surveillance element, 131–132
of waterborne disease
case-control studies of, 175–181
combined study designs for, 176–177, 181, 188
conclusions from, 181, 188, 196, 204–205
conflicting results from, 176
intervention studies of, 191–196
introduction, 175–176, 183, 191–192, 197
prospective studies of, 183–188
in developing countries, 197–205
Episys project, 22–23
Error, random, in case-control studies, 178
Error variance, in intervention studies, 194
Escherichia coli O157:H7
fecal testing for, 133
surveillance of, 18, 31, 34
United Kingdom surveillance of, 133
in United States outbreaks, 112, 114
as water quality indicator, 176
in developing countries, 202, 205
European Union, 42
European Working Group for *Legionella* Infections (EWGLI), 44–45
Exposures and exposure data
in epidemiological studies
assessment of, 187, 201
in developing countries, 200–203
as time variable, 183–184
in intervention studies, 192–196, 200
as local surveillance flaw, 18
in national surveillance systems
multiple, 37
of United States, 29–30

F

False correlations, in time series analysis
negative, 158–161
positive, 157–158
strategies for avoiding, 157–161
False negative correlations, in time series analysis, 158–161
False positive correlations, in time series analysis, 157–158
Fecal contamination, of water, 197, 199, 202, *see also* Coliforms
Fecal testing
for cryptosporidiosis, 88, 132–133
of karstic water, 160–161
for Norwalk-like viruses, 81–82
in outbreak investigations, 84, 90–91
recreational, 114, 116
in United Kingdom, 119
in United States, 114
by surveillance systems
in Sweden, 34
of United Kingdom, 14, 132
in United States, 29, 32, 114
Federation of American Scientists, 45
Feed-forward neural networks
drawbacks of, 75
forecasting with, 76
origin and function of, 74–75
in outbreak detection, 73
practical applications of, 76
training of, 74–76
Field studies, intervention studies as, 192–193
15/17-kDa antigen, in seroepidemiology, 166–171
Filtration, as water treatment, 101–103, 109, 114–115
ineffective, 116, 170–171
randomized studies of, 192, 194–195
Flexibility, of surveillance systems, 10
Fluoride poisoning, 108
Food Act, of Sweden, 33
Food poisoning, cryptosporidiosis vs. salmonellosis in, 90–91
Forecasting, in outbreak detection, 72–73
neural networks for, 76

Formal report, with outbreak investigations, 54, 64, 120–121
France, water supply surveillance, 158

G

Gastroenteritis, *see* Endemic disease; Gastrointestinal illness
Gastrointestinal illness, *see also* specific organism, e.g., *Cryptosporidium* spp.
  in epidemiology studies
    acute, 186, 195
    highly credible, 186, 195
  as global burden, 197–198, 200–201, 203
  as study design factor, 175, 179–180, 186
  syndromic surveillance of, 19, 144–145
  as waterborne outbreak, 19, 35–36, 82, 87, 112
Gel electrophoresis
  in Norwalk-like virus investigations, 82
  pulsed-field, 18
Genetic testing
  in cryptosporidiosis investigations, 88–89
    epidemiological information from, 89–92
    taxonomy and nomenclature from, 92
  in Norwalk-like virus investigations, 82–83
  in water quality testing, 21–22
Geographical incidence, of cryptosporidiosis, 137–139
Geographical information systems (GIS), 143–153
  conclusions, 151–152
  development of task-specific, 150–151
  introduction, 143–144
  for national surveillance systems, 38–39, 144
  results, 146–150
  surveillance techniques, 144–146
    analytical methods, 145–146
    public health data, 144–145
    study area and water supply data, 144–145
  utility discussion, 150–151
Geostatistical analysis, 145–146
Germany, Rhein-Berg district, water supply surveillance, 144–150
ggI virus, Lordsdale-like, outbreak of, 83–84
ggII virus, Lordsdale-like, outbreak of, 83–84
Giardia spp.
  in Australia studies, 177
  local surveillance of, 18
  United Kingdom surveillance of, 26
    age distribution from, 134
  in United States outbreaks, 107–108, 111, 115–116
Great Britain, *see* United Kingdom (U.K.)
Groundwater systems
  in Germany, 144–150
  global contamination of, 197–198, 201–202
  seroepidemiology of, 166–173
  in Sweden, 33, 35
  in United States outbreaks, 106–110, 114–115
Guinea Worm infection, as global problem, 198

H

Hawthorne effect, in epidemiological studies, 185
Hazard Analysis Critical Control Points (HACCP)
  in Germany, 144, 151
  in Sweden, 33
Hazard identification, *see also* Risk measurement
  in prospective studies, 188
Health Canada, 46
Health care facilities
  preparedness of, 42, 46
  reporting requirements of, 19, 28
Health care system, in outbreak investigations, 53–54
Health data
  real time analysis of, 21–23, 125, 138
  in surveillance system design, 5, 68–69
Health education programs, 42
Health insurance data, in disease surveillance, 145, 147
Health outcomes, in study design, 184, 193–195
  for developing countries, 200–201, 203
Helicobacter pylori, as global problem, 198
Highly credible gastrointestinal illness (HCGI), 186, 195
Hot springs, United States outbreaks associated with, 113
Howard Water Treatment Plant (HWTP), in Wisconsin outbreak investigation, 101–103
Human immunodeficiency virus (HIV) infection, *see* Acquired immunodeficiency syndrome (AIDS)
Hybridization, in Norwalk-like virus investigations, 82
Hypothesis generation, in outbreak investigations, 54, 59–60
Hypothesis testing, in outbreak investigations, 54, 61–63

I

Illinois, microsporidiosis outbreak, engineering investigation of, 100–101
Illness, measures of, in surveillance systems, 5, 68–69
Immunocompromise, as susceptibility factor, 184
  for cryptosporidiosis, 92–93, 167, 170–171
Immunodeficiency, *see* Immunocompromise
Immunofluorescent microscopy, for cryptosporidiosis identification, 88, 132
Immunoglobulin G (IgG) response, in seroepidemiology, 169
Incident room, in outbreak investigations, 57
Individual water systems, outbreaks associated with
  in Germany, 146, 149–150
  in United States, 106–107, 111
Infection control nurse, as outbreak control team member, 56, 122
Infectious disease
  definition of, 171
  environmental sources of, 33
  health outcomes of, in study design, 184, 193–195
    for developing countries, 200–201, 203
  water-related, *see* Waterborne disease
Information Direction of 1990, of United Kingdom, 120–121
Information sharing

for surveillance, *see* specific level
as surveillance barrier, 38, 42–43
International Drinking Water Supply and Sanitation Decade (1981-1990), 200
International surveillance, 41–47
of cholera, 43–44, 203
examples of, 43–46
increasing role of, 46
of Legionnaires' disease, 41, 44–45
national surveillance systems reporting to, 39, 132
principles of, 42–43
value of, 2, 41–42, 132
weaknesses of, 46
Internet, *see also* Electronic communications
as surveillance tool, 46
Interventional cohort studies, 62
Intervention options, with outbreak investigations, 1, 54, 60–61
Intervention studies, 191–196
bias in, 193–196
case study of, 194–195
conclusions from, 196
under controlled conditions, 193
designs of, 193–194
government-funded, 186, 192
introduction, 191–192
under natural conditions, 192
objectives of, 192–193
randomization of, 191, 193, 195–196
under uncontrolled conditions, 192–193
Investigation form, 16–17
Investigation(s)
analytical, *see* Analysis
international, 41, 46
local teams for, 37–38, 43–44, 56, 120
microbiological, *see* Microbiological typing
national
factors affecting, 31–32, 37
feedback on, 37
standards for, 26
steps for, 32
in Sweden, 33, 37
of outbreaks, 49–126; *see also* Outbreak investigations
of sporadic disease, 127–206; *see also* Sporadic disease investigations
stages of, 53–65
statutory authority for, 17, 38
structural, *see* Engineering investigations
Isolates, subtyping of, *see* Laboratory isolates

K

Karstic water, in time series studies, 158–191

L

Laboratory(ies)
local reporting by, 17, 147
national reporting by
in Sweden, 33–34
in United Kingdom, 26
in United States, 29, 31
surveillance role of, 131–132
test sensitivity limitations, 32
Laboratory isolates, *see also* Microbiological typing
integrated system for, 21–23
in local surveillance systems
of United Kingdom, 14
of United States, 18
in national surveillance systems
dependence on, 67–68
of United States, 32
Lake swimming, United States outbreaks associated with, 111–114
Lead poisoning, 111
Legionnaires' disease, international surveillance of, 41, 44–45
Legislation
for local surveillance systems
in United Kingdom, 14
in United States, 16–17, 19
for national surveillance systems, 38
in Sweden, 33, 37
Leptospira interrogans, in United States outbreaks, 113
Liability, as surveillance barrier, 42–43
Local competence, for investigations, 37–38, 43–44, *see also* Education; Training
Local health departments, resource limitations of, 31–32
Local surveillance systems, 13–20
functions of, 13
key components of, 1, 13
legal requirement for, 14, 16–17, 19
outbreak sensitivity of, 15, 19–20
responsibility demands for, 20, 31–32
of sporadic waterborne disease, *see* Sporadic disease surveillance
under-reporting by physicians, 19
in United Kingdom, 14–16
in United States, 16–19
Location quotients, in geographical information systems, 148, 151
Logistic function, in feed-forward networks, for outbreak detection, 75
Longitudinal data analysis, 188, 198
Lordsdale-like ggI virus, outbreak of, 83–84
Lordsdale-like ggII viruses, outbreak of, 83–84
Lovelace Clinic Foundation (LCF), 165–166, 169

M

Maps, for outbreak investigations, 57
Media, *see* Press relations
Meningococcal infections
as surveillance target, 17–18
in United States outbreaks, 113, 116
Microbiological typing, *see also* Laboratory isolates
in outbreak investigations, 34, 61
for cryptosporidium, 87–93, 119–126, 134
for Norwalk-like viruses, 79–84

Microbiologist, as outbreak control team member, 56, 122
Microbiology, as surveillance element, 131–132
Microorganisms
identification of, *see* Microbiological typing
as pathogens, *see* Pathogens; specific organism
Microscopy, immunofluorescent, for cryptosporidiosis identification, 88, 132
Microsporidiosis, Chicago, Illinois waterborne outbreak, engineering investigation of, 100–101
Missouri, salmonellosis outbreak, engineering investigation of, 98–99
Modeling techniques, in outbreak detection, 73–74
Moran I test, in geographical information systems, 146, 148, 151
Morbidity and Mortality Weekly Report (MMWR)
in outbreak detection, 69–70, 72
as surveillance system output, 7
Moving Average filters (MA)
in outbreak detection, 73
in time series analysis, 156–157
Multiple barrier concept, for drinking water systems, 98
Multiple exposures, national surveillance of, 37
Municipal drinking water
contamination case studies of, 98–103
in Germany, 144–150
in Sweden
access to, 33
outbreaks associated with, 35–36
United States outbreaks associated with
classification of, 30–31
by etiologic agent and year, 29, 107–108
reported 1991-1998, 106–111
by system deficiency, 108–110
water quality during, 110–111
by water source, 106–110, 114
by water system, 29–30, 106–110

N

National Electronic Telecommunications Surveillance System (NETSS), local systems reporting to, 17–18
National Food Administration, of Sweden, 33, 36
National investigations
factors affecting, 31–32, 37
feedback on, 37
standards for, 26
steps for, 32
support for, 37
National Rivers Authority (NRA), of United Kingdom, 120
National surveillance systems, 25–40
desirable characteristics of, 1–2
education and training for, 37–39
future strategies for, 38–39
improvement barriers of, 38
legal requirement for, 38
limitations of, 37–38
reliance on local systems, 25
reporting to international systems, 39, 132
of sporadic waterborne disease, *see* Sporadic disease surveillance
in Sweden, 32–37
in United Kingdom, 25–27
in United States, 28–32
Negative correlations, false, in time series analysis, 158–161
Negative feedback model, of public health practice, 4–5
Nephelometric turbidity units (NTU), 156
as risk measurement, 161–162
Network model, of international surveillance, 43–45
Neural networks, *see* Artificial neural networks
Neurons, in feed-forward networks, for outbreak detection, 74–75
Nitrate poisoning, 108, 111
Nomenclature, of *Cryptosporidium* spp. genetics, 92
Non-community drinking water, outbreaks associated with, 106–111, 114–116
Non-linear regression, in outbreak detection, 74
Nonparametric smoothing, in time series analysis, 157
Norwalk-like viruses (NLVs)
fecal testing for, 81–82
outbreak investigations of, 79–84
case study, 82–84
diagnostic principles, 80–82
introduction, 79–80
risk assessment, 84
surveillance of, 18, 84, 134
in United States outbreaks, 113
Notification, *see* Data reporting

O

Objectives, in surveillance system design, 5
Observational cohort studies, of interventions, 62
Office of Water Services (OFWAT), of United Kingdom, 120
Outbreak confirmation, in investigations, 54, 56, 58
Outbreak control team (OCT)
in United Kingdom, 120, 122
in United States, 37–38, 43–44, 56
Outbreak declaration, in investigations, 54, 56–57
Outbreak description, in investigations, 54, 57–59
Outbreak detection, *see also* Surveillance and surveillance systems
action thresholds, 69–70, 72
artificial neural networks for, 73–76
AutoRegressive filters, 73, 76, 156
cluster identification, 69–70
forecasting, 72–73, 76
introduction, 67–68, 132
investigations and, 54–56
measures of illness and, 68–69
Morbidity and Mortality Weekly Report, 69–70, 72
problems with, 5, 68
sporadic, *see* Sporadic disease surveillance
statistical techniques for, 69–73
strategies for early, 67–77
in Sweden, 33–36
in United Kingdom, 27–28

in United States, 31–32
Outbreak investigations, 49–126
conclusions from, 64
consistent problems of, 136
cryptosporidium typing, 87–95, 119–126, 134
early detection, 67–77
engineering considerations, 97–103
introduction, 49–51
learning curve for, 54–55
microbiology in, 34, 79–95
Norwalk-like virus typing, 79–85
systems approach, 53–65
in United Kingdom, 119–126
in United States (1991-1998), 105–117
Outbreak report, formal, with investigations, 54, 64, 120–121
Outbreak(s)
of poisoning, *see* Chemical poisoning outbreaks
of waterborne infectious disease, *see* Waterborne disease outbreaks (WBDOs)
Outbreak surveillance
for cryptosporidiosis, 136
real-time, 21–23
sensitivity of, 2, 136
innovation for increasing local, 19–20
in United Kingdom, 15, 26
in United States, 19, 32, 116
signatory states for, 4
Outcome(s)
of infections, in study design, 184, 193–195
for developing countries, 200–201, 203
of surveillance systems, 8
Output(s), of surveillance systems, 7–8
measures of, 8–9

P

Paper reports, as surveillance system flaw, 18
Parasites, *see also Cryptosporidium* spp.
as global problem, 198, 203
in United States outbreaks, 113
water quality tests for, 187
sensitivity limitations of, 32
Partial correlation coefficients, in geographical information systems, 149–151
Participation maintenance
in intervention studies, 194
in prospective studies, 184–186
Pathogens, *see also* specific organism
in endemic disease, 175
selection for case-control studies, 177
species as variable of, 184
transmission routes of, 175–176, 198
in developing countries, 204–205
Patient-identifiable date, limited access to, 38, 42
Pearson's product-moment correlation, in geographical information systems, 146, 149, 151
Perceptrons, in outbreak detection, 73–74
Phylogeny, in Norwalk-like virus investigations, 82
Physicians
as outbreak control team member, 56
reporting requirements of
in Germany, 147
in Sweden, 33
in United States, 16–17, 19
Planning, in outbreak investigations, 54–55
Point-of-entry device, in intervention studies, 193
Point-of-use device, in intervention studies, 192–194
Poisoning, from contaminated water, *see* Chemical poisoning outbreaks
Poisson probability distribution
in geographical information systems, 145, 148, 151
in prospective epidemiology studies, 185–186, 204
Poisson regression, in time series analysis, 156–157
Polyaluminum chloride (PACL), for water treatment, 102–103
Polymerase-chain reaction (PCR), *see* Reverse transcriptase-polymerase-chain reaction (RT-PCR)
Pool swimming, United States outbreaks associated with, 29–30, 113–114, 116
Population
study, *see* Study population
target, in surveillance system design, 5–6, 17–18
Positive correlations, false, in time series analysis, 157–158
Power, statistical
in outbreak investigations, 62–63, 73
in time series analysis, 158
Predictive value positive (PVP), of surveillance systems, 9
Press officer, as outbreak control team member, 56
Press relations, in outbreak investigations, 55, 57, 68
Preventive action
as international surveillance justification, 41–42
as reporting justification, 17
Private water, outbreaks associated with
in Germany, 146, 149–150
in Sweden, 33, 37
in United Kingdom, 27
in United States outbreaks, 106–107, 111, 114
Probability
in geographical information systems, 145, 148, 151
in outbreak investigations, 62–63, 73
in prospective studies, quantification of, 185–186
in syndromic surveillance, 22
Process measures, in surveillance system evaluation, 9–10
Product liability, as surveillance barrier, 42–43
Product-moment correlation, Pearson's, in geographical information systems, 146, 149, 151
ProMEDmail system, for international surveillance, 2, 42, 45–46
Prospective epidemiological studies, 183–189
bias in, 185
case ascertainment, 186
case definition, 186
conclusions from, 188
data analysis, 188
in developing countries, 197–206
age factor, 198, 201, 203–204
analytical approaches, 201, 203–204
conclusions from, 204–205
exposure assessment, 200–201

global perspective of, 197–198
health outcome measures, 200–201, 203
introduction, 197
methodological problems with, 200–204
overview, 200
study design problems, 201
transmission routes effect on, 204–205
water supplies and, 199–200
exposure assessment, 187
exposure variable of, 183–184
features of, 184–188
health outcome variable of, 184, 200, 203
introduction, 183
key design issues, 183–184
participation maintenance, 184–186
pathogen specie variable of, 184
population selection, 184–186
serological, on cryptosporidiosis, 170
time element, 188, 198, 200
Protozoa
waterborne outbreaks, in United States (1991-1998), 107, 115
as water quality indicator, 176, 187
Pseudomonas spp., in United States outbreaks, 113
Pseudo-outbreaks, 56
Public Health Intelligence Network, 46
Public Health Laboratory Service (PHLS), 25–26, 44
outbreak detection by, 70, 72
Public health measures
with outbreak investigations, 1, 54, 60–61
studies of, 192–193; *see also* Intervention studies
Public health officers, in Sweden, 33
Public health practice, negative feedback model of, 4–5
Public health professional, as outbreak control team member, 56, 122
Public health surveillance
in Germany, 144–145, 148
value of, 4, 144
Public water systems
in Germany, 144–150
outbreaks associated with
in United Kingdom, 27, 119–125
in United States, 29–30
classification of, 30–31, 106
reported 1991-1998, 106–111, 114
in Sweden, access to, 32–33
Pulsed-field gel electrophoresis (PFGE), 18
Punitive sanctions, in United Kingdom, 119, 125
Purpose, in surveillance system design, 5

Q

Quasi-experimental interventions, 193
Questionnaires
for case-control studies, 180–181
for global studies, 201

R

Random error, in case-control studies, 178
Randomization
of double-blind studies, 176–177
case-control studies with, 177–181
of prospective studies, 185
of public health intervention, 191, 193, 195–196
Real time analysis, of health and technical data, 21–23, 125, 138
Recognition, of waterborne outbreaks, *see* Outbreak detection
Recreational water
outbreaks associated with
in Sweden, 35–36
in United States, 29–30, 106–114, 116
testing criteria for, 116
Recruitment, in case-control studies
of cases, 178–179
of controls, 179–180
Reference terms, for outbreak investigations, 57
Regional variations, of cryptosporidiosis, 137–139
Regression models
for global studies, 203–204
non-linear, in outbreak detection, 74
for time series studies, 156–157, 161
Regulations, *see* Water regulations
Relative risk (RR), in time series analysis, 161–162
Remedial control, with outbreak investigations, 60–61
Reporting
formal, with outbreak investigations, 54, 64, 120–121
with surveillance, *see* Data reporting
Representativeness, of surveillance systems, 9, 31–32
Research, priority factors for, 32
Resolution, in geographical information systems, 147, 150
Resource limitations
due to decreasing outbreaks, 38
international surveillance as answer to, 41–43
of local and state health departments, 31–32
Responsibility demands
of local surveillance systems, 20
of national surveillance systems, 33, 38–39
Reverse-osmosis unit, randomized studies of, 194–195
Reverse transcriptase-polymerase-chain reaction (RT-PCR)
for cryptosporidiosis investigations, 88
for Norwalk-like virus investigations, 81–82, 84
case study, 82–84
Risk assessment, *see* Risk measurement
Risk factors, *see also* specific factor
identification by local surveillance, 15–16
including in data set, 6
Risk management
as national surveillance strategy, 37
in prospective studies, 188
Risk measurement
in intervention studies, 196
in prospective studies, 188
in time series analysis, 161–162
Risk of disease
with *Cryptosporidium,* 165–166, 171
determining acceptable, 5

factors of, *see* Risk factors
RNA concentration, in Norwalk-like virus microbiology, 81–82
"Rolling sampling" model, in outbreak investigations, 84
Rotavirus, surveillance of, 34, 145

S

Safe Drinking Water Act, 186
Salmonella spp.
fecal testing for, 133
in food poisoning, 90–91
Germany surveillance of, 145, 147
Gideon, Missouri outbreak, engineering investigation of, 98–99
surveillance of, 18, 22
United Kingdom surveillance of, 26
age distribution from, 134
data on, 133–134
Sample size
in global studies, 201
in intervention studies, 194
in outbreak investigations, 62–63
in prospective studies, 185
Sanctions, punitive, in United Kingdom, 119, 125
Sanitation, inadequate, as global burden, 197–198, 200, 205
Sapporo-like viruses (SLVs), outbreak investigations of, 80
Scan statistic, in outbreak detection, 71–72
Schistosoma spp.
as global problem, 198
in United States outbreaks, 113
Scotland, surveillance in, 26
Scottish Center for Infection and Environmental Health (SCIEH), 26
Seasonality
of *Cryptosporidium* detection, 137
as prospective study design factor, 185, 204
Sedimentation, in water treatment process, 101–103
Selection procedures
in case-control studies, 177
in outbreak investigations, 62
in prospective studies, 184–185
for study populations, *see* Study population
Self-reports, in case-control studies, 178
Sensitivity, of surveillance systems, 8–9
innovation for increasing, 19–20, 26
in United Kingdom, 15, 26
in United States, 19, 32
Sentinel surveillance
in epidemiology studies, 187
international, 42
local, 18–19, 132
Sequencing, in Norwalk-like virus investigations, 82
Seroepidemiology, 165–173
biomarkers in, 166
conclusions, 170–171
of *Cryptosporidium* spp., 165–169
introduction, 165–166
motivation for, 165
results, 169–170
statistical analysis, 169
study methods, 166–169
Western blot procedures, 165, 169
Sewage testing, *see* Fecal testing
Shigella spp.
fecal testing for, 133
Germany surveillance of, 145, 147
global incidence of, 203
United Kingdom surveillance of, age distribution from, 134
in United States outbreaks, 112–114
Signatory states, for public health surveillance, 4
Simplicity, of surveillance systems, 10
Source water, *see* Water source
Spatial data, in sporadic disease investigations, 145–146
Specialists, in national surveillance systems, improvement strategies for, 38
Sporadic disease investigations
case-control studies in, 175–182
geographical information systems for, 143–153
intervention studies in, 191–196
introduction, 127–129
prospective epidemiological studies in, 183–189
in developing countries, 197–206
seroepidemiology with, 165–173
time series analysis in, 155–163
using existing surveillance-based data, 131–141
Sporadic disease surveillance
of cryptosporidiosis, 132–138
difficulties with, 32, 127–128
using existing data for, 131–140
Sporadic waterborne disease
introduction, 127–129
investigation of, *see* Sporadic disease investigations
surveillance of, *see* Sporadic disease surveillance
Spring water, in United States outbreaks, 106–107, 114
S-pus® software, for geostatistical analysis, 146
Staining methods, for cryptosporidiosis identification, 88, 132
Standardization
of coliform analysis, 21, 110, 114
of national investigations, 26
of surveillance, 138
State health departments
resource limitations of, 31–32
statutory authority of, 17
Statistical power
in outbreak investigations, 62–63, 73
in time series analysis, 158
Statistical techniques
in geographical information systems, 145–146, 151
for global studies, 203–204
for outbreak detection, 69–74
in time series analysis, 155–157
Statutory authority
for public health reporting, 17, 38
for surveillance
in United Kingdom, 120–121, 124
in United States, 16–17
Study designs and methods
case-control, 175–181

combined, 176–177, 181, 188
conclusions from, 181, 188, 196, 204–205
conflicting results from, 176
interventional, 191–196
introduction, 175–176, 183, 191–192, 197
prospective, 183–188
in developing countries, 197–205
serological, *see* Seroepidemiology
Study population
in intervention studies, 192–193, 195
in outbreak investigations, 53–54
in prospective studies, 184–186
in time series analysis, 158–159
Subtyping, of isolates, *see* Microbiological typing
Surface water
cryptosporidiosis risks with, 165–166, 170–171
in Germany, 144–150
global contamination of, 197–198
in intervention studies, 191–192
seroepidemiology of, 166–173
in Sweden, 33, 35
in United States outbreaks, 106–109, 115
Surface Water Treatment Rule (SWTR), 115
Surveillance and surveillance systems, *see also* Outbreak detection
ascertainment with, 138–139
designing steps for, 5–8
analysis, 7
clear objectives, 5–6
data flow, 6–7
data set, 6
outcome, 8
outputs, 7–8
problem to be addressed, 5, 68
purpose, 5
system characteristics, 6–8
target population, 5–6, 17–18
epidemiology element of, 131–132
as essential, 2–3
evaluation of, 8–10
acceptability, 9–10
cost, 10
flexibility, 10
output measures, 8–9
predictive value positive, 9
process measures, 9–10
representativeness, 9, 31–32
simplicity, 10
timeliness, 9
evolutionary trends, 1
international, *see* International surveillance
introduction, 1–2, 131–132
local, *see* Local surveillance systems
microbiology element of, 131–132
national perspectives of, 1–2, 7; *see also* National surveillance systems
for outbreaks of waterborne disease, *see* Outbreak surveillance
principles, 1
of public health, 4; *see also* Public health surveillance
responsiveness, 2
by serological responses, *see* Seroepidemiology
for sporadic waterborne disease, *see* Sporadic disease surveillance
value of, 138–140
Survey methods
in case-control studies, 178
in intervention studies, 195
in seroepidemiology, 166–169
Susceptibility
in immunocompromised population, 184
in prospective studies, quantification of, 184–185
Suspended particle matter (SPM), in time series studies, 156, 161
Sweden
national surveillance systems, 2, 32–37
alternative recognition of outbreaks, 35–36
drinking water, 32–33, 37
organization of, 33
outbreak detection by, 33–35
water-related outbreaks reported by, 36–37
surveillance perspectives of, 2
Swedish Institute for Infectious Disease Control (SMI), 33
Swimming facilities, United States outbreaks associated with, 29–30, 111–114, 116
Syndromic surveillance, 19, 22

T

Tango's index, in outbreak detection, 71
Tap water
in developing countries, 199, 205
in intervention studies, 191–192, 195
in Sweden, 33, 36
Target population, in surveillance system design, 5–6, 17–18
Target variable, in time series studies, 156–157
Taxonomy, of *Cryptosporidium* spp., 92
Technical data, real time analysis of, 21–23, 125, 138
TEIS database, for geographical information systems, 144, 148, 150
Telephone questionnaires, computer-assisted, in case-control studies, 180–181
Telephone recruitment, in case-control studies, 179, 181
Telephone reports, from local surveillance systems, 18
Terrorism, biological, national surveillance of, 17, 37
Testing, *see* Laboratory(ies); Water quality testing; specific test
Third Ministerial Conference on Environment and Health of the Protocol on Water and Health, 4
Time element, in prospective studies, 188, 198, 200
Time lag, in time series analysis, 162
Timeliness, of surveillance systems, 9
as flaw in local, 17
as flaw in national, 35
improvement with integrated system, 21–23
Time series analysis, 155–163
advantages of, 162
avoiding false correlations with, 157–161
basic method of, 156–157
conclusions from, 162

disadvantages of, 162
false negative correlations with, 158–161
false positive correlations with, 157–158
introduction, 155
risk measurement, 161–162, 188
source data for, 156, 188
statistical models for, 156–157
Time series studies (TSS), 155
Time step, in time series analysis, 157
Torbay cryptosporidiosis outbreak (1995)
analysis of, 122–123
legislative response to, 123–124
Total coliform rule (TCR), 110, 114, 116
Trade, foreign, international surveillance for, 46
Training
in national surveillance systems, improvement strategies for, 37–39
on neural networks, for outbreak detection, 74–76
Transmission routes, of pathogens, with endemic disease, 175–176, 198
in developing countries, 204–205
Travel, foreign
cryptosporidiosis and, 91–92, 135, 137, 171
international surveillance for, 41, 46
as risk factor, 6, 44
Trend analysis
in local surveillance systems
integrated system for, 21–23, 144, 150
of United Kingdom, 15–16
of United States, 16–17, 19
in national surveillance systems
factors affecting, 31–32
improvement of, 38
of United Kingdom, 26
of United States, 30–31
Trihalomethanes (THM), in drinking water, 143
Turbidity, of water
measurement of, 156
pathogen occurrence raised by, 160
in time series analysis, 156, 158–162
as treatment factor, 102–103, 115
TWDB database, for geographical information systems, 144, 148, 150
27-kDa antigen, in seroepidemiology, 166, 168–171
Typhoid fever, as global problem, 18, 198

U

Underdiagnosing, 138–139
Under-reporting, by physicians, 19
United Kingdom (U.K.)
Cryptosporidium outbreaks, 119–126
analytical investigation of, 62–63
conclusions from, 125
control measures for, 64
descriptive epidemiology of, 58–59, 89
early regulations applicability to, 122
early regulatory framework, 120–121
genetic investigation of, 88–92
introduction, 119
new regulations, 124–125
surveillance-based, 136
Torbay, 122–124
Cryptosporidium surveillance in, 132–140
age distribution, 134–135
clusters, 135–136
outbreak surveillance, 136
regional variations, 137–139
screening, 132–133
seasonality, 137
surveillance data, 133–134
typing, 134
value of, 138–140
local surveillance systems, 14–16
components of, 14
data dissemination by, 15
further information collected by, 14–15
laboratory isolates of, 14
legislation governing, 14
notifications to, 14
outbreak sensitivity of, 15
risk factor identification by, 15–16
trend identification by, 15–16
national surveillance systems, 25–27
causes of outbreaks identified by, 27–28
grading water-related outbreaks in, 26
historical, 25–26
information sources of, 26
investigation standards, 26
outbreaks detected by, 27–28
private water associated with outbreaks, 27
public water associated with outbreaks, 27
surveillance perspectives of, 1, 7
Water Act (1989), 120, 124–125
Water Industry Act (1991), 120
United States (U.S.)
chemical poisoning outbreaks, 107–109, 111, 113–114
Cryptosporidium spp. outbreaks, 108, 111–112, 114–116
investigation of, 97, 101–103
engineering investigation case studies, 98–103
local surveillance systems, 16–19
authorities of, 16–17, 19
innovation for increasing sensitivity of, 19
other case data sources for, 18
outbreak sensitivity of, 19
weaknesses of, 17–18
national surveillance systems, 28–32
agencies involved, 28–29
analysis methods of, 29
characteristics of, 29–32
data sources and types for, 29–30
historical, 28
objectives of, 28–29
outbreak classification by, 30–31
representativeness of, 9, 31–32
sensitivity of, 32
strengths of, 32
usefulness of, 31–32
weaknesses of, 32

surveillance authority in, 16–17; *see also* Centers for Disease Control, U.S. (USCDC)
surveillance perspectives of, 1, 7
waterborne outbreaks detection, 31–32
waterborne outbreaks reported (1991-1998), 105–117
coliforms, 110, 115–116
distribution system contamination, 114–115
drinking water, 29–31, 106–111
groundwater systems, 106, 114
individual water systems, 111
introduction, 105–106
protozoan, 107, 115
public water systems, 29–30, 106–111, 114
recreational water, 29–30, 111–114, 116
surveillance conclusions, 116
Universal function approximators, in outbreak detection, 74–75

V

Vaccines, stockpiling of, 42
Validation, in time series analysis, 157–158
Variables, in epidemiological studies
designing for exposure, 159–161
prospective, 183–184
time series, 156, 159–161
Virus illness(es), surveillance of, 22
Virus tests, for water quality, 176, 187
sensitivity limitations of, 32
Volatile organic compounds (VOCs), in groundwater reservoirs, 143
Volunteers, for prospective studies, 185

W

Wading pools, United States outbreaks associated with, 111, 113–114
Wales, *see* United Kingdom (U.K.)
Water Act of 1989, of United Kingdom, 120, 124–125
Waterborne disease
epidemiology of
case-control studies of, 175–181
conclusions from, 181, 188, 196, 204–205
conflicting results from, 176
intervention studies of, 191–196
introduction, 175–176, 183, 191–192, 197
prospective studies of, 183–188
in developing countries, 197–205
global burden of, 197–198
health outcomes of, in study design, 184, 193–195
in developing countries, 200–201, 203
investigation of, 49–126; *see also* Investigation(s)
with sporadic incidence, 127–206
microorganism identification, 26, 34; *see also* specific organism
outbreaks of, *see* Waterborne disease outbreaks (WBDOs)
sporadic, *see* Sporadic waterborne disease
surveillance of, 1–47; *see also* Surveillance and surveillance systems
Waterborne disease outbreaks (WBDOs)
causes of
in Sweden, 35–37
in United Kingdom, 27–28
in United States (1991-1998), 105–117
classification of, in United States, 30–31
criteria for, 30
detection of, *see* Outbreak detection
dose response relationship in, 63
investigations of, *see* Outbreak investigations
private water associated with
in Sweden, 33, 37
in United Kingdom, 27
public water associated with
in Sweden, 35–37
in United Kingdom, 27
in United States, 29–30
classification of, 30–31
reported 1991-1998, 106–111, 114
sporadic, *see* Sporadic waterborne disease
surveillance for, *see* Outbreak surveillance
Water contamination
deficiency classification, 30
engineering investigations of
case studies of, 98–103
discussion on, 97–98, 103
fecal, 197, 199; *see also* Coliforms
GIS linking to disease, 143–152
global perspectives of, 197, 199, 202–205
local surveillance of, 68
multiple barrier prevention of, 98
national surveillance of
in United Kingdom, 26
in United States, 30
time series studies of, 155–162
Water cycle, 119
Water Industry Act 1991 (WIA), of United Kingdom, 120
Water intervention trials, *see* Intervention studies
Water parks, United States outbreaks associated with, 112
Water Quality Regulations, of United Kingdom, 120, 124
Water quality testing
in cryptosporidiosis investigations, 90–91, 93
in developing countries, 199, 202, 204–205
with geographical information systems
conclusions, 151–152
development of task-specific, 150–151
introduction, 143–144
methods, 144–146
results, 146–150
utility discussion, 150–151
integrated system for, 21–23, 144, 150
in national surveillance systems
of Sweden, 35–36
of United Kingdom, 26
of United States, 29–31, 110–*111
in Norwalk-like virus investigations, 81–82, 84
case study, 82–84
pathogen indicators in, 176, 184
for recreational water, 116

in time series analysis, 156
Water regulations, *see also* specific act
in Sweden, 33
in United Kingdom, 120, 122, 124–125
in United States, *see* Environmental Protection Agency, U.S. (EPA)
Water source
global perspectives of, 197–200, 203
protection of, as pathogen barrier, 98
in Sweden, 33, 35
in United States outbreaks, 106–110, 114
Water Supply and Water Resources Division (WSWRD), of United States EPA, in outbreak investigations, 99, 101
Water supply engineers, as outbreak control team member, 56, 122
Water Supply Regulations, of United Kingdom, 120, 124
Water supply systems
for drinking, *see* Drinking water
multiple barrier concept of, 98
outbreaks associated with
engineering investigations of, 97–103
intervention options for, 1, 54, 60–61
investigation stages of, 53–54, 57, 60
in Sweden, 32–33, 35
in United States, 29–30, 105–111, 114–116
in Rhein-Berg, Germany, surveillance of, 144–145
Water treatment facilities
in developing countries, 199–201, 203, 205
as pathogen barrier, 98
turbidity and, 160
United Kingdom case study of, 122–124
United States case study of, 101–103
randomized studies of, 191–196
Water Undertakers (Information) Direction of 1990, of United Kingdom, 120–121
Weather patterns, national surveillance of, 37
Weekly Epidemiological Record (WHO), 43
Weighting, of neural networks, for outbreak detection, 74–75
Well water, *see* Private water
Western blot test, for cryptosporidiosis identification, 88, 165, 169
Wisconsin, cryptosporidiosis outbreak, engineering investigation of, 97, 101–103
World Health Organization (WHO)
cholera surveillance by, 43–44
coliform guidelines of, 199
surveillance system, 2, 198

Y

Yersinia spp., Germany surveillance of, 145

Z

Ziehl-Neelsen test, for fecal screening, 132–133
Zoonotic infections, 203